Questions for the Final FFICM Structured Oral Examination

Questions for the Final FFICM Structured Oral Examination

Kate Flavin
The Central London School of Anaesthesia

Clare Morkane
The Central London School of Anaesthesia

Sarah Marsh (Editor)
Harrogate and District NHS Foundation Trust

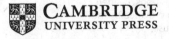
CAMBRIDGE
UNIVERSITY PRESS

CAMBRIDGE
UNIVERSITY PRESS

University Printing House, Cambridge CB2 8BS, United Kingdom

One Liberty Plaza, 20th Floor, New York, NY 10006, USA

477 Williamstown Road, Port Melbourne, VIC 3207, Australia

314-321, 3rd Floor, Plot 3, Splendor Forum, Jasola District Centre, New Delhi - 110025, India

79 Anson Road, #06-04/06, Singapore 079906

Cambridge University Press is part of the University of Cambridge.

It furthers the University's mission by disseminating knowledge in the pursuit of education, learning and research at the highest international levels of excellence.

www.cambridge.org
Information on this title: www.cambridge.org/9781108401425
DOI: 10.1017/9781108233712

© Cambridge University Press 2018

First published 2018

A catalogue record for this publication is available from the British Library

Library of Congress Cataloging in Publication data
Names: Flavin, Kate, author. | Morkane, Clare, author. | Marsh, Sarah, editor.
Title: Questions for the final FFICM structured oral examination / Kate Flavin, Clare Morkane ; Sarah Marsh, editor.
Description: Cambridge, United Kingdom ; New York, NY : Cambridge University Press, [2018] | Includes bibliographical references and index.
Identifiers: LCCN 2017055390 | ISBN 9781108401425 (paperback : alk. paper)
Subjects: | MESH: Critical Care | Emergencies | Study Guide
Classification: LCC RC86.9 | NLM WX 18.2 | DDC 616.02/8076–dc23
LC record available at https://lccn.loc.gov/2017055390

ISBN 978-1-108-40142-5 Paperback

Contents

Foreword

In the same year that we celebrate 100 years of women in medicine I cannot think of a better way for Intensive Care Medicine (ICM) to be recognised than with this publication, the first revision aid I am aware of for the Fellow of the Faculty of Intensive Care Medicine (FFICM) exam created by an all-woman team. It started off as Kate's brain child; Kate and Clare, currently dual trainees, revised together for most of their exams and passed all of them the first time so they are an experienced team to advise future candidates. Add in Sarah, Consultant in ICM, as editor and hey presto, a winning combination. I don't know Kate and Clare personally, but I have known Sarah since her second year of medical school when I became her personal tutor. I am proud of all her achievements and now it is her turn to become the role model. All three are highly driven individuals seeking perfection and this is reflected in the book you are about to use to help you pass the exam.

As a current FFICM examiner I am often asked about the availability, or lack of, revision aids for exam preparation so now I can direct them to this new resource. Kate and Clare have done an incredible job, bringing together relevant material and presenting it in a user-friendly manner. I particularly like the way each of the 91 topics is presented in the format of a structured oral exam (SOE). Having been masterly edited by Sarah it will be of interest, not only to those of you sitting the exam but also those wanting to create lifelike exam scenarios. All three have first-hand experience of the FFICM by sitting the exam and, in Sarah's case, creating and continuing to run the Faculty's exam preparation course. The book is not meant to be used in isolation and the reader is directed to other appropriate resources where available. As both Kate and Clare have said, I hope this makes your journey a little easier and I look forward to seeing some of you in person at The Faculty.

Dr Alison J Pittard MBChB MD FRCA FFICM
Consultant in Anaesthesia and Intensive Care Medicine
Examiner FFICM

Preparation for the Viva

Revising for the Final FFICM SOE proved a rather onerous task for Clare and me. The exam was in its infancy: there was limited information available from the Faculty at that stage and revision resources were rather scant. However, a few of our friends and colleagues had taken it, and they provided us with advice and some fabulous resources. Clare and I decided to work together, spending days revising pre-planned topics which we would then quiz each other on. The single best piece of advice we could give you is to get yourself a revision buddy.

Whilst we have written this book in an effort to provide a useful resource for SOE revision, it is not intended to be used in isolation: the topic list and questions within them are by no means exhaustive. We tried to focus on the big topics, but also wanted to include some of the more unusual areas (certainly, there are several that we would not have thought to revise had we not been told they had come up in previous sittings).

Below is a list of the resources that we found useful in our revision. We hope that it will save you some time!

Steve Mathieu's excellent website, **The Bottom Line**, provides neat summaries of all the important papers and is kept very current. A great resource!

ICU Trials is an app available on iOS and Android that summarises succinctly most of the important ICU trials you should be aware of. It's free and pretty useful to have on hand when you're at work too.

For the anaesthetists among you, we are sure you will be aware of **BJA Education**, formerly **Continuing Education in Anaesthesia, Critical Care and Pain**. We used this journal a lot while we were revising and in preparing the model answers for this book. The articles are usually about four pages long, well-written, and factually sound.

Finally, **e-ICM** is the latest e-Learning for Health (e-lfh) programme, and is dedicated to Intensive Care Medicine. It is mapped to the syllabus and contains approximately 700 interactive e-learning sessions as well as review articles and links to relevant guidelines. It is free to access for anyone who works within the NHS.

In addition to the above, there are also many fantastic revision courses across the country, with more springing up all the time. They often base their questions on previous questions that have come up in the actual exam or 'hot topics' that they suspect might feature. Most run both a mock SOE and OSCE and vary between one and two days in length. Well worth the money!

There are certain topics that we elected not to cover; for example, muscle relaxants and problems with suxamethonium in ICU patients (a question that has been asked in previous exam sittings). Whilst questions on topics like this will be fairly straightforward for the anaesthetists, we would recommend that the non-anaesthetists source a **Final FRCA Viva book** or two to review the ICM-themed topics within (I'm sure you will be able to borrow them from your anaesthetist peers). We have tried to stay away from repeating subject matter that can be found in these books for fear of creating a huge, unmanageable tome!

Useful books

Cook S-C, Thomas M, Nolan J, Parr M. *Key Topics in Critical Care*. London: JP Medical Ltd, 2014 (amazing book, well worth the purchase).

Parsons P, Wiener-Kronish JP, eds. *Critical Care Secrets*. Missouri: Elsevier Mosby, 2013 (this is an American book but it has a lot of really useful content).

Final FRCA SOE books

Barker JM, Mills SJ, Maguire SL. The Clinical Anaesthesia Viva Book. Cambridge: Cambridge University Press, 2009

Bricker S. The Anaesthesia Science Book. Cambridge: Cambridge University Press, 2008

Leslie RA, Johnson EK, Thomas G, Goodwin APL. Dr Podcast Scripts for the Final FRCA. Cambridge: Cambridge University Press, 2011

It is a daunting task and we appreciate that, but we hope that this book will make the experience slightly less stressful. Good luck!

Kate and Clare

From the Editor

The FFICM is a daunting and challenging exam. The syllabus is as deep as it is wide and incorporates many varied aspects of medicine. The exam reflects this, featuring subjects as diverse as life threatening skin conditions, ethical dilemmas and complex resuscitation scenarios.

In view of this, Kate and Clare have written model answers to 91 different topics that have featured previously in the exam. The question style reflects that seen in the SOE and succinct but comprehensive answers are presented in a practical format. Where possible the latest evidence base is discussed and pertinent guidelines included, providing an accessible, up-to-date and user-friendly training tool.

Although primarily written as a key revision aid, this book will also be a resource that will be useful on a daily basis for the intensive care trainee of any level when working on a critical care unit.

We hope that this publication will give the reader a real flavour of the depth and range of what to expect in the exam, and thus arm them with the necessary experience and knowledge to pass the FFICM.

All that remains to be said is good luck, and remember *faber est suae quisque fortunae*.

Dr Sarah Marsh

Acknowledgements

First and foremost, I would like to thank Clare for agreeing to help write this book. You're an absolute star, and I certainly wouldn't have passed this exam if it was not for all our revision sessions!

Huge thanks to our editor, Sarah, for her patience, guidance, kindness and hard work throughout this venture, especially since she was on maternity leave and juggling editing with a new baby!

Thank you to PJ Zolfaghari, my long-suffering Educational Supervisor, for being an incredible support during this project and throughout my ICM training.

And to 'The Other Sarah Marsh', Melissa Asaro and Neil Ryan, our publishers and mentors, thank you for guiding us through this foreign land of writing and publishing.

Clare and I would also like to thank the various people who lent us notes and provided us with the topics from their vivas, which helped us in our revision and in writing this book. Jon Brammall, Ele Galtry, Caroline Moss and Rachel Baumber: you are all stars, thanks a million!

Last, but certainly not least, I would like to thank my incredible family and friends for their love and support.

Kate

Firstly, I would like to thank Kate and Clare for their tireless efforts in bringing this book to life. They have been dedicated, diligent and incredibly industrious over the last twelve months, and always with a smile. It has been a pleasure to work with these talented young women who have such an enthusiasm for Intensive Care Medicine.

Secondly, I would like to thank my three boys for their patience, support and encouragement throughout this process. You'll have me back soon!

Sarah

Thank you to our various colleagues and friends for their help in reviewing topics and supplying figures for us:

Dr Rasha K Al-Lamee MA (Oxon) MB BS (Lond) MRCP
Consultant Cardiologist
Imperial College Healthcare NHS Trust
Dr Bara Erhayiem BMedSci BMBS MRCP
ST7 in Cardiology
Nottingham University Hospitals NHS Trust

Mr Thomas König BSc (Hons) MB BS FRCS (Gen Surg) RAMC
Vascular and Trauma Surgeon
Defence Medical Services
Royal London Hospital

Dr Dan G Nevin MBBCh, Dip PEC, DA, Dip IMC RCSEd, FCA (SA), MSc Med
Consultant in Anaesthesia and Pre-Hospital Care
Royal London Hospital

Dr Andrew Retter MBBS MRCP FRCPath DICM
Consultant in ICU and ECMO
Guys and St Thomas' NHS Foundation Trust

Dr Andrew Taylor MBChB MRCP
ST8 in Renal and Intensive Care Medicine

Dr Claire Tordoff MBChB (Hons) BSc (Hons) FRCA FFICM
Consultant in Anaesthesia and Intensive Care Medicine
St James's University Hospital

Abbreviations

AAA	Abdominal aortic aneurysm
ABG	Arterial blood gas
ACA	Anterior cerebral artery
ACE	Angiotensin converting enzyme
ACEi	Angiotensin converting enzyme inhibitor
ACh	Acetylcholine
AChR	Acetylcholine receptor
ACS	Acute coronary syndrome
ACTH	Adrenocorticotrophic hormone
ADEM	Acute disseminated encephalomyelitis
ADH	Antidiuretic hormone
AECOPD	Acute exacerbation of chronic obstructive pulmonary disease
AED	Anti-epileptic drug
AF	Atrial fibrillation
AFE	Amniotic fluid embolism
AgPC	Antigen-presenting cell
AIDP	Acute inflammatory demyelinating polyneuropathy
AIDS	Acquired immunodeficiency syndrome
AIS	Abbreviated injury scale
AKI	Acute kidney injury
ALF	Acute liver failure
ALI	Acute lung injury
ALS	Advanced life support
ALT	Alanine aminotransferase
AMAN	Acute motor axonal neuropathy
AMSAN	Acute motor and sensory axonal neuropathy
ANP	Atrial natriuretic peptide
APACHE	Acute Physiology and Chronic Health Evaluation
APC	Activated protein C
APP	Abdominal perfusion pressure
APS	Antiphospholipid syndrome
ARB	Angiotensin receptor blocker
ARDS	Acute respiratory distress syndrome
ARP	Absolute refractory period
ARR	Absolute risk reduction
ARV	Antiretroviral (drug)
ASD	Atrial septal defect
AST	Aspartate aminotransferase

AT	Anaerobic threshold (CPET)
ATC	Acute traumatic coagulopathy
ATIII	Antithrombin III
ATLS	Advanced Trauma Life Support
ATN	Acute tubular necrosis
ATP	Adenosine triphosphate
AUROC	Area under receiver-operating characteristic curve
AV	Atrioventricular
AVNRT	Atrioventricular nodal re-entrant tachycardia
AVRT	Atrioventricular re-entrant tachycardia
AXR	Abdominal X-ray
BAL	Bronchoalveolar lavage
BBB	Blood-brain barrier
BE	Base excess
BiVAD	Biventricular assist device
BMI	Body mass index
BMR	Basal metabolic rate
BNP	Brain natriuretic polypeptide
BP	Blood pressure
BPF	Bronchopleural fistula
BSA	Body surface area
BTF	Brain Trauma Foundation
CAD	Coronary artery disease
CAM-ICU	Confusion Assessment Method-ICU
cAMP	Cyclic adenosine monophosphate
CAP	Community-acquired pneumonia
CBF	Cerebral blood flow
CCB	Calcium channel-blocker
CCF	Congestive cardiac failure
CDC	Centers for Disease Control and Prevention
CDT	Clostridium difficile toxin
CF	Cystic fibrosis
CI	Cardiac index
CI-AKI	Contrast-induced acute kidney injury
CIM	Critical illness myopathy
CINM	Critical illness neuromyopathy
CIPN	Critical illness polyneuropathy
CJD	Creutzfelt-Jacob disease
CK	Creatine kinase
CKD	Chronic kidney disease
CMAP	Compound muscle action potential
CMACE	Centre for Maternal and Child Enquiries
$CMRO_2$	Cerebral oxygen requirement
CMV	Cytomegalovirus
CN	Cranial nerve
CNS	Central nervous system
CO	Cardiac output

COM	Cardiac output monitoring
COPD	Chronic obstructive pulmonary disease
CPAP	Continuous positive airway pressure
CPB	Cardiopulmonary bypass
CPET	Cardiopulmonary exercise testing
CPP	Cerebral perfusion pressure
CPR	Cardiopulmonary resuscitation
CPS	Child-Turcotte-Pugh Score
CRBSI	Catheter-related bloodstream infection
CRE	Carbapenem-resistant enterococci
CRH	Corticotrophin-releasing hormone
CRP	C reactive protein
CRT	Capillary refill time
CSA	Cross-sectional area
CSF	Cerebrospinal fluid
CSHT	Context-sensitive half-time
CSWS	Cerebral salt-wasting syndrome
CT	Computed tomography
CTPA	Computed tomography pulmonary angiography
CVC	Central venous catheter
CVP	Central venous pressure
CVS	Cardiovascular system
CVVHD	Continuous veno-venous haemodialysis
CVVHDF	Continuous veno-venous haemodiafiltration
CVVHF	Continuous veno-venous haemofiltration
CXR	Chest X-ray
DAH	Diffuse alveolar haemorrhage
DAI	Diffuse axonal injury
DBD	Donation after brain death
DBP	Diastolic blood pressure
DC	Decompressive craniectomy
DCCV	Electrical (direct current) cardioversion
DCD	Donation after cardiac death
DCI	Delayed cerebral ischaemia
DCR	Damage control resuscitation
DCT	Distal convoluted tubule
DDAVP	Deamino-delta-arginine vasopressin, desmopressin
DHF	Dihydrofolate
DI	Diabetes insipidus
DIC	Disseminated intravascular coagulation
DKA	Diabetic ketoacidosis
DLCO	Diffusing capacity of the lungs for carbon monoxide
DLT	Double lumen (endotracheal) tube
DM	Diabetes mellitus
DNA	Deoxyribonucleic acid
DND	Delayed neurological deficit
DOC	Disorder of consciousness

DOLS	Deprivation of liberty safeguard
DSM-IV	Diagnostic and Statistical Manual of mental disorders, 4th edition
DVT	Deep vein thrombosis
EBV	Epstein-Barr virus
ECCO$_2$R	Extracorporeal carbon dioxide removal
ECG	Electrocardiogram
ECLS	Extracorporeal life support
ECMO	Extracorporeal membrane oxygenation
ED	Emergency Department
EEG	Electroencephalogram
EGDT	Early goal-directed therapy
eGFR	Estimated glomerular filtration rate
EMG	Electromyography
EN	Enteral nutrition
EPAP	Expiratory positive airway pressure
EPO	Erythropoeitin
ERCP	Endoscopic retrograde cholangiopancreatography
ESBL	Extended spectrum beta-lactamase
ESR	Erythrocyte sedimentation rate
ESRD	End-stage renal disease
ETT	Endotracheal tube
EVAR	Endovascular aneurysm repair
EVD	Extraventricular drain
EVLW	Extravascular lung water
FAST	Focussed assessment with sonography for trauma
FBC	Full blood count
FDP	Fibrin-degradation product
FEV1	Forced expired volume in one second
FFP	Fresh frozen plasma
FHF	Fulminant hepatic failure
FPM	First-pass metabolism
FRC	Functional residual capacity
FTc	Flow time corrected
FVC	Forced vital capacity
FWI	Functional warm ischaemia
GABA	Gamma-aminobutyric acid
GAS	Group A Streptococci (*Strep. pyogenes*)
GBS	Guillain-Barré syndrome
GCS	Glasgow Coma Score
GEDV	Global end-diastolic volume
GFR	Glomerular flow rate
GI	Gastrointestinal
GMC	General Medical Council
GOSE	Extended Glasgow Outcome Scale
GTN	Glyceryl trinitrate
GU	Genitourinary

GvHD	Graft vs host disease
H$_2$RA	H$_2$-receptor antagonist
HAART	Highly active antiretroviral therapy
HAP	Hospital-acquired pneumonia
HAS	Human albumin solution
HbCO	Carboxyhaemoglobin
HBOT	Hyperbaric oxygen therapy
HbO$_2$	Oxyhaemoglobin
HBV	Hepatitis B virus
HCC	Hepatocellular carcinoma
HCT	Haematopoietic cell transplantation
HCV	Hepatitis C virus
HDU	High Dependency Unit
HELLP	Haemolysis, elevated liver enzymes, low platelets
HES	Hydroxyethyl starch
HFOV	High-frequency oscillatory ventilation
HFV	High-frequency ventilation
HHS	Hyperglycaemic hyperosmolar state
HILU	High Level Isolation Unit
HIT	Heparin-induced thrombocytopenia
HIV	Human immunodeficiency virus
HIV	HIV-associated nephropathy
HME	Heat and moisture exchanger
HMG-CoA	3-hydroxy-3-methyl-glutaryl-CoA
HPA	Hypothalamo-pituitary-adrenal (axis)
HPVC	Hypoxic pulmonary vasoconstriction
HR	Heart rate
HRCT	High-resolution CT
HRS	Hepatorenal syndrome
HSV	*Herpes simplex* virus
HUS	Haemolytic uraemic syndrome
IABP	Intra-aortic balloon pump
IAH	Intra-abdominal hypertension
IAP	Intra-abdominal pressure
IBD	Inflammatory bowel disease
IBP	Invasive blood pressure
IBW	Ideal body weight
ICDSC	Intensive Care Delirium Screening Checklist
ICD-10	International Statistical Classification of Diseases and Related Health Problems, 10th edition
ICH	Intracerebral haemorrhage
ICP	Intracranial pressure
ICU	Intensive Care Unit
ICUAW	Intensive Care Unit-acquired weakness
IE	Infective endocarditis
IFN	Interferon
Ig	Immunoglobulin

IHD	Ischaemic heart disease
IJV	Internal jugular vein
IL	Interleukin
ILD	Interstitial lung disease
IM	Intramuscular
IMCA	Independent mental capacity advocate
IMV	Invasive mechanical ventilation
INR	International normalised ratio
IPAP	Inspiratory positive airway pressure
IPF	Idiopathic pulmonary fibrosis
IPPV	Invasive positive pressure ventilation
IRS	Immune reconstitution syndrome
ISS	Injury severity score
IV	Intravenous
IVC	Inferior vena cava
IVDU	Intravenous drug user
IVIg	Intravenous immunoglobulin
JAMA	Journal of the American Medical Association
JVP	Jugular venous pressure
LA	Left atrium
LACS	Lacunar syndrome
LAP	Left atrial pressure
LDH	Lactate dehydrogenase
L-DOPA	L-3,4-dihydroxyphenylalanine
LEMS	Lambert-Eaton Myasthenic Syndrome
LFTs	Liver function tests
LMWH	Low molecular weight heparin
LOS	Length of stay
LP	Lumbar puncture
LPS	Lipopolysaccharide
LPV	Lung protective ventilation
LRTI	Lower respiratory tract infection
LSD	Lysergic acid diethylamide
LTA	Lipotechoic acid
LTOT	Long-term oxygen therapy
LV	Left ventricle
LVAD	Left ventricular assist device
LVEDV	Left ventricular end-diastolic volume
LVF	Left ventricular failure
LVH	Left ventricular hypertrophy
MAHA	Microangiopathic haemolytic anaemia
MAOI	Monoamine oxidase inhibitor
MA	Maximum amplitude (TEG®)
MAP	Mean arterial pressure
MBRRACE-UK	Mothers and Babies: Reducing Risk through Audits and Confidential Enquiries across the UK
MC+S	Microbiology, culture and sensitivity

MCA	Middle cerebral artery
MCS	Minimally conscious state
MDMA	3,4-methylenedioxy-methamphetamine
MDR	Multi-drug resistant
MDT	Multi-disciplinary team
MELD	Model for End-stage Liver Disease
MEOWS	Modified early obstetric early warning score
MET	Metabolic equivalent
MG	Myasthenia gravis
MH	Malignant hyperthermia
MHC	Major histocompatibility complex
MI	Myocardial infarction
MIC	Minimum inhibitory concentration
MILS	Manual in-line stabilisation
MPAP	Mean pulmonary arterial pressure
MRA	Magnetic resonance angiography
MRCP	Magnetic resonance cholangiopancreatography
MRI	Magnetic resonance imaging
MRSA	Methicillin-resistant *Staphylococcus aureus*
MSH	Melanocyte-stimulating hormone
MSSA	Methicillin-sensitive *Staphylococcus aureus*
MW	Molecular weight
NAC	N-acetyl cysteine
NAFLD	Non-alcoholic fatty liver disease
NAP	National Audit Project of the Royal College of Anaesthetists
NCEPOD	National Confidential Enquiry into Patient Outcome and Death
NCS	Nerve conduction studies
NCSE	Non-convulsive status epilepticus
NEJM	New England Journal of Medicine
NF	Necrotising fasciitis
NG	Nasogastric
NHS	National Health Service
NHSBT	NHS Blood and Transplant
NICE	National Institute for Health and Care Excellence
NIHSS	National Institute of Health Stroke Scale
NIV	Non-invasive ventilation
NJ	Nasojejunal
NMBA	Neuromuscular blocking agent
NMDA	N-methyl-D-aspartate
NMJ	Neuromuscular junction
NMS	Neuroleptic malignant syndrome
NNH	Number needed to harm
NNRTI	Non-nucleoside reverse transcriptase inhibitor
NNT	Number needed to treat
NO	Nitric oxide
NOAC	Novel oral anticoagulant

NOS	Nitric oxide synthase
NPSA	National Patient Safety Agency
NRLS	National Reporting and Learning System
NRTI	Nucleoside reverse transcriptase inhibitor
NSAID	Non-steroidal anti-inflammatory drug
NSMS	Neurogenic stunned myocardium syndrome
NSTEMI	Non-ST elevation myocardial infarction
ODC	Oxygen dissociation curve
ODM	Oesophageal Doppler monitoring
OER	Oxygen extraction ratio
OOHCA	Out-of-hospital cardiac arrest
OSA	Obstructive sleep apnoea
PA	Pulmonary artery
PAC	Pulmonary artery catheter
PACS	Partial anterior circulation syndrome
PAH	Pulmonary arterial hypertension
PAMP	Pathogen-associated molecular pattern
PAP	Pulmonary artery pressure
PBM	Patient blood management
PCA	Patient-controlled analgesia
PCC	Prothrombin complex concentrate
PDE	Phosphodiesterase
PCI	Percutaneous coronary intervention
PCP	Pneumocystis pneumonia
PCR	Polymerase chain reaction
PCT	Proximal convoluted tubule
PCWP	Pulmonary capillary wedge pressure
PDE	Phosphodiesterase
PE	Pulmonary embolus
PEA	Pulseless electrical activity
PEEP	Positive end-expiratory pressure
PEFR	Peak expiratory flow rate
PEG	Percutaneous endoscopic gastrostomy
PET	Pre-eclampsia (toxaemia)
PEx	Plasma exchange
PG	Prostaglandin
pK_a	Dissociation constant
PN	Parenteral nutrition
PoCA	Posterior cerebral artery
POCS	Posterior circulation syndrome
POSSUM	Physiological and Operative Severity Score for the enUmeration of Mortality and morbidity
PPE	Personal protective equipment
PPi	Proton pump inhibitor
P_{plat}	Plateau pressure
PPR	Pattern-recognition receptors
PPV	Positive pressure ventilation

PRBCs	Packed red blood cells
PRES	Posterior reversible encephalopathy syndrome
PRIS	Propofol infusion syndrome
PT	Prothrombin time
PTH	Parathyroid hormone
PTSD	Post-traumatic stress disorder
PVL	Panton Valentine leucocidin
PVR(I)	Pulmonary vascular resistance (index)
QoL	Quality of life
QTc	QT interval (corrected)
RA	Right atrium
RAA(S)	Renin-angiotensin-aldosterone (system)
RAP	Right atrial pressure
RAS	Renal artery stenosis
RASS	Richmond Agitation-Sedation Score
RAST	Radioallergosorbent test
RBBB	Right bundle branch block
RBC	Red blood cell
RBF	Renal blood flow
RCA	Right coronary artery
RCT	Randomised controlled trial
REBOA	Resuscitative endovascular balloon occlusion of the aorta
rFVIIa	Recombinant activated factor VII
RNA	Ribonucleic acid
ROS	Reactive oxygen species
ROSC	Return of spontaneous circulation
ROTEM®	Rotational Thromboelastometry
RR	Respiratory rate
RRT	Renal replacement therapy
RSBI	Rapid shallow breathing index
RSI	Rapid sequence induction
RTA	Renal tubular acidosis
rTPA	Recombinant tissue plasminogen activator
RUQ	Right upper quadrant
RV	Right ventricle
RVAD	Right ventricular assist device
RVEDP	Right ventricular end-diastolic pressure
RVEDV	Right ventricular end-diastolic volume
RVF	Right ventricular failure
RVP	Right ventricular pressure
RWMA	Regional wall motion abnormality
SA	Sinoatrial
SAH	Subarachnoid haemorrhage
SaO$_2$	Arterial oxygen saturation
SAP	Severe acute pancreatitis
SARS	Severe acute respiratory syndrome
SBOT	Short-burst oxygen therapy

SBP	Systolic blood pressure
SBT	Spontaneous breathing trial
SC	Subcutaneous
SCD	Sickle cell disease
SCCDs	Sequential calf compression devices
SCUF	Slow continuous ultrafiltration
$ScvO_2$	Central venous oxygen saturation
SDD	Selective decontamination of the digestive tract
SIADH	Syndrome of inappropriate antidiuretic hormone
SIRS	Systemic inflammatory response syndrome
$SjvO_2$	Jugular bulb oxygen saturation
SLE	Systemic lupus erythematosis
SLEDD	Sustained low-efficiency daily dialysis
SMR	Standardised mortality rate
SNP	Sodium nitroprusside
SO_2	Oxygen saturation
SOFA	Sequential Organ Failure Assessment
SPM	Semi-permeable membrane
SpO_2	Peripheral capillary oxygen saturation
SSEP	Somatosensory evoked potential
SSRI	Selective serotonin reuptake inhibitor
SV(I)	Stroke volume (index)
SVC	Superior vena cava
SvO_2	Mixed venous oxygen saturation
SVR(I)	Systemic vascular resistance (index)
SVT	Supraventricular tachycardia
TACO	Transfusion-associated circulatory overload
TACS	Total anterior circulation syndrome
TAPSE	Tricuspid annular plane systolic excursion
TB	Tuberculosis
TBI	Traumatic brain injury
TBSA	Total body surface area
TCA	Tricyclic antidepressant
TCD	Transcranial Doppler
TEG®	Thromboelastography
TFTs	Thyroid function tests
TH	Therapeutic hypothermia
THF	Tetrahydrofolate
THR	Total hip replacement
TIA	Transient ischaemic attack
TIC	Trauma-induced coagulopathy
TIF	Tracheo-innominate fistula
TIPSS	Transjugular intrahepatic porto-systemic shunt
TKR	Total knee replacement
TLR	Toll-like receptor
TLS	Tumour lysis syndrome
TNF	Tissue necrosis factor

TOE	Transoesohageal echocardiography
tPA	Tissue plasminogen activator
TR	Tricuspid regurgitation
TRALI	Transfusion-related acute lung injury
TSH	Thyroid stimulating hormone
TSS	Toxic shock syndrome
TTE	Transthoracic echocardiography
TTP	Thrombotic thrombocytopenic purpura
TXA	Tranexamic acid
TXA_2	Thromboxane A_2
U+Es	Urea and electrolytes
UC	Ulcerative colitis
UFH	Unfractionated heparin
UGI	Upper gastrointestinal
UKELD	UK Model for End-Stage Liver Disease
URTI	Upper respiratory tract infection
UTI	Urinary tract infection
VAD	Ventricular assist device
VAP	Ventilator-associated pneumonia
VATS	Video-assisted thoroscopic surgery
VBG	Venous blood gas
VC	Vital capacity
Vd	Volume of distribution
VF	Ventricular fibrillation
VHA	Viscoelastic haemostatic assay
VHF	Viral haemorrhagic fever
VILI	Ventilator-induced lung injury
VO_2	Oxygen consumption
V/Q	Ventilation/perfusion
VRE	Vancomycin-resistant enterococcus
VS	Vegetative state
VSD	Ventricular septal defect
Vt	Tidal volume
VT	Ventricular tachycardia
VTE	Venous thromboembolism
vWD	von Willebrand disease
vWF	von Willebrand Factor
vWF-CP	von Willebrand factor-cleaving protease
VZV	Varicella-Zoster virus
WCC	White cell count
WHO	World Health Organisation
WPW	Wolff-Parkinson-White syndrome
2,3-DPG	2,3-diphosphoglycerate

Chapter 1

Abdominal Aortic Aneurysm

What is the mortality and morbidity associated with ruptured abdominal aortic aneurysm?

A ruptured abdominal aortic aneurysm (AAA) is one of the most commonly fatal surgical emergencies with only approximately 50% of patients reaching hospital alive; of those who do reach the hospital, up to 50% die before having surgery, and a further 50% do not survive surgical repair.

What are the risk factors for AAA?

Risk factors for AAA include:

1 Male gender
2 Age >65 years
3 Smoking
4 Hypertension
5 Myocardial and/or cerebrovascular disease
6 Genetic/familial disposition (e.g. inherited connective tissue disorders such as Marfans and Ehlers-Danlos)

How does a ruptured AAA present?

The majority of AAAs will rupture into the retroperitoneal cavity, resulting in the classical triad of:

– Pain (typically severe and usually located in the back)
– Signs of circulatory compromise (often the patient is shocked)
– Pulsatile abdominal mass

However, patients may present with atypical symptoms and signs that can lead to misdiagnosis including:

– Back pain (may mimic renal colic)
– +/– radiation to the legs (mimicking sciatica)
– Chronic severe back pain (contained rupture)
– Transient lower limb paralysis

Massive gastrointestinal (GI) haemorrhage raises the suspicion of an aortoenteric fistula (usually in the context of a previous AAA graft that has eroded into the GI tract).

How would you treat a patient with AAA rupture?

Ruptured AAA is a surgical emergency and transfer for definitive surgical management should not be delayed by unnecessary investigations or procedures. Management should follow an ABCDE approach, and abnormalities should be treated as they are found.

1 Resuscitation
   - Two large bore peripheral intravenous (IV) cannulae, attached to giving sets with hand pumps or rapid infusion systems
   - Crossmatch ≥6 units of blood and activate massive transfusion protocol as necessary
   - Target systolic blood pressure (SBP) ~90 mmHg to maintain end organ perfusion
   - Provide titrated analgesia (e.g. fentanyl or morphine)
2 Investigations
   - Full blood count (FBC), urea and electrolytes (U+Es), coagulation profile, venous gas
   - Electrocardiogram (ECG, massive MI is a differential diagnosis)
   - Imaging as necessary (see below)
3 Transfer to the operating theatre for definitive treatment

Both open and endovascular approaches are currently used to repair ruptured AAA. There is some evidence to suggest that perioperative (30-day) outcomes for endovascular aneurysm repair (EVAR) following ruptured AAA may be better than for open AAA repair; however, significant differences in mortality rates have not definitively been demonstrated and studies are ongoing.

Contained rupture still requires urgent repair, but less acutely than an uncontained rupture.

What imaging may be used and what are the advantages and disadvantages of each?

Imaging should *never* delay potentially lifesaving abdominal surgery when such surgery is immediately available and the diagnosis is strongly suspected. Table 1.1 describes advantages and disadvantages of each modality.

Table 1.1 Imaging modalities used to characterise aortic aneurysms

Imaging modality	Advantages	Disadvantages
CT	Best investigation if diagnosis is uncertain Detailed analysis of the extent of aneurysmal disease Can confirm and localise the site of rupture Evaluate aortic wall morphology and extra-aortic structures	Haemodynamic stability required for transfer Can result in a delay to surgery Nephrotoxicity of the contrast media
Ultrasound	Can be rapidly performed at the bedside (i.e. suitable for unstable patients) Can detect aneurysm and free fluid Simple Economical	Imperfect sensitivity (~95%)
MRI	Highly specific and sensitive Lack of nephrotoxicity of the contrast media Tissue characterisation using pulsed sequences	Long scanning time – not appropriate in AAA rupture Higher cost Inferior spatial resolution

CT – computed tomography; MRI – magnetic resonance imaging

What complications can arise following emergency surgery for AAA rupture?

A number of complications can occur following emergency AAA repair as highlighted in Table 1.2.

How can you prognosticate in ruptured AAA?

Emergency surgery for ruptured AAA is associated with a high mortality. The Acute Physiology and Chronic Health Evaluation (APACHE) II and Physiological and Operative Severity Score for the enUmeration of Mortality and morbidity (POSSUM) scoring widely used in other settings do not accurately predict outcome in ruptured AAA, hence specific tools for this purpose exist. The Hardman index for ruptured AAA was published in 1996 and consists of five preoperative variables with a range of possible scores from 0–5 (Table 1.3). Recent studies have predicted a mortality of 80% with Hardman index scores ≥2.

The Glasgow Aneurysm Score is also used in predicting outcome after both elective and emergency aneurysm surgery (Table 1.4). A value of 84 indicates a predicted mortality of 65%.

Table 1.2 Complications following emergency surgery for ruptured AAA

	Early complications	Late complications
Graft-related	Massive transfusion	Infection
	Distal embolisation (trash foot)	Graft occlusion
	Aortic branch involvement resulting in ischaemia i.e. pancreatitis, AKI	Aorto-enteric fistula
	Endoleak	Anastomotic pseudoaneurysm
Non-graft related	Renal failure	Prolonged respiratory wean
	Myocardial infarction	Small bowel obstruction
	Paraplegia	Sexual dysfunction
	Hepatic dysfunction	Incisional herniae
	HAP/VAP	DVT/PE
	ARDS	
	Abdominal compartment syndrome	
	Ileus	

AKI – acute kidney injury; HAP – hospital-acquired pneumonia; VAP – ventilator-associated pneumonia; ARDS – Acute Respiratory Distress Syndrome; DVT – deep vein thrombosis; PE – pulmonary embolus

Table 1.3 The Hardman index for predicting immediate outcome after surgery for ruptured AAA

Variable	Points
Age >76	1
Serum creatinine >190 μmol/l	1
Haemoglobin <90 g/l	1
Myocardial ischaemia on ECG	1
A history of loss of consciousness after arrival to hospital	1

Table 1.4 Glasgow Aneurysm Score for predicting immediate outcome after surgery for ruptured AAA

Variable	Points
Age of patient	= age in years
Shock	17
Myocardial disease	7
Cerebrovascular disease (all grades of stroke including TIA)	10
Renal disease (urea >20 μmol/l and/or creatinine >150 μmol/l)	14

TIA – transient ischaemic attack

Age is an important independent risk factor for post-operative mortality after AAA rupture as highlighted by both systems.

What interventions may help reduce the mortality from ruptured AAA?

1 Abdominal ultrasound screening
  Elective repair should be undertaken in:
   i Male with AAA >5.5 cm
   ii Female with AAA >5 cm
   iii Rapid growth >1 cm/year
2 Advances in endovascular techniques
3 National audit
4 Vascular teamwork with standardisation of care pathways and treatments

What are the indications for spinal drain insertion?

Indications for spinal drain insertion in patients undergoing aneurysm repair include:

1 To reduce cerebrospinal fluid (CSF) pressure following complex abdominal EVARs where patients are considered to be at particular risk of spinal cord ischaemia
2 Rescue therapy for delayed paraplegia postoperatively.

Other indications for CSF drainage:

1 Reduce intracranial pressure (ICP), e.g. pre-, intra-, or post-neurosurgery
2 Monitor CSF chemistry, cytology, and physiology
3 Provide temporary CSF drainage in patients with infected cerebrospinal fluid shunts

How do lumbar spinal drains work?

Spinal drainage of CSF can be used to prevent or treat spinal cord ischaemia. The physiological basis for lumbar CSF drainage is that spinal cord perfusion pressure is a function of the mean arterial pressure (MAP) minus the lumbar CSF pressure.

Cord perfusion pressure = MAP – CSF pressure

Draining CSF by percutaneous insertion of a catheter into the subarachnoid space between lumbar spinal processes has the potential to increase spinal cord perfusion pressure by decreasing the CSF pressure.

What are the contraindications to spinal drain insertion?

Absolute contraindications are:

1 Patients receiving anticoagulants
2 Bleeding diathesis

Lumbar drainage is *not recommended* in the following (use for external drainage and monitoring is at the discretion of the physician):

1 Non-communicating hydrocephalus
2 Presence of large intracranial mass lesions, e.g. tumours, haematomas or cysts
3 Infection in the surrounding area, i.e. skin, subcutaneous tissue, bone and epidural space

Further Reading

Kent K C. Clinical practice. Abdominal aortic aneurysms. *New Engl J Med* 2014; **371**(22): 2101–2108

Li Y, Li Z, Wang S, et al. Endovascular versus open surgery repair of ruptured abdominal aortic aneurysms in hemodynamically unstable patients: Literature review and meta-analysis. *Ann Vasc Surg* 2016; **32**: 135–144

Thompson J. Anaesthesia for ruptured abdominal aortic aneurysm. *Contin Educ Anaesth Crit Care Pain* 2008; **8**(1): 11–15

Chapter 2

Abdominal Compartment Syndrome and the Open Abdomen

What is the normal intra-abdominal pressure?

Normal intra-abdominal pressure (IAP) is 5–7 mmHg.

How are intra-abdominal hypertension and abdominal compartment syndrome defined?

Abdominal perfusion pressure (APP) is calculated using the following formula:

$$APP = MAP - IAP$$

The following are definitions from the World Society for Abdominal Compartment Syndrome (WSACS):

Intra-abdominal hypertension (IAH) is defined as sustained or repeated pathological elevations in IAP >12 mmHg.

Abdominal compartment syndrome is a sustained IAP >20 mmHg (with or without an APP <60 mmHg) that is associated with new organ dysfunction or failure.

Intra-abdominal hypertension may be graded according to severity:

Grade 1	12–15 mmHg
Grade 2	16–20 mmHg
Grade 3	21–25 mmHg
Grade 4	≥26 mmHg

Abdominal compartment syndrome may be *primary* (due to abdominal pathology) or *secondary* to one or more extra-abdominal processes.

What risk factors are associated with the development of intra-abdominal hypertension and abdominal compartment syndrome?

There are many risk factors associated with the development of IAH and abdominal compartment syndrome:

1 Diminished abdominal wall compliance
   i Abdominal surgery with tight primary closure
   ii Trauma, burns, obesity
   iii Prone positioning
2 Increased abdominal contents
   – Intraluminal: ileus, gastroparesis, pseudo-obstruction
   – Extraluminal: ascites, haemoperitoneum, pneumoperitoneum
3 Capillary leak
   i Severe sepsis, trauma, pancreatitis, burns
   ii Hypothermia
   iii Acidosis
   iv Massive transfusion
   v Fluid resuscitation, positive fluid balance
4 Other/miscellaneous
   i Mechanical ventilation
   ii Positive end-expiratory pressure (PEEP) >10 cmH$_2$O
   iii Increased head of bed angle
   iv Shock or hypotension

How is intra-abdominal pressure measured?

Clinical examination has a low sensitivity for diagnosing IAH, hence IAP measurements are key. It can be measured directly or indirectly:

1 Direct method
   – Via the introduction of a needle into the abdomen (e.g. during laparoscopy)
2 Indirect method
   – Transduction of pressure via an intra-abdominal viscus can be used to measure IAP using a non-invasive technique (bladder, stomach, colon, uterus)
   – Intra-vesical pressure is the most commonly used method and is performed via a urinary bladder catheter
   – 25 ml of sterile saline is introduced into the bladder and the drainage bag is reconnected and cross-clamped
   – A 16 G needle is connected to a pressure transducer and introduced via the culture port site of the catheter

Outline the pathophysiological effects of IAH on other organ systems

Respiratory

– Raised IAP causes basal atelectasis and collapse due to diaphragmatic splinting and reduced chest wall and lung compliance
– There is increased ventilation/perfusion (V/Q) mismatch, hypoxaemia and hypercapnia

- The application of PEEP and use of positive pressure ventilation (PPV) will worsen venous return and cardiac output (CO)

Cardiovascular

- The raised IAP is transmitted directly to the abdominal vasculature
- There is a reduction in cardiac output secondary to reduced venous return to the right ventricle (due to venous compression) and increased afterload (due to arterial compression)
- The reduction in CO will further reduce the APP
- Increased intra-thoracic pressure due to diaphragmatic splinting may compromise CO further

Neurological

- Increased ICP can occur secondary to the impedance of cerebral venous return due to raised intra-thoracic pressure
- The ICP may be increased further due to cerebral vasodilatation caused by concomitant hypoxaemia and hypercapnia

Renal

- There is direct transmission of the raised IAP to the renal vasculature, which in combination with a reduction in CO reduces renal blood flow
- The raised IAP is also transmitted to the renal outflow tract, causing increased pressure within the tubules and reducing the filtration gradient
- Compensatory activation of the renin-angiotensin-aldosterone (RAA) system further worsens the renal insult

Gastrointestinal and hepatic

- The hypoperfusion caused by critical illness is exacerbated by venous hypertension, which results in bowel wall oedema
- This may cause bowel ischaemia and bacterial translocation, increasing the risk of developing sepsis
- There is reduced flow in the hepatic artery, vein and portal system, which contributes to liver dysfunction
- Biliary stasis resulting from increased pressure within the biliary tree

What are the principles of managing abdominal compartment syndrome?

Abdominal compartment syndrome should be managed with an ABCDE approach, treating abnormalities as they are found. Specific management priorities are optimisation of the patient's physiological and metabolic status alongside restoring vital organ function. The WSACS have produced an algorithm for the treatment of IAH (Figure 2.1). The principles of management are:

1 Serial monitoring of IAP in at-risk patients
2 Medical management to reduce IAP
   i Improve abdominal wall compliance
      – Adequate sedation, analgesia and muscle relaxation to avoid coughing/ straining
      – Optimal positioning (avoid prone position)
   ii Optimise fluid administration and correct positive fluid balance
      – Avoid excessive fluid resuscitation
      – Consider renal replacement therapy
   iii Evacuation of intraluminal contents
      – Gastric decompression
      – Use of prokinetics and laxatives
   iv Evacuation of abdominal fluid collections
      – Drainage of intra-abdominal collections
      – Paracentesis
   v Organ support
      – Optimal ventilator settings to deliver adequate ventilation with alveolar recruitment
      – Maintain APP >60 mmHg with vasopressors
3 Surgical decompression
   i Laparotomy decompression is the definitive treatment for refractory abdominal compartment syndrome
   ii The use of negative pressure wound therapy to manage open abdominal wounds (laparostomy) is recommended by the National Institute for Health and Care Excellence (NICE)

What are the complications of abdominal compartment syndrome?

Untreated abdominal compartment syndrome is associated with a mortality approaching 100%.

Multi-organ failure will result and is a consequence of the severity and duration of IAH.

Why might a patient on the ICU require an open abdomen?

The recent WSACS consensus statement has defined the open abdomen as one that requires a temporary abdominal closure due to the skin and fascia not being closed after laparotomy. The necessity for an open abdomen has progressed from a last resort treatment strategy in abdominal catastrophes, to a preferred management (and indeed preventative) strategy in abdominal compartment syndrome in both trauma and non-trauma patients.

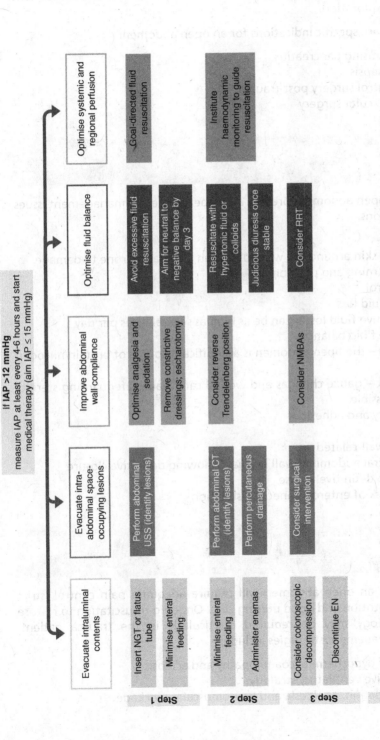

Figure 2.1 Intra-abdominal hypertension/abdominal compartment syndrome medical management algorithm
Adapted with permission from Kirkpatrick AW, et al. (*Intensive Care Med* 2013)

If IAP >12 mmHg
measure IAP at least every 4-6 hours and start medical therapy (aim IAP ≤ 15 mmHg)

| Evacuate intraluminal contents | Evacuate intra-abdominal space-occupying lesions | Improve abdominal wall compliance | Optimise fluid balance | Optimise systemic and regional perfusion |

Step 1
- Insert NGT or flatus tube
- Minimise enteral feeding
- Perform abdominal USS (identity lesions)
- Optimise analgesia and sedation
- Avoid excessive fluid resuscitation
- Goal-directed fluid resuscitation

Step 2
- Minimise enteral feeding
- Administer enemas
- Perform abdominal CT (identity lesions)
- Perform percutaneous drainage
- Remove constrictive dressings; escharotomy
- Aim for neutral to negative balance by day 3
- Institute haemodynamic monitoring to guide resuscitation

Step 3
- Consider colonoscopic decompression
- Discontinue EN
- Consider surgical intervention
- Consider reverse Trendelenberg position
- Resuscitate with hypertonic fluid or colloids
- Judicious diuresis once stable
- Consider NMBAs
- Consider RRT

Step 4
If IAP >20 mmHg + new organ dysfunction/failure and patient's IAP is refractory to medical treatment surgical decompression should be strongly considered

An open abdomen surgical approach will enable initial control of haemorrhage and/or contamination, any necessary intra-peritoneal packing, facilitation of resuscitation to normal physiology on the intensive care unit and subsequent definitive re-exploration.

The following are specific indications for an open abdomen:

1 Severe necrotising pancreatitis
2 Abdominal sepsis
3 Damage control surgery post-trauma
4 Emergent vascular surgery

What issues and complications are associated with open abdomens?

Patients with open abdomens present a number of specific management issues and complications:

1 Nursing issues
   i Skin care; skin around the wound is often moist and prone to damage
   ii Patient turning and positioning
   iii Pain control
2 Significant fluid loss
   i Postoperative fluid losses can be as high as several litres per day
   ii Unreliable fluid balance
3 Malnutrition – the open abdomen is a significant source of protein/nitrogen loss
4 Infection risk – gauze changes and wound care make safeguarding sterility almost impossible
5 Visceral injury and adhesions
6 Ileus
7 Abdominal wall-related
   i Large ventral abdominal wall hernias following definitive closure
   ii Inability to definitively close
8 Significant risk of enterocutaneous fistulation

How should the patient with an open abdomen be managed on the ICU?

A patient with an open abdomen will require adequate pain control, strict attention to nutrition and good nursing care. Ongoing resuscitation to restore normal physiology may be required, particularly in the trauma patient. Additional management strategies include:

1 Correction of hypothermia, coagulopathy and acidosis
2 Lung protective ventilatory strategy
3 Adequate sedation, analgesia and neuromuscular blockade

    i Target Richmond Agitation-Sedation Score (RASS) –4 during the acute resuscitation phase

    ii Paralysis

4 Nutritional support and fluid resuscitation

    i Enteral feeding is safe in a patient with an intact GI tract

    ii Supplement protein – an estimate of 2 g of nitrogen per litre of abdominal fluid output should be included in the nitrogen balance calculations of any patient with an open abdomen

5 Antibiotics tailored to the clinical situation

6 Monitoring for abdominal compartment syndrome

7 Adequate source control with bedside washouts as necessary

The aim is for definitive closure within eight days of initial laparostomy.

What devices/techniques are employed for temporary abdominal closure?

The options for temporary abdominal closure are many and include:

1 The Bogota bag (a 3-litre urological irrigation bag fixed to the fascia or skin – essentially a ready to use 'bowel bag')

2 Negative pressure therapy techniques such as vacuum pack devices

3 Synthetic mesh devices/patches (absorbable or non-absorbable)

4 Velcro-type sheath – 'Whittmann patch'

Further Reading

Berry N, Fletcher S. Abdominal compartment syndrome. *Contin Educ Anaesth Crit Care Pain* 2012; 12(3): 110–117

Dutton W D, Diaz J J. Critical care issues in managing complex open abdominal wound. *Journal of Intensive Care Medicine* 2012; 27(3): 161–171

Kirkpatrick A W, Roberts D J, De Waele J, et al. Intra-abdominal hypertension and the abdominal compartment syndrome: updated consensus definitions and clinical practice guidelines from the World Society for Abdominal Compartment Syndrome. *Intensive Care Med* 2013; 39: 1190–1206

Chapter 3

Acute Ischaemic Stroke

How would you recognise an acute ischaemic stroke?

The clinical presentation of a stroke depends on the site of ischaemia or infarction (Table 3.1). In the UK, NICE has recommended the Face, Arms, Speech and Time test (FAST) for use by paramedics as a screening tool.

How do you classify acute ischaemic stroke?

One commonly used classification system is the Oxford Community Stroke Project classification (also known as the Bamford classification). This is detailed in Table 3.2.

What imaging is required?

Initial imaging is typically a non-contrast CT brain. This will exclude haemorrhage, but may not reliably demonstrate infarction. MRI (or diffusion-weighted MRI) is more superior in this regard; however, this modality may not be readily available in all centres.

Later imaging includes carotid Doppler and magnetic resonance angiography (MRA). A transthoracic echocardiogram (TTE) should be considered in all young patients if more than one territory is involved, there is an audible murmur or there is an abnormal ECG. If a right to left intracardiac shunt is suspected, a transoesophageal echocardiogram (TOE) and bubble-contrast echocardiogram or transcranial Doppler (TCD) should be considered.

NICE recommend urgent imaging within one hour if the patient meets any of the following criteria:

1 Thrombolysis or early anticoagulation treatment indicated
2 Taking anticoagulation therapy
3 Known bleeding tendency
4 Glasgow Coma Score (GCS) <13
5 Progressive or fluctuating symptoms
6 Papilloedema, neck stiffness or fever
7 Severe headache at onset of symptoms

Table 3.1 Clinical features of stroke according to territory

Site of Ischaemia/Infarction	Clinical Features
Anterior cerebral artery (ACA)	Weakness of contralateral leg Behaviour changes
Middle cerebral artery (MCA)	Weakness of contralateral face and arm Aphasia, dysarthria Hemianopia Inattention to stimuli Sensory deficit
Posterior cerebral artery (PoCA)	Visual field deficits Sensory deficits
Vertebrobasilar system	Dizziness, ataxia, impaired balance Pupil and eye movement abnormalities Changes in voice and swallowing Weakness and sensory changes Decreased consciousness
Cerebral vein and sinuses	Decreased consciousness Headache Vomiting

Table 3.2 Bamford classification of stroke

	Features	Anatomy
Total anterior circulation syndrome (TACS)	All three of: i Unilateral motor, sensory deficit or both affecting at least two of face, arm or leg ii Higher cerebral dysfunction (e.g. dysphasia, dyspraxia) iii Homonymous hemianopia	Occlusion of MCA
Partial anterior circulation syndrome (PACS)	Two of the three components of TACS	Occlusion of MCA / branch of ACA
Lacunar syndrome (LACS)	i Pure motor or sensory deficit affecting at least two of face, arm or leg ii Sensorimotor deficit not meeting TACS/PACS criteria iii Ataxic hemiparesis iv Dysarthria and clumsy hand	Occlusion of small, deep penetrating artery causing subcortical stroke
Posterior circulation syndrome (POCS)	i Isolated homonymous hemianopia or cortical blindness ii Brainstem or cerebellar syndromes / cranial nerve palsy iii Loss of consciousness	Brainstem / cerebellum / occipital lobe

How would you manage a patient suffering an acute ischaemic stroke?

Recognition, rapid assessment and distinguishing between ischaemic and haemorrhagic stroke are key management elements. The overall aims of treatment are to restore cerebral blood flow and maintain normal physiology to avoid secondary brain injury.

Patients should be managed with an ABCDE approach, treating abnormalities as they are found. Specific management involves:

1 Investigations
   - Imaging as above
   - Blood tests: FBC, U+Es, C-reactive protein (CRP), erythrocyte sedimentation rate (ESR), thyroid function tests (TFTs), lipid profile
   - ECG
   - TTE, TOE +/- bubble-contrast echocardiogram

2 Maintain **normal physiology**
   The following parameters should be maintained in the normal range:
   i Blood glucose (4–10 mmol/l)
   ii Blood pressure (BP)
      - There is uncertainty about when to treat hypertension as it represents a compensatory mechanism to maintain cerebral perfusion pressure (CPP) in the face of raised ICP and disordered autoregulation
      - BP should be treated in the presence of a hypertensive emergency; in the absence of end-organ dysfunction, a BP of up to 220/120 mmHg may be tolerated
      - In patients suitable for thrombolysis, the Intercollegiate Stroke Working Party guidelines (2016) recommends a BP <185/110 mmHg
      - If necessary BP should be lowered *cautiously* under careful observation for neurological deterioration
   iii Oxygenation (peripheral capillary oxygen saturation (SpO$_2$) >94%)
   iv Temperature

3 Consider **thrombolysis**
   Thrombolysis should be administered if the following criteria are met, and contraindications excluded.

   IV alteplase (recombinant tissue plasminogen activator, rTPA) should be given as soon as possible at a weight dependant dose. The **IST-3** trial (Lancet, 2012) demonstrated a clear time-dependent benefit when rTPA was administered within 4.5 hours of onset of symptoms.

   The following contraindications to thrombolysis for acute ischaemic stroke originate from the expert consensus for the National Institute of Neurological Disorders and Stroke (NINDS) trial:
   i Acute or previous intracranial haemorrhage
   ii Severe uncontrolled hypertension
      - SBP >185 mmHg or diastolic BP (DBP) >110 mmHg

iii Serious head trauma/stroke in the last 3 months
iv Thrombocytopenia and coagulopathy
  - Platelets <100 x 10^9/l
  - International Normalised Ratio (INR) >1.7
  - Prothrombin time (PT) >15 sec
v Current use of oral anticoagulants or treatment dose heparin in the last 48 hours
vi Major surgery within the preceding 14 days
vii Recent gastrointestinal or genitourinary haemorrhage within the previous 21 days
viii Severe hypoglycaemia or hyperglycaemia
ix Seizure at the onset of stroke
x Central nervous system structural lesions
xi Isolated mild neurological deficits
xii Recent myocardial infarction

4 Administer **aspirin**
All patients in whom haemorrhage has been excluded should be administered 300 mg aspirin (per rectum [PR] or nasogastric [NG] if dysphasic) with gastric protection as necessary.

5 Consider **decompressive craniectomy** (DC) in patients at high risk of malignant MCA syndrome, i.e.:
  i >50% MCA territory stroke on CT
  ii >82 ml infarct volume at 6 hours on MRI
  iii >145 ml infarct volume at 14 hours on MRI
The **DESTINY, DECIMAL** and **HAMLET** trials (2007–2009) looked at DC patients <60 years old within 48 hours of MCA infarct. There was a reduction in mortality from 71% to 21%. No individual study showed an increase in good outcome in survivors, although the pooled analysis did. The **DESTINY II** trial (2014) looked at DC in appropriate patients over the age of 60. Almost all survivors were severely disabled.

On this basis, DC should be *considered* in patients who have sustained an MCA infarct (malignant MCA infarction) and meet the following criteria:
  i <60 years of age
  ii Clinical neurological deficits in keeping with MCA infarct
  iii National Institute of Health Stroke Scale (NIHSS) of >15
  iv CT demonstrating evidence of an infarct of at least 50% of the MCA territory

6 **Therapeutic hypothermia**
A Cochrane review found no significant effect on reducing the risk of poorer outcome or death. **EuroHYP-1**, a phase III randomised controlled trial (RCT) is underway to further assess the impact of cooling to 34°C following moderate to severe ischaemic stroke. Hyperthermia should be avoided.

7 **Interventional radiology**
Recanalisation therapy with clot retrieval +/– intra-arterial rTPA may be considered in patients who present >6–8 hours after onset of symptoms. Additionally, it may be useful in the subset of patients with carotid or MCA occlusion who do badly with IV rTPA alone.

8 General measures:
  i Thromboprophylaxis
  ii Physiotherapy for weak/immobile limbs
  iii Nutritional support
  iv Pressure area care

Which patients would you admit to the ICU?

The following are some potential indications for admission to ICU:

1 Seizures
2 Deteriorating neurological status and airway compromise
3 Mass effect secondary to large space occupying infarcts
4 Respiratory failure (secondary to neurogenic pulmonary oedema, depressed central respiratory drive, aspiration etc.)
5 To facilitate interventions

Which patients are most at risk of pneumonia following stroke?

Pneumonia after stroke is associated with:

1 Old age
2 Dysarthria, aphasia
3 Severity of post-stroke disability
4 Cognitive impairment
5 Abnormal water swallow test result

When does focal cerebral ischaemia result in coma?

Only in the following situations:

1 Brainstem stroke: basilar artery occlusion causes ischaemia of the reticular activating system
2 Malignant MCA syndrome: cerebral oedema leading to transtentorial herniation
3 Cerebral venous thrombosis: causes intracranial hypertension, cerebral oedema and seizures

How would you assess the swallow of a patient following an acute ischaemic stroke?

Swallowing impairment is common following a stroke and is associated with an increased risk of aspiration pneumonia. Guidelines support the use of a bedside swallow test before eating or drinking but do not provide specifics on test administration and interpretation. If there is coughing or a wet voice after swallowing a small glass of water, then oral intake should be withheld. Input from a speech and language therapy specialist will be required.

Bedside tests used include a simple two-step swallowing provocation test and the repetitive saliva swallowing test.

Further Reading

BMJ Best Practice, 2015. Ischaemic stroke [online]. London: British Medical Association. Available at: http://bestpractice.bmj.com/best-practice/monograph/1078/treatment/step-by-step.html [Accessed: 26 November 2016]

Intercollegiate Stroke Working Party, 2016. National clinical guideline for stroke, 5th edition [online]. London: Royal College of Physicians. Available at: www.strokeaudit.org/SupportFiles/Documents/Guidelines/2016-National-Clinical-Guideline-for-Stroke-5 t-(1).aspx (Accessed: 25 February 2017)

Raithatha A, Pratt G, Rash A. Developments in the management of acute ischaemic stroke: implications for anaesthetic and critical care management. *Contin Educ Anaesth Crit Care Pain* 2013; 13(3): 80–86

Chapter 4

Acute Kidney Injury and Renal Replacement Therapy

What systems do you know of to classify kidney injury?

The KDIGO (Kidney Disease: Improving Global Outcomes) classification is the most recent (Table 4.1). It harmonises the differences between the RIFLE (Risk Injury Failure Loss End-stage renal disease) and AKIN (Acute Kidney Injury Network) definitions.

What do you understand by the term contrast-induced acute kidney injury?

Contrast-induced acute kidney injury (CI-AKI) is the development of AKI within 48 hours of a contrast load.

The exact underlying mechanisms are unclear but likely to be a combination of:

1 Direct nephrotoxicity of reactive oxygen species (ROS)
2 Imbalance of vasoconstriction vs vasodilation
3 Increased oxygen consumption
4 Contrast-induced diuresis
5 Increased viscosity of urine

What are the risk factors for CI-AKI?

1 Increasing age >75
2 Presence of underlying renal impairment (eGFR <60 ml/min/1.73 m^2)
   - Pre-renal: hypovolaemia, hypoxaemia, e.g. sepsis, cardiac failure
   - Renal: diabetes mellitus (DM), vascular disease including hypertension and renal artery stenosis (RAS)
   - Post-renal: renal calculi, other obstructive nephropathy
3 Nephrotoxic drugs
   - Non-steroidal anti-inflammatory drugs (NSAIDs)
   - Aminoglycosides, amphotericin
   - Angiotensin-converting-enzyme inhibitors (ACEis), angiotensin-receptor blockers (ARBs)
   - Tacrolimus (nephrotoxic in supra-therapeutic levels)
4 IV contrast is more likely to be associated with CI-AKI than oral, and risk is directly proportional to contrast load

Table 4.1 The KDIGO classification of acute kidney injury

KDIGO Stage	Serum Creatinine	Urine Output
1	1.5–2-fold increase in baseline $\geq$26.5 µmol/l increase	<0.5 ml/kg/hr for 6–12 hours
2	2–3-fold increase in baseline	<0.5 ml/kg/hr for $\geq$12 hours
3	$\geq$354 µmol/l $\geq$3-fold increase in baseline Requirement for RRT	<0.3 ml/kg/hr for $\geq$24 hours Anuria for $\geq$12 hours

What strategies do you know of that can help prevent CI-AKI?

1 General strategies:
  i Avoid contrast in high-risk patients
    – Consider alternative imaging modalities that don't necessitate contrast use
  ii If contrast is mandatory:
    – Use diluted, low osmolality or non-ionic contrast media
    – Use lowest dose possible
    – Avoid repetitive dosing
  iii Stop other nephrotoxins
2 Intravenous volume expansion, i.e. *pre-hydration*:
  – e.g. IV normal saline 1 ml/kg/hour pre- and post-contrast procedure
3 N-acetyl cysteine:
  – 600 mg orally bd for two days prior to contrast
  – No definitive evidence
  – May decrease creatinine release from muscle rather than actually provide renal protection
4 IV sodium bicarbonate:
  – It is postulated that alkalinisation of renal tubular fluid reduces production of ROS in addition to its volume expansion effect
  – An example protocol may be:
    3 ml/kg 1.26% $NaHCO_3$ over 1 hour prior to contrast + 1 ml/kg/hour 1.26% $NaHCO_3$ for 6 hours post contrast (there may be a local protocol in your trust)
  – There is some evidence to suggest a small benefit over 0.9% saline
5 Other approaches:
  i Diuretics – may actually worsen nephropathy
  ii Vasodilators (dopamine, fenoldopam, atrial natriuretic peptide (ANP), calcium-channel blockers (CCBs)) – no benefit shown with any
  iii Renal replacement therapy (RRT) – dialysis is effective in removing contrast media from the circulation; however, there is no evidence to suggest that it works prophylactically

How do you diagnose CI-AKI?

A rise in serum creatinine of ≥ 44 μmol/l or an increase in serum creatinine by 25% from baseline value within 48 hours of precipitating procedure (KDIGO).

How do you manage a patient with AKI?

The patient with AKI should be managed with an ABCDE approach, treating abnormalities as they are found. Specific management should involve treating the underlying cause and stopping any precipitants. The London AKI Network have produced the STOP-AKI acronym:

S Sepsis and hypoperfusion
  – Treat Sepsis
  – Ensure euvolaemia, optimise cardiac output
T Toxins
  – Remove nephrotoxic drugs including contrast
O Obstruction
  – Rule out obstruction with renal tract ultrasound +/– catheterisation
P Primary renal
  – Screen for intrinsic renal disease
  – Urine dip +/– immunological/viral infection screen

If renal function continues to deteriorate, RRT may then need to be considered.

There is no evidence that converting oliguric AKI into polyuric AKI with diuretics leads to prognostic benefit. Therefore, they should be used only in the presence of hyperkalaemia or fluid overload.

What are the indications for RRT on the ICU?

1 Metabolic acidaemia
2 Hyperkalaemia (life-threatening or unresponsive to medical therapy)
3 Symptomatic uraemia
4 Fluid overload unresponsive to medical therapy
5 Treatment of overdose with dialysable toxins, e.g. lithium and salicylates most commonly

What are the modes of RRT used on the ICU?

1 **CVVHF** (continuous veno-venous haemofiltration)
  – Utilises the principle of *convection* and mimics glomerular filtration
  – There is bulk flow of solute and water down a hydrostatic pressure gradient, across a semi-permeable membrane (SPM)

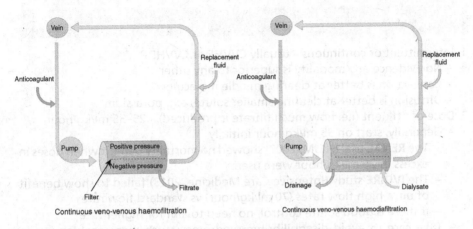

Figure 4.1 Schematic diagram comparing CVVHF and CVVHD

- Rate of fluid removal is proportional to blood flow rate, hydrostatic pressure gradient and membrane surface area
2 **CVVHD** (continuous veno-venous haemodialysis)
   - Utilises the principle of *diffusion* (not widely used in the UK)
   - There is countercurrent flow of blood and dialysate, with diffusion of solutes down a concentration gradient, across a SPM
   - The higher the dialysate (up to 500 ml/minute) and blood flow (up to 200–300 ml/minute) rates, the better maintained the concentration gradient, and the more effective the solute removal
   - Application of a pressure difference across the SPM allows for fluid removal
3 **CVVHDF** (continuous veno-venous haemodiafiltration)
   - Combines convective and diffusive clearance of solutes
4 **SCUF** (slow continuous ultrafiltration)
   - Ultrafiltration only, i.e. solely fluid removal
   - Does not alter the patient's biochemistry
5 Intermittent haemodialysis
   - Used in patients with pre-existing end-stage renal disease (ESRD)
   - Poorly tolerated with haemodynamic instability due to larger blood volumes in the extracorporeal circuit and high blood pump speeds
6 Others, e.g. **SLEDD** (sustained low-efficiency daily dialysis)
   - Can be performed for 8–10 hours per day, usually overnight
   - Hybrid method: benefits from being intermittent, but also associated with less haemodynamic and osmotic disturbance than intermittent HD, and good solute control

Figure 4.1 illustrates the difference between CVVHF and CVVHD.

How do you prescribe RRT?

1 Intermittent or continuous – usually CVVHF or CVVHDF
   - No evidence any modality is superior to any other
   - Convection is better at clearing middle molecules
   - Diffusion is better at clearing smaller solute, e.g. potassium
2 Dose of effluent (i.e. how much filtrate is produced) – 25–35 ml/kg/hour
   - Generally, start on 35 ml/kg/hour initially
      - The **RENAL** trial (NEJM, 2009) showed no mortality benefit when doses in excess of 25 ml/kg/hour were used
      - The **IVOIRE** study (Intensive Care Medicine, 2013) failed to show benefit of ultra-high flow rates (70 ml/kg/hour) vs standard flow rates
      - If there is good solute control, no need to aim for higher rate
   - Take care to avoid disequilibrium syndrome (much more problematic in dialysis than CVVHF)
      - Aim to reduce urea by 30% or less within the first 24 hours in uraemic patients
   - Consider dose prescribed vs dose actually received
      - Time on filter may be less than prescribed due to transfers and technical issues
3 Pre- or post-dilution fluid replacement
   - A pre-dilution regime adds the fluid to the circuit before the filter
      - This reduces the blood's viscosity and reduces the risk of clotting inside the filter
      - However, also reduces solute clearance
   - A post-dilution regime adds the replacement fluid to the blood after the filter
      - This is the ideal, but a compromise is often made to prolong the lifespan of the filter
   - Prescribed as a pre:post ratio, e.g 30:70
4 Fluid balance target
5 Anticoagulation (see Table 4.2 for comparison of the different methods of anticoagulation)
6 Other factors:
   - Ensure good blood flow rates – titrate up fairly quickly to 250 ml/min
   - IV access is the usual rate-limiting step

Table 4.2 Methods of anticoagulation in RRT

Method of Anticoagulation	Advantages	Disadvantages
None	Minimises bleeding risk	Shortened filter life / increased time off RRT
UFH (Usually only used to anticoagulate the filter circuit, i.e. regional anticoagulation)	Titratable Easily monitored Readily available reversal agent	Risk of HIT
LMWH		Not titratable No definitive reversal agent
Prostcyclin	Reduced bleeding risk	Shorter filter life Hypotension
Citrate	Good regional anticoagulation Decreased risk of bleeding as anticoagulation effects limited to extra-corporeal circuit Pre-mixed solutions with established protocols to follow	Large sodium load with trisodium citrate Hypocalcaemia (need to monitor and replace) Metabolic alkalosis (citrate metabolised to lactate in liver) Special dialysate required (hyponatraemic, no buffer, calcium-free) Contraindicated in liver failure (citrate is acidic, so causes a metabolic acidosis in liver failure)

UFH – unfractionated heparin; LMWH – low molecular weight heparin; HIT – heparin-induced thrombocytopenia

Further Reading

Gemmell L, Docking R, Black E. Renal replacement therapy in critical care. *BJA Educ* 2017; **17**(3): 88–93

Kidney Disease: Improving Global Outcomes (KDIGO) Acute Kidney Injury Work Group. KDIGO Clinical practice guideline for acute kidney injury. *Kidney Inter, Suppl* 2012; **2**: 1–138

London Acute Kidney Injury Network, 2015. STOP AKI and checklist [online]. Available at: www.londonaki.net/clinical/guidelines-pathways.html (Accessed: 9 January 2017)

Chapter 5

Acute Liver Failure and Paracetamol Overdose

How is acute liver failure defined?

Acute liver failure (ALF) is a rare life-threatening illness occurring most frequently in patients without pre-existing liver disease. It presents with jaundice, encephalopathy and coagulopathy and may progress to multi-organ failure and death in up to half of cases.

Modern definitions recognise disease phenotypes and quantify interval between onset of symptoms and development of encephalopathy. Multiple classification systems exist. The *O'Grady* system categorises ALF based on the interval between onset of jaundice to development of encephalopathy:

Hyperacute	<1 week
Acute	1–4 weeks
Subacute	4–12 weeks

What are the causes of ALF?

Causes of ALF are listed in Table 5.1. In the developing world viral infections are the commonest cause (Hepatitis A, B and E), whereas paracetamol toxicity is the most common cause in the developed world.

What are the King's College criteria? Describe the components.

The King's College criteria (Table 5.2) are the most well characterised and widely accepted prognostic tool for patients who present with acute liver failure. The criteria identify patients who have a high risk of mortality and are useful in helping to ascertain the suitability of a patient for transplantation.

How does ALF present?

Patients present with malaise, nausea and jaundice, with encephalopathy developing over a variable period of time. The condition is characterised by a high cardiac output state with reduced systemic vascular resistance (SVR), making it a differential for septic shock. The liver necrosis that develops triggers an

Table 5.1 Causes of acute liver failure

Infective	Hepatitis A-E HSV, CMV, VZV, EBV
Drugs	Paracetamol Anti-epileptic drugs, e.g. phenytoin Anti-tuberculous drugs, e.g. isoniazid St. John's Wort Chemotherapy agents Recreational drugs, e.g. ecstasy, amphetamines
Toxins	Amanita phalloides (mushroom)
Malignancy	Primary / secondary
Vascular	Budd-Chiari syndrome (hepatic vein thrombosis) Ischaemic hepatitis (hypotension, hypoperfusion, hypoxia-related)
Pregnancy-related	HELLP syndrome Acute fatty liver of pregnancy
Metabolic disease	Wilson's disease
Other	Seronegative hepatitis Autoimmune

HSV – *Herpes simplex virus*; CMV – Cytomegalovirus; VZV – Varicella-Zoster virus; EBV – Epstein-Barr virus; HELLP – Haemolysis, Elevated Liver enzymes, Low Platelets

Table 5.2 King's College selection criteria for liver transplantation in acute liver failure

Paracetamol toxicity	1. pH <7.30
	Or
	2. All three of:
	   i INR >6.5 (PT >100 seconds)
	   ii Serum creatinine >300 μmol/l
	   iii Grade 3 or 4 hepatic encephalopathy

Non-paracetamol-induced ALF	1.INR >6.5 (PT >100 seconds)
	Or
	2. Any three of the following:
	   i Age <11 or >40 years
	   ii Aetiology non-A, non-B hepatitis, or idiosyncratic drug reaction
	   iii Time from onset of jaundice to encephalopathy >7 days (i.e. not hyperacute)
	   iv INR >3.5 (PT >50 seconds)
	   v Serum bilirubin >300 μmol/l

inflammatory cascade, resulting in vasoplegic cardiovascular collapse, a subsequent AKI and cerebral oedema.

How is encephalopathy graded?

Encephalopathy is a clinical diagnosis, graded by the *West Haven* criteria as shown in Table 5.3. The development of encephalopathy has a central place in the definition of acute liver failure which reflects its key prognostic importance. In the later stages of encephalopathy, elevation in ICP is common due to the development of cerebral oedema (80% of patients with grade IV encephalopathy develop cerebral oedema, of which approximately 25% will die).

Table 5.3 West Haven grading of encephalopathy

Grade I	Trivial lack of awareness, euphoria or anxiety, shortened attention span, impaired performance of addition or subtraction
Grade II	Lethargy or apathy, disorientation in time, personality change, inappropriate behaviour
Grade III	Somnolence to semi-stupor, confusion, gross disorientation, remains responsive to verbal stimuli
Grade IV	Coma (unresponsive to stimuli)

What are the potential mechanisms of renal failure in ALF?

There are four potential mechanisms contributing to the development of renal failure in patients with ALF:

1 Acute tubular necrosis (most commonly)
   - Hypovolaemia, hypotension, hypoperfusion
   - Nephrotoxins, e.g. paracetamol
2 Secondary to underlying disease process, e.g. glomerulonephritis in hepatitis B (HBV) and hepatitis C (HCV)
3 Intra-abdominal hypertension due to ascites
4 Hepatorenal syndrome (see page 128)

What is the ICU management of acute liver failure?

Early referral to a tertiary centre is mandatory.

Respiratory

Grade III or IV encephalopathy is often an indication for intubation and ventilation. Avoid excessive PEEP if possible as this will increase hepatic venous pressure and ICP.

Cardiovascular

Reduced systemic vascular resistance is characteristic of ALF. This may result in hepatic hypoperfusion despite an elevated cardiac output. Fluid resuscitation is an important early management step. Targeted fluid management is important (avoiding external lactate load), taking care not to overload the intravascular space and worsen cerebral oedema. The addition of a vasopressor is often required to maintain MAP 60–65 mmHg and CPP 60–80 mmHg.

Neurological

Simple neuroprotective measures should be implemented:

  i Elevate head to improve CPP
  ii Appropriate sedation
  iii Avoid hypotension (aim CPP 60–80 mmHg, targeting MAP >75 mmHg)
  iv Avoid hypoxia and hypercapnia
  v Avoid fever; maintain core body temp 35–36°C
  vi Glycaemic control with blood sugar 4–10 mmol/l

Mannitol or hypertonic saline can be used to treat intracranial hypertension associated with cerebral oedema.

The role of ICP monitoring devices in ALF is controversial. The benefits of targeted vasopressor and fluid therapy to CPP must be carefully weighed up against the risks of insertion in this coagulopathic population.

Other less commonly used therapies to manage ALF-induced intracranial hypertension include therapeutic hypothermia to core temperature 34–35°C, barbiturates (in resistant cases as a bridge to liver transplant) and indomethacin (used when cerebral hyperaemia is present).

Renal

Renal replacement therapy should be initiated early when necessary to prevent fluid overload and worsening acidosis.

Coagulation

The liver synthesises all the coagulation factors apart from factor VIII. Abnormal synthesis of these factors, in addition to protein C and antithrombin III deficiency, mean severe coagulopathy and disseminated intravascular coagulation (DIC) are common in ALF. Active bleeding will necessitate appropriate product replacement, but routine coagulopathy correction is not advised as prothrombin time is used as a prognostic marker.

Liver transplantation remains the only effective treatment for patients with ALF in whom prognostic indicators suggest a high likelihood of death.

What is the mechanism of liver injury in paracetamol overdose?

The reactive metabolite N-acetyl-p-benzoquinone imine (NAPQI) is responsible for paracetamol's hepatotoxicity.

Under usual therapeutic conditions, paracetamol is metabolised by glucuronidation and sulphation in the liver. A small amount is metabolised by the cytochrome P450 system into the highly reactive intermediary metabolite NAPQI. This is then detoxified by the antioxidant effects of hepatic glutathione. In paracetamol overdose, the sulphate and glucuronide pathways become saturated, and more paracetamol is shunted to the cytochrome P450 system to produce NAPQI. The glutathione stores are rapidly depleted, allowing NAPQI to cause widespread hepatocyte damage leading to acute hepatic necrosis.

What are the risk factors for developing paracetamol toxicity?

These can be divided into two main groups:

1 Cytochrome enzyme induction
   - Chronic excessive alcohol consumption
   - Concomitant use of enzyme-inducing drugs, e.g. carbamazepine, barbiturates, rifampicin, isoniazid, St John's Wort
2 Glutathione depletion
   - Malnutrition, eating disorders
   - Patients with other factors causing liver injury, e.g. viral hepatitis, alcoholic hepatitis

What is the specific treatment for paracetamol overdose?

N-acetylcysteine (NAC) is a precursor to glutathione and replenishes hepatic stores. It is an effective antidote if administered within 8 hours of an acute overdose and has been shown to improve prognosis if administered beyond 8 hours.

All patients with serum paracetamol levels above the paracetamol treatment nomogram (modified Rumack-Matthew nomogram) line should be given NAC.

Further Reading

Bernal W, Wendon J. Acute Liver Failure. *New Engl J Med* 2013; **369**(26): 2525–2534

Lee W M, Larson A M, Stravitz R T. AASLD position paper: The management of acute liver failure: Update 2011. *Hepatology* 2011; **55**: 965–967

O'Grady J G, Alexander G J, Hayllar K M, et al. Early indicators of prognosis in fulminant hepatic failure. *Gastroenterology* 1989; **97**: 339–345

Chapter 6

Acute Respiratory Distress Syndrome

Define *ARDS*

This condition was first described as 'shocked lung' or 'Adult Respiratory Distress Syndrome' in the 1960s. It was soon realised that the condition could affect all ages and the term acute respiratory distress syndrome (ARDS) was introduced by Ashbaugh in 1967.

In 1994 the American-European Consensus Conference (AECC) published a new definition for ARDS to include clinical, radiological and physiological parameters. The term acute lung injury (ALI) was also introduced to denote a less severe presentation of ARDS. The parameters for diagnosis were as follows:

1. Acute onset
2. Hypoxaemia
   – ALI PaO_2/FiO_2 ratio $\leq$ 300 mmHg
   – ARDS PaO_2/FiO_2 ratio $\leq$ 200 mmHg
3. Bilateral pulmonary infiltrates on chest X-ray (CXR)
4. Pulmonary capillary wedge pressure (PCWP) $\leq$ 18 mmHg, i.e. not attributable to left ventricular failure (LVF)

However, it was recognised that there were a number of limitations associated with the AECC definition:

1. Lack of clarity of the term *acute*
2. No formal inclusion of known risk factors for ARDS
3. Inter-observer variability in CXR interpretation
4. Increasingly rare measurement of PCWP
5. Sensitivity of PaO_2/FiO_2 to ventilator settings, particularly PEEP

The Berlin Definition was subsequently published in 2012 and aimed to overcome these limitations:

> *ARDS is an acute diffuse, inflammatory lung injury, leading to increased pulmonary vascular permeability, increased lung weight and loss of aerated lung tissue with hypoxaemia and bilateral radiographic opacities, associated with increased venous admixture, increased physiological dead space and decreased lung compliance.*

The term ALI was abandoned and the condition was divided into mild, moderate and severe ARDS. This new categorisation has shown improved correlation with observed mortality as compared with the AECC definition.

Table 6.1 Oxygenation criteria with associated mortality and outcome data

	Mild	Moderate	Severe
Oxygenation criteria	PaO_2/FiO_2 200–300 mmHg (PaO_2/FiO_2 26.7–40 kPa) + PEEP/CPAP ≥5 cmH$_2$O	PaO_2/FiO_2 100–200 mmHg (PaO_2/FiO_2 13.3–26.7 kPa) + PEEP ≥5 cmH$_2$O	PaO_2/FiO_2 ≤100 mmHg (PaO_2/FiO_2 ≤13.3 kPa) + PEEP ≥5 cmH$_2$O
Mortality (%)	27	32	45
Median ventilator-free days	20	16	1
Median duration of ventilation in survivors (days)	5	7	9

Data from The ARDS Definition Taskforce (*JAMA* 2012)
CPAP – continuous positive airway pressure

The essential components required to diagnose ARDS are:

1 Development within one week of insult/worsening respiratory symptoms – *acute*
2 Bilateral opacities on CXR not explained by effusions, collapse or nodules
3 Respiratory failure not explained by LVF or fluid overload
   – Necessitates echo if no risk factors for ARDS are present
4 Oxygenation criteria (see Table 6.1)
5 Patient has to be ventilated (invasive/non-invasive with a PEEP of ≥5 cmH$_2$O) for a diagnosis of ARDS to be considered

What are the causes of ARDS?

The causes can be divided into pulmonary and extra-pulmonary, and are listed in Table 6.2.

Table 6.2 Causes of ARDS

Pulmonary causes	Extra-pulmonary causes i.e. systemic inflammation
Pneumonia	Sepsis
Pulmonary contusion	Severe burns
Aspiration pneumonitis	Major trauma
Inhalational injury	Transfusion-associated lung injury
Pulmonary vasculitis	Severe acute pancreatitis
Submersion/drowning	Cardiopulmonary bypass (pump lung)

Can you outline the pathophysiology of ARDS?

The pathophysiology is thought to be triphasic:

1 Exudative stage (days 2–4)
   - Inflammatory insult to epithelium
   - Leakage of protein-rich fluid and inflammatory cells into alveoli and interstitium
   - Destruction of the pulmonary vascular bed
   - Dysregulation of coagulation and fibrinolysis leading to microthrombus formation
   - This causes:
     i V/Q mismatch, leading to hypoxic hypoxia
     ii Reduction in lung compliance, causing increased work of breathing
2 Proliferative stage (days 4–7)
   - Proliferation of type II pneumocytes and fibroblasts, with alveolar fibrin deposition
   - Organisation of exudate leading to scar formation
3 Fibrotic stage (days 7–14) – does not occur in all patients
   - Fibrosis of lung tissue and global damage to underlying lung structure

How does ARDS present?

The patient will usually present with increasing respiratory distress (dyspnoea and increased work of breathing), hypoxia and tachycardia, with or without an altered conscious level. The presentation may vary depending on the underlying aetiology. In addition, patients with ARDS will typically have some level of multi-organ dysfunction during their illness; this is the usual cause of death.

How would you investigate the patient with ARDS?

In addition to confirming the presence of ARDS, investigations should be targeted towards identification of the underlying cause if it is unclear.

1 Blood tests including inflammatory markers, serum amylase/lipase, cultures
2 Arterial blood gas to quantify the severity of the ARDS
3 CXR (or CT chest)
4 Echocardiography – performed in the absence of a known risk factor for ARDS

What ventilatory strategies are you aware of in ARDS? Is there any evidence to support their use?

Mechanical ventilation is now known to be injurious to the lungs and can exacerbate ARDS by causing ventilator-induced lung injury (VILI) via several mechanisms:

1 Volutrauma (overdistension of healthy alveoli)
2 Barotrauma (high pressure injury to alveoli)
3 Atelectrauma (shearing forces due to repeated collapse and expansion of alveoli)
4 Biotrauma (release of inflammatory mediators in response to high-volume ventilation)

The ventilatory strategies are as follows:

1 *Lung-protective ventilation*
The **ARDSNet** trial (NEJM, 2000) randomised patients with early ARDS to receive either traditional (12 ml/kg) or low (6 ml/kg) tidal volume ventilation. The trial was stopped prematurely because mortality and number of ventilator-free days during the first 28 days was significantly reduced in the lower tidal volume group. The number needed to treat (NNT) was 12. Additionally, the incidence of extra-pulmonary organ failure was lower in the intervention group.

ARDSNet protocol:
  i Low tidal volumes (5–7 ml/kg ideal body weight (IBW)) with a higher than physiological respiratory rate (≤35) to minimise volutrauma
     – Allow permissive hypercapnia – tolerate higher than usually acceptable levels of $PaCO_2$ providing pH ≥7.2 (unless there is concurrent brain injury)
  ii Aim SpO_2 88–95% to reduce oxygen toxicity
     – Consider increasing the I:E ratio or using inverse ratios if oxygenation is a problem
  iii Use PEEP ≥ 5 cmH_2O to minimise atelectrauma
     – Aim to find the *optimum PEEP*, i.e. the point at which the lung is the most compliant
     – Consider using incremental FiO_2/PEEP combinations
     – There is evidence of mortality benefit to using high PEEP in severe ARDS
  iv Maintain plateau pressures (P_{plat}) ≤30 cmH_2O to minimise barotrauma

2 *Use of neuromuscular blocking agents* (NMBAs)
The **ACURASYS** trial (NEJM, 2010) randomised patients with severe ARDS to receive either a cisatracurium infusion or placebo for 48 hours. They demonstrated a 90-day mortality benefit for patients with a PaO_2/FiO_2 ratio ≤120 mmHg in the intervention arm and an increase in ventilator-free days, with no increase in the development of ICU-acquired weakness (ICU-AW).

3 *Recruitment manoeuvres and decremental PEEP*
In 2016, **Kacmarek, et al** (Critical Care Medicine) conducted a pilot study in patients with moderate-severe ARDS, which demonstrated improvement in oxygenation, lung mechanics and peak pressure with the introduction of a recruitment manoeuvre and decremental PEEP trial. There was no mortality benefit, although the study was underpowered to detect this. Importantly, there was no significant difference in the incidence of adverse effects between the groups.

4 *Prone ventilation*
Prone ventilation has gained popularity following the results of the **PROSEVA** trial (NEJM, 2013), which demonstrated a considerable (>50%) reduction in mortality in patients who were ventilated in the prone position for at least 16 hours per day, compared to those who were ventilated supine. The NNT was 6 for both 28-day and 90-day mortality. Importantly, all centres involved in this trial had at least five years proning experience, which brought into question its external validity given the complexity and resources necessary for prone positioning. A subsequent meta-analysis has corroborated these findings.

5 *High frequency oscillatory ventilation* (HFOV)
High frequency oscillatory ventilation was evaluated in two trials in 2013. The **OSCAR** (NEJM, 2013) trial showed no mortality benefit to HFOV, and no improvement in the number of ventilator-free days. Neuromuscular blocking agents were used for a longer duration in the intervention group. The **OSCILLATE** (NEJM, 2013) trial demonstrated evidence of harm (number needed to harm [NNH] was 9), and was stopped early. Patients who were randomised to receive oscillation were more likely to need vasopressor support and NMBAs. Interestingly, the OSCILLATE trial reported a lower mortality rate compared to the OSCAR trial in the 'conventional' arms. This may be because OSCILLATE mandated the use of lung protective ventilation (LPV), whereas OSCAR only suggested it.

What pharmacological strategies have been used in ARDS?

1 *Steroids*
ARDS is an inflammatory disease, and so it has been hypothesised that corticosteroid therapy may be helpful. The evidence is somewhat conflicted but suggests a potential benefit to longer courses of low-dose steroids later in the disease process.

Two meta-analyses in 1995 looked at the use of high-dose steroids in early ARDS, and concluded that there was evidence of increased harm with no associated benefit.

In 2006, **Steinberg, et al** (NEJM) randomised patients with persistent ARDS (for 7–28 days) to receive either methylprednisolone or placebo for at least 7 days. Methylprednisolone increased the number of ventilator-free days in the first 28 days, but no difference was seen in 60-day mortality. Importantly, there was an increased incidence of myopathy or neuropathy in the intervention arm, and the patients who were randomised after 14 days had significantly higher mortality rates with methylprednisolone.

Meduri, et al (Chest, 2007) randomised patients with severe ARDS to receive either low-dose methylprednisolone infusion (1 mg/kg/day) or placebo, within the first 72 hours of diagnosis. The trial demonstrated a significant improvement in pulmonary and extra-pulmonary organ dysfunction, and reduced duration of mechanical ventilation and length of stay (LOS) on ICU. However, there were several limitations to the study design: there were twice as many patients with vasopressor-dependent shock in the placebo group (which was a confounder), there was open label use of methylprednisolone to non-responders at day 7–9 and the study was underpowered to detect a significant difference in mortality.

2 *Inhaled nitric oxide* (NO)

Inhaled NO reduces V/Q mismatch by causing localised vasodilation in pulmonary capillaries adjacent to ventilated lung units. There is a transient improvement in oxygenation, although this has not been shown to translate into a reduction in mortality. Inhaled NO may sometimes be used as a bridge to other therapy.

What else would you consider in cases of refractory hypoxaemia?

Patients that have failed to respond to conventional therapy and have a Murray score of ≥3 should be considered for referral to a specialist centre for veno-venous extracorporeal membrane oxygenation (ECMO). The Murray score was developed in 1988 and uses four criteria to grade the severity of the patient's clinical condition (see Table 6.3).

Table 6.3 Murray score

Score	0	1	2	3	4
PaO_2/FiO_2 ratio (kPa)	≥40	30–30.9	23.3–29.9	13.3–23.2	<13.3
PEEP (cmH_2O)	≤5	6–8	9–11	12–14	≥15
Compliance (ml/cmH_2O)	≥80	60–79	40–59	20–39	≤19
CXR (quadrants infiltrated)	0	1	2	3	4

In 2009, the **CESAR** trial (Lancet) demonstrated improved survival without severe disability in patients with ARDS who were transferred to a single tertiary centre with the intent to initiate ECMO if there was no improvement following the instigation of an ARDS ventilation protocol for 12 hours. However, there were a number of issues with the study: there was no protocol in place for the control arm of the trial (30% did not receive LPV), 6% of patients died before or during transfer, and 19% of the patients who were transferred did not go on to receive ECMO. Importantly, this trial was *not* a comparison of LPV versus ECMO.

How does ECMO work and what types are there?

ECMO is the use of modified cardiopulmonary bypass to provide respiratory or cardiorespiratory support at the bedside. Following its introduction in the 1970s, ECMO was initially associated with poor survival rates. However, recent techno-logical advances alongside improved understanding of the benefits of ECMO (following its widespread use as a rescue therapy for patients with ARDS during the 2009 H1N1 infection) have resulted in a reduction in complication rates.

There are a number of different forms of ECMO. The two most commonly used are veno-venous and veno-arterial ECMO:

1 *Veno-arterial ECMO (VA ECMO)*
   – Blood is pumped from the venous to the arterial circulation
   – Facilitates gas exchange and provides haemodynamic support
2 *Veno-venous (VV ECMO)*
   – Blood is removed from and returned to the venous circulation (via the same or an alternative vein)
   – Facilitates gas exchange
   – Does not provide haemodynamic support
3 A variant of VV ECMO is *extracorporeal CO_2 removal (ECCO$_2$R)*
   – The ECMO circuit acts to remove CO_2 whilst oxygenation is provided by ventilation of the lungs

The flow through an ECMO circuit is typically 25–75% of the cardiac output. This high flow requires the placement of large catheters into the vasculature. The circuit setup for VA and VV ECMO is almost identical (see Figure 6.1) and the following summarises the main components used in both circuits:

1 Cannulae (peripheral or central)
2 Tubing (heparin bonded)
   – Systemic heparin is used, but is not essential for successful ECMO use in the bleeding/polytrauma patient
3 Pump
   – Blood movement is facilitated by an external pump with a centrifugal or roller mechanism of action
4 Membrane oxygenator and heat exchanger
5 Gas blender

Veno-arterial ECMO bypasses the patient's heart and lungs, and part or all of the blood flow is diverted through the ECMO circuit. In contrast, VV ECMO returns the blood to the circulation before it enters the pulmonary vasculature.

What are the indications and contraindications for ECMO?

Table 6.4 describes the indications for both VA and VV ECMO.

The following are absolute contraindications to ECMO:

1 Irreversible organ damage, multi-organ failure, or those who are not candidates for transplantation
2 Advanced malignancy
3 Chronic severe pulmonary hypertension

Of note, the inability to anticoagulate a patient is not an absolute contraindication to extracorporeal support.

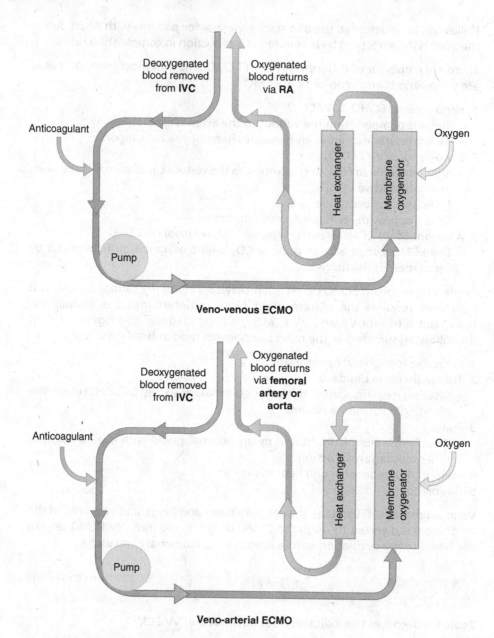

Figure 6.1 Schematic representation of ECMO circuits
IVC – inferior vena cava; RA – right atrium

Table 6.4 Indications for ECMO

VA-ECMO	VV-ECMO
Cardiogenic shock secondary to almost any cause: – Acute myocarditis – Intractable arrhythmia – Drug overdose with profound cardiac depression (e.g. local anaesthetic toxicity) – Pulmonary embolism – Acute anaphylaxis	Any potentially **reversible** acute respiratory failure
Weaning from cardiopulmonary bypass after cardiac surgery	ARDS associated with bacterial or viral pneumonia
Heart transplant – Bridge to lung transplant – Primary graft failure after heart or heart-lung transplant	Lung transplant – Bridge to transplant – Primary graft failure – Intraoperative ECMO
Chronic cardiomyopathy – As a bridge to longer term VAD support – Or as a bridge to a decision	Extracorporeal assistance to provide lung rest – Lung contusion (trauma) – Smoke inhalation – Airway obstruction
Pulmonary hypertension (after pulmonary endarterectomy)	Pulmonary haemorrhage or massive haemoptysis
Extra-corporeal life support (ECLS)	Lung hyperinflation – Status asthmaticus

Relative contraindications include:

1 Age >75
2 Polytrauma with multiple bleeding sites
3 Cardiopulmonary resuscitation (CPR) >60 minutes
4 Multiple organ failure
5 CNS injury

Specific contraindications for VA ECMO:

1 Severe aortic regurgitation
2 Aortic dissection

Specific contraindications for VV ECMO:

1 Unsupportable cardiac failure
2 Severe pulmonary hypertension
3 Cardiac arrest

An ECMO specialist should be involved in discussing indications and contra-indications on a case by case basis as the speciality is constantly evolving.

What are the complications of ECMO?

ECMO complications include those associated with cannulation, anticoagulation and equipment:

1 Cannulation
   - Pneumothorax
   - Vascular disruption
   - Infection
   - Emboli
   - Bleeding
2 Systemic anticoagulation
   - Haemorrhage including intracranial and gastrointestinal bleeding
   - Heparin-induced thrombocytopenia
3 Equipment
   - Exsanguination resulting from circuit disruptions
   - Oxygenator failure
   - Pump failure

Figure 6.2 summarises which interventions are indicated as the severity of the ARDS increases.

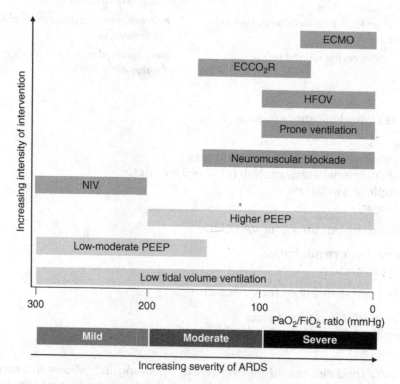

Figure 6.2 Increasing intensity of interventions in ARDS
Adapted with permission from Ferguson ND, et al. (*Intensive Care Med* 2012)
NIV – non-invasive ventilation

Further Reading

The ARDS Definition Task Force. Acute respiratory distress syndrome: The Berlin definition. *J Am Med Assoc* 2012; **307**(23): 2526–2533

Ferguson N D, Fan E, Camporota L, et al. The Berlin definition of ARDS: an expanded rationale, justification and supplementary material. *Intensive Care Med* 2012; **38**(10): 1573–1582

Martinez G, Vuylsteke A. Extracorporeal membrane oxygenation in adults. *Contin Educ Anaesth Crit Care Pain* 2012; **12**(2): 57–61

Chapter 7

Adrenal Insufficiency in the ICU

What are the causes of adrenal insufficiency?

Adrenal failure can result from insufficiency of any part of the hypothalamo-pituitary-adrenal (HPA) axis. Table 7.1 illustrates a number of causes that can be classified according to the endocrine organ involved: *primary* (adrenal gland, decreased cortisol secretion), *secondary* (pituitary gland, decreased adrenocorticotrophic hormone (ACTH) secretion) and *tertiary* (hypothalamus, decreased corticotrophin-releasing hormone (CRH) secretion).

What is Addison's disease?

Addison's disease is a disorder of the adrenal glands whereby the adrenal cortex fails, leading to reduced or absent glucocorticoid (cortisol) secretion. It was first described in 1855 by Thomas Addison, who identified a syndrome of long-term adrenal insufficiency. Common causes include autoimmune processes, infection or surgery. It is often associated with concomitant mineralocorticoid deficiency and does not usually present until over 90% of the cortex has been destroyed.

Cortisol deficiency results in failure of negative feedback to the pituitary gland and continual production of ACTH in an attempt to stimulate cortisol production (so ACTH levels are high). Melanocyte stimulating hormone (MSH) and ACTH share the same precursor molecule pro-opiomelanocortin, hence MSH production is also increased, leading to the characteristic hyperpigmentation of the skin and buccal mucosa seen in Addisonian patients.

How is adrenal insufficiency diagnosed?

1 Cortisol and ACTH levels
  – In primary adrenal failure, cortisol will be inappropriately low with very high serum concentrations of ACTH
  – In secondary or tertiary failure, both cortisol and ACTH will be inappropriately low
  – Exogenous steroids will impact results
2 The standard test of adrenal function is the *Synacthen test*
  – Cortisol concentrations are measured before and after injection of synthetic ACTH

Table 7.1 Causes of adrenal insufficiency

Type	Cause	Details
Primary (Addison's Disease)	Autoimmune	70–90% of cases are caused by autoimmune conditions
	Infectious causes	Tuberculosis with bilateral adrenal infiltration
		Disseminated fungal infection e.g. from histoplasmosis
		Patients with HIV are at risk of:
		– Necrotising adrenalitis secondary to CMV infection
		– Infiltration by Mycobacterium avium-intracellulare or Kaposi's sarcoma
	Cancer	Metastatic infiltration of the adrenal glands
		Primary adrenal gland tumours
	Drugs	Examples include:
		– Etomidate
		– Ketoconazole
		– Metyrapone
	Others	Critical illness-related corticosteroid insufficiency (relative adrenal insufficiency)
		Surgical adrenalectomy
		Adrenal gland haemorrhage e.g. Waterhouse-Friderichsen syndrome (following meningococcal septicaemia)
		Granulomatous and amyloid infiltration
		Irradiation of the adrenals
		Iron deposits secondary to haemochromatosis
Secondary / tertiary	HPA axis suppression secondary to exogenous steroids	Prolonged administration of glucocorticoids leads to HPA axis suppression – adequate replacement is required to prevent adrenal crisis
	Hypothalamic or pituitary failure	Malignancy
		Haemorrhage
		Infarction (e.g. Sheehan's syndrome)

HIV – Human Immunodeficiency Virus

- Failure of cortisol to increase beyond a threshold value at 30 minutes indicates adrenal insufficiency
- This test can run alongside emergency treatment for adrenal crisis as it is not affected by dexamethasone
- A negative result can rule out primary hypoadrenalism, but not secondary or tertiary

3 Adrenal antibodies and radiological imaging may be useful in determining the cause

How might an acute Addisonian crisis present?

A hypoadrenal crisis is a life-threatening condition that is difficult to diagnose but easily treated once recognised. In contrast to the chronic condition, which has an insidious onset with fatigue, anorexia, weight loss and postural hypotension (due to salt and water loss), an acute adrenal crisis can manifest with the following signs and symptoms:

Cardiovascular

- High-output distributive shock (hypotension, tachycardia, profound vasoplegia)

Neurological

- Lethargy, fatigue, extreme weakness
- Headache, dizziness
- Confusion
- Loss of consciousness

Gastrointenstinal

- Vomiting and diarrhoea
- Abdominal pain

Cutaneous

- Hyperpigmentation of light-exposed skin in primary hypoadrenalism (as a result of increased concentrations of MSH)

Biochemical abnormalities

- Hyponatraemia, hyperkalaemia, metabolic acidosis
- Hypoglycaemia

Other

- Autoimmune Addison's disease may be associated with other autoimmune diseases such as pernicious anaemia and Grave's disease

What is the management of an acute Addisonian crisis?

An acute hypoadrenal crisis would present with signs of a high output shock state that is dependent on vasopressors. It can be initially misdiagnosed as septic shock. A high-index of suspicion for adrenal failure is necessary and treatment should not be delayed to make a diagnosis. Initial management should follow an ABCDE approach, treating abnormalities as they are found. The focus is correction of hypotension, electrolyte imbalance and cortisol deficiency.

1 **Initial resuscitation**
   - Large bore IV access
   - Send bloods including electrolytes, glucose, cortisol and ACTH
   - Fluid resuscitation
   - Monitor blood glucose and correct with dextrose as necessary
2 **Replacement of glucocorticoids and mineralocorticoids**
   - High-dose IV hydrocortisone should be initiated: an initial dose of 200 mg is followed by 100 mg every 6 hours until oral supplements can be taken
   - Mineralocorticoids are not required acutely, as the crystalloid infused replaces the sodium (they also take several days to act)
   - Consideration to fludrocortisone administration should be given following fluid resuscitation under the advice of an endocrinologist
3 **Invasive monitoring** in a level 2/3 environment
4 **Identification of likely cause** to guide treatment after the acute crisis has been treated
    i Severe stress, e.g. sepsis, surgery
    ii Steroid use: dose and duration
    iii Other autoimmune conditions
    iv Travel/contact with infectious diseases
    v Drugs that interfere with steroid metabolism or synthesis
    vi History of cancer
    vii Pregnancy

What is the significance of adrenal insufficiency in the critically ill?

Relative hypoadrenalism in the critically ill is a common occurrence. The term critical illness-related corticosteroid insufficiency has been proposed to describe relative and absolute adrenal failure in this population. It is a particular issue in septic shock, with widely differing cortisol measurements. *Surviving Sepsis* guidelines suggest using steroids in patients who remain hypotensive despite fluid resuscitation and increasing doses of vasopressor. There is no evidence that treating patients based on measurements of adrenal function improves outcome (see page 415).

Further Reading

Davies M, Hardman J. Anaesthesia and adrenocortical disease. *Contin Educ Anaesth Crit Care Pain* 2005; **5**(4): 122–126

Miller T, Gibbison B, Russel G M. Hypothalamo-pituitary-adrenal function during health, major surgery and critical illness. *BJA Educ* 2017; **17**(1): 16–21

Chapter 8

Amniotic Fluid Embolism

What is amniotic fluid embolism?

Amniotic fluid embolism (AFE) is a rare, catastrophic obstetric emergency that can present with sudden maternal collapse, associated with hypoxaemia, shock and coagulopathy. It occurs when amniotic fluid or cells enter the maternal circulation.

What is the incidence of AFE?

Studies estimate an incidence between 1 and 12 cases per 100,000 deliveries.

What are the pathogenic mechanisms of AFE?

The pathophysiology of AFE is still poorly understood. The syndrome was previously thought to have an embolic mechanism, due to fetal tissue/amniotic fluid forcibly entering the maternal circulation and resulting in physical consequences similar to that of a pulmonary embolus. However, it is now thought to be a two-phase immune response to the antigens contained in fetal tissue, resulting in a systemic response similar to that of anaphylaxis:

Phase 1

Vasoactive substances are produced in response to fetal tissue antigens. This results in pulmonary artery vasospasm leading to acute right heart failure, hypotension and hypoxaemia. This phase may last up to 30 minutes.

Phase 2

Right ventricle recovers, but left ventricular failure and pulmonary oedema occur. Biochemical mediators and severe hypoxaemia lead to increased capillary permeability, DIC, uterine atony and massive haemorrhage.

What are the clinical features of AFE?

The classical triad of an AFE is hypoxaemia, cardiovascular collapse and coagulopathy. It may present with breathlessness, cyanosis, hypotension, dysrhythmias,

DIC or sudden maternal collapse. However, presentation may be more subtle, with non-specific symptoms including vomiting and anxiety.

What are the risk factors for AFE?

There are no proven risk factors, but the following are associated with an increased risk of AFE:

1 Advanced maternal age
2 Placental pathology (praevia/abruption)
3 Induction of labour
4 Operative delivery
5 Multiparity
6 Polyhydramnios
7 Uterine rupture
8 Intrauterine death
9 Trauma (cervical lacerations etc.)

The syndrome is considered to be largely unpredictable and unpreventable.

What are the principles of management of AFE?

The key features of the management of AFE focus on early recognition with prompt resuscitation of the mother, and expedited delivery of the fetus. Treatment is predominantly supportive.

1 **Rapid intravenous filling** and the use of directly acting **vasopressors** are usually required
   - **Left lateral tilt** is essential in the antenatal patient to reduce aortocaval compression by the gravid uterus
2 **Rapid delivery** of the fetus (do not delay delivery by transferring to theatre)
3 Activation of the **major haemorrhage protocol** should be considered as plasma, cryoprecipitate and platelets are frequently required alongside packed red cells (DIC is likely, secondary to activation of tissue factor and factor X)
   - Surgical intervention may be necessary for haemorrhage control
   - Maintenance of uterine tone with oxytocin, ergometrine and prostaglandins is essential
4 Establishing invasive monitoring can be hazardous due to rapidly developing consumptive coagulopathy

What are the differential diagnoses?

There are a number of differential diagnoses that can be divided into obstetric and non-obstetric in aetiology.

Obstetric causes:

1 Placental abruption
2 Eclampsia
3 Uterine rupture
4 Peripartum haemorrhage

Non-obstetric causes:

1 Anaphylaxis
2 Total spinal anaesthesia
3 Septic shock
4 Massive pulmonary embolus

Further Reading

Dedhia J, Mushambi M. Amniotic fluid embolism. *Contin Educ Anaesth Crit Care Pain* 2007; 7(5): 152–156

Tuffnell D, Brocklehurst P, Spark P, Kurinczuk J J. Incidence and risk factors for amniotic-fluid embolism. *Obstet Gynecol* 2010; 115(5): 910–917

Chapter 9

Anaphylaxis

How are hypersensitivity reactions classified?

Hypersensitivity reactions are classified into four groups (Gell and Coombs, 1963 (Table 9.1)).

A fifth type of reaction, termed *idiopathic*, was added to the classification system several years later.

What is anaphylaxis?

The European Academy of Allergy and Immunology redefined anaphylaxis as:

A severe, life-threatening, generalised, or systemic hypersensitivity reaction, sub-divided into allergic and non-allergic reactions:

1 *Allergic* anaphylaxis implies an immunological reaction (usually IgE-mediated)
   – Histamine, pro-inflammatory cytokines (e.g. tumour necrosis factor (TNF)), prostaglandins and leukotrienes are released causing vasodilatation with resultant hypotension and a reflex tachycardia
   – Oedema and urticaria can develop due to increased vascular permeability
   – Bronchoconstriction, increased secretions and airway oedema can also occur
2 *Non-allergic* reactions are caused by direct drug action
   – Mast cell and basophil degranulation occur with no immune trigger

Anaphylaxis is defined by a number of signs and symptoms, occurring alone or in combination:

– Awake patients may experience a metallic taste and a sense of impending doom
– The commonest symptoms are:
   – Hypotension (80%)
   – Rash/erythema (50%)
   – Bronchospasm (35%)
– SVR is decreased by as much as 80% due to the direct effect of histamine
– Other symptoms include:
   Respiratory: Oedema of the tongue, oropharynx or larynx, rhinitis, pulmonary oedema
   Cardiovascular: Arrhythmias, syncope, pulmonary oedema
   Gastrointestinal: Abdominal pain, nausea, vomiting, diarrhoea

Table 9.1 Classification of hypersensitivity reactions

Type	Name	Mediators	Disease examples
Type I	Immediate hypersensitivity	IgE	Anaphylaxis Allergic rhinitis Asthma
Type II	Antibody-mediated hypersensitivity	IgG or IgM and complement	Autoimmune haemolytic anaemia Rheumatic heart disease Goodpasture's disease
Type III	Immune complex-mediated hypersensitivity	IgG and complement	Lupus nephritis Rheumatoid arthritis Serum sickness
Type IV	Delayed hypersensitivity	T cells, macrophages, histocytes	Contact dermatitis Chronic transplant rejection Coeliac disease

Ig – immunoglobulin

List some of the common trigger agents that are used in intensive care

1 Neuromuscular blocking agents
   - Reported incidence of anaphylaxis due to each specific agent differs, but the most common precipitants are rocuronium, suxamethonium and atracurium
2 Antibiotics
   - Predominantly penicillins containing a beta lactam ring
   - There is an 8% cross reactivity with cephalosporins which is often incomplete
3 Thiopentone
4 Latex
   - Particularly common in patients who have had repeated interventions, e.g. urinary catheterisation
   - Also more common in healthcare professionals
   - Cross-reactivity with kiwi and strawberry
5 Plasma expanders
   - Dextrans
   - Starches
   - Gelatins
6 Antiseptics and disinfectants
   - Chlorhexidine is a particular problem in ICU
   - Betadine
7 Iodine-containing contrast used for diagnostic radiological imaging

THE ASSOCIATION OF ANAESTHETISTS
of Great Britain & Ireland

Management of a Patient with Suspected Anaphylaxis During Anaesthesia
SAFETY DRILL

(Revised 2009)

Immediate management

- Use the ABC approach (Airway, Breathing, and Circulation). Team-working enables several tasks to be accomplished simultaneously.

- Remove all potential causative agents and maintain anaesthesia, if necessary, with an inhalational agent.

- CALL FOR HELP and note the time.

- Maintain the airway and administer oxygen 100%. Intubate the trachea if necessary and ventilate the lungs with oxygen.

- Elevate the patient's legs if there is hypotension.

- If appropriate, start cardiopulmonary resuscitation immediately according to Advanced Life Support Guidelines.

- Give adrenaline i.v.

  ○ Adult dose: 50 μg (0.5 ml of 1:10 000 solution).
  ○ Child dose: 1.0 μg.kg^{-1} (0.1 ml.kg^{-1} 1:100 000 solution).

- Several doses may be required if there is severe hypotension or bronchospasm. If several doses of adrenaline are required, consider starting an intravenous infusion of adrenaline.

- Give saline 0.9% or lactated Ringer's solution at a high rate via an intravenous cannula of an appropriate gauge (large volumes may be required).

  ○ Adult: 500 - 1 000 ml
  ○ Child: 20 ml.kg^{-1}

- Plan transfer of the patient to an appropriate Critical Care area.

CONTINUED OVERLEAF

Figure 9.1 Safety drill for anaphylaxis
Reproduced with kind permission from the AAGBI

Secondary management

- Give chlorphenamine i.v.

Adult:	10 mg
Child 6 - 12 years:	5 mg
Child 6 months - 6 years:	2.5 mg
Child <6 months:	250 µg.kg⁻¹

- Give hydrocortisone i.v.

Adult:	200 mg
Child 6 - 12 years:	100 mg
Child 6 months - 6 years:	50 mg
Child <6 months:	25 mg

- If the blood pressure does not recover despite an adrenaline infusion, consider the administration of an alternative i.v. vasopressor according to the training and experience of the anaesthetist, e.g. metaraminol.

- Treat persistent bronchospasm with an i.v. infusion of salbutamol. If a suitable breathing system connector is available, a metered-dose inhaler may be appropriate. Consider giving i.v. aminophylline or magnesium sulphate.

Investigation

- Take blood samples (5 - 10 ml clotted blood) for **mast cell tryptase:**

  ○ Initial sample as soon as feasible after resuscitation has started – do not delay resuscitation to take the sample.

  ○ Second sample at 1 - 2 h after the start of symptoms.

  ○ Third sample either at 24 h or in convalescence (for example in a follow-up allergy clinic). This is a measure of baseline tryptase levels as some individuals have a higher baseline level.

- Ensure that the samples are labelled with the time and date.

- Liaise with the hospital laboratory about analysis of samples.

Later investigations to identify the causative agent

The anaesthetist who gave the anaesthetic or the supervising consultant anaesthetist is responsible for ensuring that the reaction is investigated. The patient should be referred to a specialist Allergy or Immunology Centre (see www.aagbi.org for details). The patient, surgeon and general practitioner should be informed. Reactions should be notified to the AAGBI National Anaesthetic Anaphylaxis Database (see www.aagbi.org).

This guideline is not to be construed as a standard of medical care. Standards of medical care are determined on the basis of all clinical data available for an individual case and are subject to change as knowledge advances. The ultimate judgement with regard to a particular clinical procedure or treatment plan must be made by the clinician in light of the clinical data presented and the diagnostic and treatment options available.

© The Association of Anaesthetists of Great Britain & Ireland 2009

Figure 9.1 (cont.)

How should an acute anaphylactic reaction be managed?

The patient with suspected anaphylaxis should be managed with an ABCDE approach, and abnormalities treated as they are found. Specific management is as follows:

1 Immediate management
  i Stop the administration of all potentially offending agents
  ii Secure the airway, administer 100% oxygen and lie the patient flat with legs elevated
  iii Give adrenaline:
    – Intramuscular (IM) at a dose of 0.5–1 mg (0.5–1 ml of 1:1000)
    – IV at a dose of 50–100 mcg (0.5–1 ml of 1:10 000)
  iv Resuscitate with IV fluid (crystalloid preferable as colloids have a higher incidence of allergy)
2 Subsequent management
  i Give antihistamine: chlorpheniramine 10–20 mg IV
  ii Administer steroids: hydrocortisone 100–200 mg IV
  iii Bronchodilators (salbutamol, ipratropium, aminophylline, magnesium) may be required for ongoing bronchospasm
  iv Catecholamine infusion as cardiovascular instability may persist for hours
  v Consider bicarbonate for severe metabolic acidosis
3 Immediate investigation
  – Take three blood samples for mast cell tryptase:
    i Immediately after the reaction has been treated
    ii Approximately 1 hour after the reaction has been treated
    iii 6 to 24 hours after the reaction
  – Normal tryptase results do not exclude anaphylaxis and can be seen in serious reactions

The Association of Anaesthetists of Great Britain and Ireland (AAGBI) have produced a Safety Drill for suspected anaphylaxis under anaesthesia (Figure 9.1).

What further actions are required following a suspected drug mediated anaphylactic reaction?

Subsequent investigations to identify the causative agent (where the cause is unknown or unclear):

1 The patient should be referred to a *Regional Allergy Centre* for specialist investigation by an allergy specialist
  – Skin prick testing can be performed 4–6 weeks after the reaction (to allow replenishment of histamine in mast cell granules) to identify the presence of IgE–mediated reactions
  – Paired tests are performed on the volar aspect of the forearm
  – Skin prick testing is less helpful for NSAIDs, dextrans or radiocontrast media

2 Other tests:
  i Radioallergosorbent test (RAST)
     – Measures antigen-specific IgE antibodies in the serum
  ii ImmunoCAP® test
     – Fluorescent enzyme immunoassay
     – More sensitive than RAST
     – Detects specific IgE to known allergens and may provide additional evidence by indicating specific IgE sensitisation

These tests have a low sensitivity, therefore negative results still require skin prick testing

Reporting reactions:

1 All suspected reactions should be reported on a *yellow card*
2 The reaction should be documented clearly in the notes with a copy to the GP
3 The patient should be given a written record of the reaction and encouraged to wear a *Medic-Alert* bracelet

Further Reading

The Association of Anaesthetists of Great Britain and Ireland (AAGBI), 2009. Suspected Anaphylactic Reactions: AAGBI Safety Guideline [online]. London: AAGBI. Available at: www .aagbi.org/sites/default/files/anaphylaxis_2009.pdf (Accessed: 25 February 2017)

Mills A T D, Sice P J A. Anaesthesia-related anaphylaxis: investigation and follow-up. *Contin Educ Anaesth Crit Care Pain* 2014; **14**(2): 57–62

Chapter 10

Antibiotic Therapy

What factors influence antibiotic choice in critically ill patients?

Patients often require empirical antimicrobial therapy before microbiological diagnosis. There should be close collaboration with the microbiology team, with the choice of agents influenced by:

1 Likely site of infection and causative organism(s)
2 Likelihood of resistant organisms as assessed by:
   - Recent courses of antibiotics
   - LOS in hospital/ICU
   - Whether they were admitted from home or another institution
   - Recent travel, e.g. some parts of Spain have high rates of carbapenem-resistant enterococci (CRE)
   - Occupation
   - Results from screening (e.g. methicillin-resistant *S. aureus* [MRSA]) and surveillance (e.g. vancomycin-resistant enterococci [VRE]) cultures
   - Local and national patterns of resistance
3 Severity of infection (fulminant infection should be treated aggressively with broad-spectrum antibiotics that should cover more unusual organisms)
4 Patient allergy status
5 Risk of side effects including *C. difficile* infection
6 Potential drug interactions
7 Pharmacokinetic considerations, e.g. need for blood-brain barrier penetration in meningitis, poor lung penetration with aminoglycosides (should be used in conjunction with another agent in pseudomonal pneumonia)

Broadly speaking, how do antibiotics work?

Antibacterial drugs may be:

1 *Bacteriostatic* – limit bacterial growth allowing the immune system to remove the bacteria from the body
2 *Bactericidal* – cause bacterial death whilst the host cells remain undamaged; rely on intact immune system to clear the infection

Table 10.1 details which antibiotics are bactericidal and bacteriostatic.

Table 10.1 Bactericidal and bacteriostatic antibiotics*

Bactericidal	Bacteriostatic
Penicillins	Macrolides
Cephalosporins	Tetracyclines
Aminoglycosides	Lincosamides
Glycopeptides	Sulphonimides
Quinolones	Trimethoprim
Nitroimidazoles	
Rifampicin	
Nitrofurantoin	

What mechanisms are involved in antibiotic activity?

There are three principal mechanisms of antibacterial drug action:

1 *Inhibition of cell wall synthesis*
 These drugs act on bacteria that have a cell wall consisting of a lattice work of murein, by preventing cross linkage (mammalian cells lack these cell walls so are unaffected)
2 *Inhibition of DNA synthesis or function*
3 *Inhibition of tetrahydrofolate (THF) synthesis*
4 *Inhibition of protein synthesis*

Table 10.2 classifies antimicrobial agents by mechanism of action.

What is time-dependent and concentration-dependent killing?

Time-dependent killing refers to agents whose activity depends on the amount of time the serum concentration is above the minimum inhibitory concentration (MIC). These agents include β-lactams, erythromycin, clindamycin, linezolid, vancomycin. They are therefore dosed regularly to keep the serum levels above MIC as long as possible. Their half-life may be increased by the addition of a drug that reduces elimination of the antibiotic, e.g. probenecid given in penicillin treatment. Infusions may also be useful.

Concentration-dependent killing refers to agents whose activity correlates with peak serum concentration. Such agents include aminoglycosides and quinolones. High doses are used, with lower frequency of administration. However, this may impact on toxicity, e.g. aminoglycoside toxicity relates to tissue accumulation (i.e. trough levels) rather than peak serum concentration and they work best at 10–12 times MIC.

Table 10.2 Mechanism of action of antimicrobial agents

Classification	Drug	Examples	Mechanism	Spectrum of activity, uses, notes
Inhibition of cell wall synthesis	Penicillins	Penicillin	Transpeptidase inhibition (enzyme that forms cross-links in cell wall)	Streptococci, enterococci, Neisseria, spirochetes
		Flucloxacillin	β-lactam ring confers anti-transpeptidase activity	β-lactamase resistant – covers MSSA
		Amoxicillin		Improved Gram-negative cover, first-line for CAP
		Co-amoxiclav	β-lactamase-producing organisms are penicillin-resistant	Clavulanic acid prevents the action of β-lactamase
		Piperacillin/ tazobactam		Gram-positive, Gram-negative and pseudomonal cover
				Used as first-line in HAP, VAP and neutropenic sepsis
		Carbapenems, e.g. meropenem		β-lactamase resistant
				Increased activity against Gram-negatives and anaerobes, may be combined with another drug for improved Gram-positive cover
				Can be used for ESBL
				Emerging resistance of enterococci (CRE)
				No activity against MRSA, atypicals or stenotrophomonas
	Cephalosporins	1st generation, e.g. cephalexin	Contain β-lactam ring as per penicillins	Gram-positive
		2nd generation, e.g. cefuroxime		Some Gram-negative cover, e.g. E.coli, Klebsiella
		3rd generation, e.g. ceftriaxone, cefotaxime, ceftazidime		Improved Gram-negative, reduced Gram-positive cover
				CNS penetration – can be used for meningitis
				Ceftazidime has pseudomonal cover

	Class	Mechanism	Drug	Notes
	Glycopeptides	Vancomycin Teicoplanin	Exhibit slow, time-dependent killing (vancomycin is used as an infusion)	Vancomycin is highly polar and not absorbed from GI tract – used in C. difficile colitis; vancomycin has poor chest penetration (teicoplanin better) / Aerobic and anaerobic Gram-positive cover including MRSA
	Polymixin E	Colistin	Binds to lipopolysaccharide in the cell wall of Gram-negative organisms	Used in treatment of Acinetobacter and Pseudomonas, especially in CF / Nebulised preparations exhibit less nephrotoxicity and ototoxicity
Inhibition of DNA synthesis/ function	Nitroimidazoles	Metronidazole	Inhibits DNA synthesis – forms complexes with DNA and causes strand breakage	Activity against anaerobes and protozoa / First-line for C. difficile colitis (oral or IV)
	Rifamycins	Rifampicin	Inhibits DNA-dependent RNA polymerase	Has anti-staphylococcal (including MRSA) and anti-streptococcal activity / Mycobacterial infection (TB and leprosy) / Used as post-exposure prophylaxis in Neisseria/Haemophilus meningitis
	Quinolones	Ciprofloxacin	Inhibits DNA gyrase and topoisomerase-4 (DNA synthesis)	Active against Gram-negatives, atypicals and some streptococci
Inhibition of THF synthesis	Trimethoprim			Uncomplicated UTI
	Sulphonamides	Co-trimoxazole	Inhibit conversion of dihydrofolate (DHF) to tetrahydrofolate by blocking DHF reductase THF is a co-enzyme required for the synthesis of DNA and RNA	Sulfamethoxazole affects a different step in the folate metabolic pathway and is combined with trimethoprim synergistically to provide increased efficacy / First-line for PCP, Stenotrophomonas maltophilia, Burkholderia cephacia / Associated with neutropenia and epidermolysis
	Dapsone			Leprosy, acinomycoses, toxoplasmosis

Table 10.2 (cont.)

Classification	Drug	Examples	Mechanism	Spectrum of activity, uses, notes
Inhibition of protein synthesis	Tetracyclines	Tetracycline Oxytetracycline	Reversibly bind to 30s ribosomal subunit Prevent tRNA binding with mRNA	Gram-positive and Gram-negative cover Used for atypicals, Ricketsiae and protozoa
		Tigecycline		Broad spectrum of activity but not anti-pseudomonal
	Aminoglycosides	Gentamicin Amikacin	Cause insertion of incorrect amino acid, producing false proteins and causing cell death	Gram-negative cover (also enterococci and MRSA) No activity against anaerobes (oxygen needed for uptake of aminoglycoside into cell), poor anti-streptococcal activity Peak levels are associated with efficacy and trough levels with toxicity
	Chloramphenicol		Inhibits peptide synthetase, preventing amino acid linking	Bacterial meningitis
	Macrolides	Erythromycin Clarithromycin Azithromycin	Reversibly inhibit 50s ribosomal subunit Prevents ribosome moving along mRNA strand	Atypicals (mycoplasma has no cell wall, chlamydia is intracellular) Streptococcal and MSSA cover Clarithromycin is used first-line in CAP in combination with a penicillin
	Lincosamides	Clindamycin	Acts on 50s ribosomal subunit (may compete with macrolides)	Used in necrotising soft tissue infections Mixed aerobic/anaerobic infections, especially in penicillin-resistance Anti-exotoxin effect, so used in Group A streptococcal infections
	Oxazolidinones	Linezolid	Inhibit 50s ribosomal subunit	Gram-positive cover including MRSA and VRE Has high oral bioavailability (approaching 100%) Associated with myelosuppression, thrombocytopenia, peripheral and optic neuropathy, lactic acidosis and MAOi-like effects

MSSA – methicillin-sensitive *S. aureus*; CAP – community-acquired pneumonia; ESBL – extended spectrum beta-lactamase; CNS – central nervous system; CF – cystic fibrosis; TB – tuberculosis; DNA – deoxyribonucleic acid; RNA – ribonucleic acid; MAOi – monoamine oxidase inhibitor; UTI – urinary tract infection; PCP – *Pneumocystis jirovecii pneumonia*

Table 10.3 Gram staining of bacteria

Gram-positive cocci		Gram negative cocci

Staphylococci	Streptococci
	  i β-haemolytic
	    – Group A strep (*Str. pyogenes*)
	    – Group B strep (*Str. agalactiae*)
	  ii γ-haemolytic – enterococci
	  iii α-haemolytic
	    – *Str. Pneumoniae*
	    – *Str. viridans*
		Neisseria
		Moraxella

Gram positive bacilli		**Gram negative bacilli**
Actinomyces *Bacillus* Clostridia Diptheria (Corynebacterium) *Listeria*		Everything else

Table 10.3 provides a summary of Gram-positive and Gram-negative bacteria.

Further Reading
Varley A J, Sule J, Absalom A R. Principles of antibiotic therapy. *Contin Educ Anaesth Crit Care Pain* 2009; 9(6): 184–188

Chapter 11

Antimicrobial Resistance

What mechanisms do you know that confer antibiotic resistance to bacteria?

1 Intrinsic
  i Lack of molecular target
  ii Lack of transport mechanism required for the antibiotic to enter the cell
  iii Membrane impermeability, e.g. Gram-negative bacteria have a thick cell wall
2 Acquired
  i Drug inactivation e.g. Beta-lactamases
    – Initially found in Gram-positive organisms, e.g. staphylococci
    – Now in Gram-negative organisms, e.g. *Pseudomonas*
    – Increased spectrum: plasmid-encoded ESBL
  ii Reduced permeability
    – Usually in combination with other mechanisms of resistance
    – E.g. *Pseudomonas* has a relatively impermeable outer membrane and subsequent additional loss of porin channel confers carbapenem resistance
  iii Efflux of drugs
    – Primarily Gram-negative bacteria
    – Active transport of antibiotic out of organism via pump
    – Can be highly specific or broad ranging
    – E.g. *Pseudomonas* has a pump for penicillins, cephalosporins, chloramphenicol, tetracyclines and fluoroquinolones
  iv Alteration of molecular target/creation of alternative pathway
    – E.g. production of low-affinity penicillin binding protein by MRSA and coagulase-negative staphylococci
    – E.g. Genetic modification resulting in altered cell wall substrate in VRE

How do bacteria acquire resistance to antimicrobial drugs?

Table 11.1 summarises the mechanisms of acquisition of antimicrobial resistance.

Table 11.1 Mechanisms by which bacteria acquire antibiotic resistance

Intrinsic		Innate resistance
Sporadic mutation		May have adverse effect on bacteria, otherwise will be passed on to progeny
Horizontal gene transfer	Transformation	Free DNA released from lysed bacteria
	Transduction	Bacteriophages (viruses that infect bacteria) can transfer DNA from one bacteria to another
	Conjugation	Plasmids cannot move independently of a bacterium – requires direct contact of two bacteria
	Transposition	Transposons are small segments of bacterial DNA that can move independently between plasmids or bacterial chromosomes

Why is antibiotic resistance a particular problem in the ICU?

1 Use of broad spectrum antibiotics leading to selection pressure
2 Immunocompromised patients
3 Invasive devices breaching normal defences
4 Area of high intensity care with potential for cross-contamination in a busy unit

What interventions do we use to try to minimise antibiotic resistance?

1 Antimicrobial stewardship is the mainstay
  i Selecting the correct drug, dose and duration
  ii Close monitoring of antibiotic use by doctors and pharmacists
  iii De-escalating broad spectrum antibiotic at earliest opportunity – use narrow spectrum antibiotics where possible
  iv Minimising length of courses of antibiotics
  v Monitoring for toxicity
  vi Avoidance of drugs likely to contribute to *C. difficile* infection where possible
  vii Cycling antibiotics
2 Using local microbiological guidance to guide empirical therapy when considering:
  i Site of suspected infection
  ii Community-acquired vs hospital-acquired infection
  iii Recent antibiotic use
  iv Knowledge of common organisms locally
3 Aim to obtain microbiological samples *prior* to initiating empirical antibiotic therapy whenever possible

4 Rigorous infection control
   i Side rooms for patients with resistant bugs
   ii Barrier nursing, signs
   iii Alcohol gel and hand washing
   iv Audit
5 **Selective decontamination of the digestive tract** (SDD)
   – SDD involves the administration of non-absorbable oral and enteral antibiotics, and short-term intravenous antibiotics
   – The objective is to reduce/prevent colonisation or overgrowth of potentially pathogenic commensal bacteria (either the patient's own flora or those acquired following admission) thereby preventing endotoxin translocation and infection
   – A typical regime includes:
      i Topical oral paste containing tobramycin, polymixin E and amphotericin B
      ii Gastrointestinal tract decontamination with above paste administered via NG tube
         – If MRSA cover is required, enteral vancomycin is added
      iii Systemic high dose cefotaxime for four days from time of admission
   – Regular microbiological surveillance using throat and rectal swabs to monitor efficacy
   – Studies have consistently shown it to reduce both mortality and the incidence of VAP and bacteraemia
   – However, there is conflicting evidence surrounding the emergence of resistance as a result of SDD; concerns about selecting out resistant organisms have prevented its widespread use in the UK

What resistant bacteria are you aware of that represent a concern in the ICU? How do we treat these bacteria?

Table 11.2 outlines the commonest resistant bacteria.

Table 11.2 Resistant bacteria common in the ICU

Bacteria	Microbiology	Infection Control	Treatment
MRSA	MEC-A gene carried by transposon codes for low affinity penicillin-binding protein in cell wall **Panton Valentine leucocidin (PVL)** – Present in community-acquired MRSA – Causes necrotising skin and soft tissue infections and pneumonia – Treated with linezolid + rifampicin + clindamycin + IVIg	**Eradication therapy (5 days)** Mupirocin 2% tds (nasal) + Octenisan / chlorhexidine wash	First line: glycopeptides Second line: linezolid

Table 11.2 (cont.)

Bacteria	Microbiology	Infection Control	Treatment
C. difficile	Gram-positive bacillus, anaerobic, spore-forming Produces two toxins: i Toxin A (enterotoxin) causes bowel fluid sequestration ii Toxin B (cytotoxin) – detected with CDT	Increased risk with broad spectrum antibiotics (clindamycin, cephalosporins, ciprofloxacin) Must wash hands with soap and water – spores not killed by alcohol gel	First line: oral (or IV) metronidazole Second line: oral vancomycin
VRE	Enterococci – gram-positive coccus (γ-haemolytic) Previously called group D strep *E. faecalis* – usually sensitive *E. faecium* – usually resistant Six different resistance genes identified (VAN A-F) conferring multi-drug resistance		Linezolid / daptomycin
Pseudomonas	Gram-negative bacillus Acquires resistance easily Forms biofilms Common cause of late-onset VAP		Antipseudomonal penicillins (piperacillin/tazobactam) *or* Gentamicin (poor chest penetration so not monotherapy for VAP) *or* Ceftazidime *Usually dual therapy*
ESBL	Typically Klebsiella (but other coliforms as well) Resistance transferred by plasmids		Meropenem
Acinetobacter baumannii	Gram-negative cocco-bacillus Ubiquitous in soil and water Resistant to desiccation for weeks Intrinsic resistance to multiple antibiotics	May require closure of the ICU and disinfection with chlorhexidine and colistin	Colistin

IVIg – intravenous immunoglobulin; CDT – *C. difficile* toxin

Further Reading

Johnson I, Banks V. Antibiotic stewardship in critical care. *BJA Educ* 2017; **17**(4): 111–116

Varley A J, Williams H, Fletcher S. Antibiotic resistance in the intensive care unit. *Contin Educ Anaesth Crit Care Pain* 2009; **9**(4): 114–118

Chapter 12

Aortic Dissection

How is aortic dissection classified?

The *Stanford* and *DeBakey* systems are most commonly used to classify aortic dissection.

The Stanford Classification

Type A: Involves the ascending aorta
Type B: Involves the descending aorta only, distal to the origin of left sub-
          clavian artery

The DeBakey Classification

Type I: Originates in the ascending aorta and propagates at least to the
          aortic arch
Type II: Involves the ascending aorta only
Type III: Originates in the descending aorta and has two subtypes:

- Type IIIA: limited to the thoracic aorta (above the diaphragm)
- Type IIIB: extends below the diaphragm

What are the risk factors for aortic dissection?

Risk factors include:

1 Hypertension
2 Advanced age
3 Male gender
4 Smoking
5 Family history
6 Pregnancy
7 Trauma (deceleration injury)
8 Congenital disorders, e.g. Marfan syndrome, Ehlers-Danlos syndrome,
  aortic coarctation, Turner's syndrome, congenital aortic stenosis, bicuspid
  valve

What are the presenting symptoms/signs of aortic dissection?

1 Pain
   - Type A dissection classically presents with sudden onset, severe anterior chest pain, often with extension into the back
   - Type B dissection classically presents with back pain alone
2 Differential or absent pulses in the extremities
3 Aortic regurgitation (early diastolic murmur heard best between the scapulae in expiration) may be present
4 Syncope
   - This is a recognised feature of dissection, resulting from impairment of cerebral blood flow
   - Stroke and other neurological manifestations may also be present

What are the complications of aortic dissection?

Table 12.1 illustrates the complications associated with aortic dissection.

Table 12.1 The complications of aortic dissection

Cardiovascular	Acute aortic regurgitation
	Myocardial ischaemia or infarction
	Cardiac tamponade
	Hypertension (more common with distal disease)
	Hypotension or shock secondary to: tamponade, dissection of the coronary arteries, acute AR, blood loss, intra-abdominal catastrophe etc.
	Limb ischaemia
Neurological	Ischaemic stroke
	Acute paraplegia secondary to spinal cord hypoperfusion
Pulmonary	Pleural effusions (usually on the left)
Renal	Acute kidney injury
Haematological	Major transfusion requirement
	Coagulopathy
Gastrointestinal	Mesenteric ischaemia

What imaging modalities are used in the diagnosis?

Multiple imaging modalities may be used to establish a diagnosis, depending on availability. These are outlined in Table 12.2.

Table 12.2 Imaging modalities for aortic dissection

Modality	Findings
CXR	Widened mediastinum Cardiomegaly secondary to pericardial effusion Blunting of the costophrenic angle as a result of haemothorax It may be possible to see separation of calcified intima at the aortic knuckle
TTE	May allow visualisation of intimal flap in some cases, but may also be inadequate to exclude diagnosis in others Presence and severity of aortic regurgitation; dynamic assessment of cardiac function
TOE	True and false lumens may be identified with colour flow mapping. Semi-invasive, requires sedation and strict blood pressure control
CT	Confirms diagnosis and enables surgical planning via 3D reconstruction Will reveal the extent of the dissection flap
MRI	Confirms diagnosis and reveals extent of dissection flap Not suitable for unstable patients
Aortography	Historical gold standard (rarely performed nowadays) Visualisation of the dissection flap, false lumen and origin of branch arteries Can visualise the aortic valve and LV function Contrast required, slow image acquisition

LV – left ventricle

What are the principles of management for a patient with aortic dissection?

The patient with suspected aortic dissection should be managed with an ABCDE approach, treating abnormalities as they are found. The specific goals of medical management in confirmed dissection are to aggressively treat hypertension, manage pain and establish the need for surgical intervention.

1 Initial investigation and management
   i Administer oxygen
   ii Insert two large-bore IV cannulae and take bloods (FBC, U&E, clotting, crossmatch, troponin, venous gas)
   iii Establish invasive BP monitoring
   iv Insert a urinary catheter
   v 12-lead ECG
   vi Parenteral analgesia

2 Management of *hypotension*:
  i Judicious volume resuscitation as necessary to achieve systolic pressure adequate for organ perfusion whilst avoiding over-resuscitation (aim SBP 100–120 mmHg)
  ii Search for underlying aetiology including tamponade, myocardial dysfunction and acute haemorrhage
  iii Urgent surgical review with a view to emergency surgery
3 Management of *hypertension*:
  Aim to lower SBP to 100-120 mmHg or MAP to 60–65 mmHg, *or* the lowest level compatible with perfusion of the vital organs
  i First line:
    It is important to reduce shear force around the origin of the dissection flap by avoiding tachycardia, therefore adequate beta-blockade must be established before the vasodilator is initiated
    – Beta-blockers, e.g. IV esmolol, metoprolol, labetalol
    – Vasodilators, e.g. glyceryl trinitrate (GTN), sodium nitroprusside (SNP)
  ii Second line: CCBs
4 Imaging and ongoing care
  i Imaging studies at the earliest opportunity
  ii Transfer to definitive care (theatre/regional cardiothoracic centre as appropriate)

How does the management of Stanford type A and type B dissections differ?

1 Both type A and complicated type B dissections should be managed in a cardiothoracic centre
2 Type A dissections are a surgical emergency
  – Medical management is essential to halt the progression of the dissection whilst the diagnostic work-up takes place
  – Surgery is usually performed through a median sternotomy and necessitates cardiopulmonary bypass (CPB)
3 Complicated type B dissections will require a left lateral thoracotomy
4 Uncomplicated type B dissections are managed medically with beta-blockers and anti-hypertensives
  – There is a developing role for endovascular intervention in the treatment of some acute type B dissections

Further Reading

Erbel R, Aboyans V, Boileau C, et al. 2014 ESC Guidelines on the diagnosis and treatment of aortic diseases. *Eur Heart J* 2014; **35**(41): 2873–2926

Hagan P G, Nienaber C A, Isselbacher E M, et al. The International Registry of Acute Aortic Dissection (IRAD): new insights into an old disease. *J Am Med Assoc* 2000; **283**: 897–903

Chapter 13

Arrhythmias

How can you classify arrhythmias?

Arrhythmias may be classified according to:

1 Heart rate – tachycardia >100 bpm, bradycardia <60 bpm
2 Where they originate within the heart – supraventricular tachycardia (SVT), ventricular tachycardia (VT)
3 Regularity – regular or irregular

The ALS approach classifies tachyarrhythmias into narrow- or broad-complex tachycardias.

Sinus tachycardia is common in critically ill patients and is seen as a result of increased sympathetic tone, as compensation for vasodilatation (via the baroreceptor reflex), low CO, anaemia or hypoxia and in hyperthermia. It resolves once the underlying cause is treated.

Atrial tachycardia may be seen as a result of increased automaticity, channelopathy or structural abnormalities.

Atrioventricular tachycardias include nodal and non-nodal re-entrant tachycardias.

Ventricular tachycardia is most often seen in electrolyte abnormalities, especially hypokalaemia and hypomagnesaemia, and following myocardial ischaemia. It may also occur in long QT syndrome.

What is the most common tachyarrhythmia seen in critically ill patients?

Atrial fibrillation (AF).

What are the causes of AF?

Atrial fibrillation is most commonly seen in:

1 Hypovolaemia
2 Sepsis
3 Metabolic disturbance, e.g. hypokalaemia, hypomagnesaemia
4 Hypoxia
5 Ischaemia

6 Thyrotoxicosis
7 PE

How is it managed?

The patient with AF should be managed with an ABCDE approach, treating abnormalities as they are found. Specific management involves:

1 **Synchronised electrical (direct current) cardioversion** (DCCV) should be performed if there are any adverse signs:
   i Hypotension (SBP <90 mmHg)
   ii Evidence of pulmonary oedema
   iii Reduced GCS/syncope
   iv Chest pain
2 Treatment of the underlying cause, e.g. sepsis
   – Correction of hypovolaemia with fluid resuscitation
   – Correction of electrolyte disturbance – magnesium is often effective even in the absence of significant hypomagnesaemia
3 Decision whether to rate control or attempt cardioversion
   i Rate-control with beta-blocker or rate-limiting CCB, e.g. diltiazem or verapamil
      – Often used if duration of AF >48 hours, as there is increased risk of embolism of atrial thrombus
   ii Chemical cardioversion with amiodarone
      – May be unsuccessful if underlying cause not treated effectively
   iii Electrical cardioversion

If chemical or electrical cardioversion is considered in the non-emergency setting, TOE must be performed to exclude the presence of intra-atrial or left atrial appendage thrombus prior to cardioversion if AF onset is unknown or is known to be >48hr prior to presentation.

The CHA_2DS_2VASc score is used to determine whether anticoagulation should be instituted in paroxysmal or persistent AF, and is outlined in the 'Scoring Systems' topic (see page 399).

What is atrial flutter and how is it managed?

Atrial flutter is a type of SVT that is caused by the presence of a re-entry circuit within the right atrium (RA). The atrial rate approaches 300 bpm, and the atrioventricular (AV) node physiologically blocks the rapid flutter waves, producing a lower ventricular rate, e.g. 2:1 block (rate ~150 bpm, Figure 13.1), 3:1 block (rate ~100 bpm). Flutter waves may be seen in the inferior leads (Figure 13.2). Atrial flutter is usually unresponsive to vagal manoeuvres. Adenosine may reveal the underlying rhythm in cases of doubt, but will not cardiovert it. Rate control to increase the AV block, or chemical or electrical cardioversion may be required.

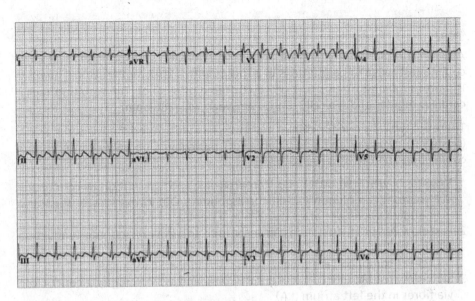

Figure 13.1 Atrial flutter with 2:1 block

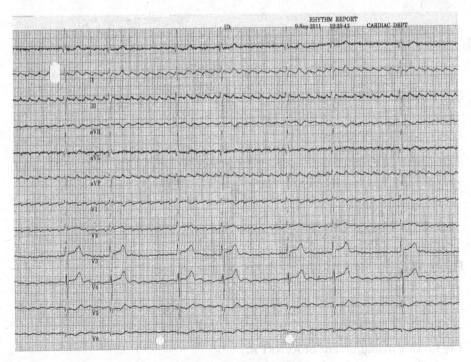

Figure 13.2 Atrial flutter with slow variable block

What is atrioventricular nodal re-entrant tachycardia?

Atrioventricular nodal re-entrant tachycardia (AVNRT) is a type of SVT and is the commonest cause of palpitations in patients with a structurally normal heart. It is paroxysmal and often provoked by caffeine or alcohol. The resulting tachycardia is regular and typically ranges between 140–280 bpm.

There are typically two functional pathways located around the AV node: a slow (posterior) pathway and a fast (anterior) pathway. One allows anterograde conduction and the other retrograde:

1 Slow-fast AVNRT (80–90%) – slow anterograde and fast retrograde conduction
   - P waves often hidden within corresponding QRS complexes or seen as a 'pseudo-R wave' just after the QRS in V1 or V2
2 Fast-slow AVNRT (~10%) – fast anterograde and slow retrograde conduction (Figure 13.3)
   - QRS-P-T complexes are seen (P waves within the ST segment)
3 Slow-slow AVNRT (≤5%) – slow anterograde and slow retrograde conduction via fibres in the left atrium (LA)
   - P wave seen in mid-diastole, often just before the QRS complex meaning it may be mistaken for sinus tachycardia

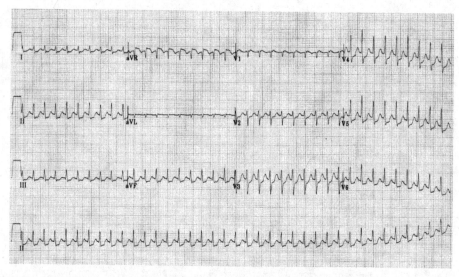

Figure 13.3 Fast-slow AVNRT with QRS-P-T morphology

How do you manage AVNRT?

The specific management of AVNRT is:

1 Vagal manoeuvres
2 Adenosine may cardiovert the rhythm

3 Beta-blockers or rate-limiting CCBs are first-line if adenosine unsuccessful
4 Flecainide or amiodarone are second-line

What is atrioventricular re-entrant tachycardia?

Atrioventricular re-entrant tachycardia (AVRT) is another type of SVT caused by a re-entrant circuit that is anatomically distinct from the AV node, and can cause pre-excitation of the ventricles. This can degenerate into tachycardia because there is no AV node to delay conduction. The commonest cause of AVRT is Wolff-Parkinson-White (WPW) syndrome.

Tell me about Wolff-Parkinson-White syndrome.

Wolff-Parkinson-White syndrome is caused by aberrant conduction via the *Bundle of Kent*, a congenital accessory pathway. Impulses may be conducted in an anterograde or retrograde fashion, but more commonly they are bidirectional. The ECG changes (which may only be present intermittently) include:

1 *Delta wave* (slurred upstroke of the QRS complex) due to pre-excitation of the ventricles by the accessory pathway
2 PR interval <120 ms
3 QRS-T wave discordance (i.e. the T wave deflection is in the opposite direction to the QRS)
4 Presence of tall R waves and T wave inversion in the precordial leads mimicking either right ventricle (RV, leads V1-V3) or LV (leads V4-V6) hypertrophy

WPW is described as type A or B:

Type A – positive delta wave in precordial leads, dominant S wave in V1 (left-sided pathway, Figure 13.4)

Type B – negative delta wave in V1 (right-sided pathway)

AVRT is often triggered by premature beats and the features of pre-excitation are lost. Conduction through the AV node may be either:

1 *Orthodromic* (~95%) – antegrade, with retrograde conduction through the accessory pathway
   - Narrow complexes
   - Rate 200–300 bpm
   - No visible P waves
   - Pattern mimics AVNRT
2 *Antidromic* – retrograde, with antegrade conduction through the accessory pathway
   - Broad complexes
   - Rate 200–300 bpm

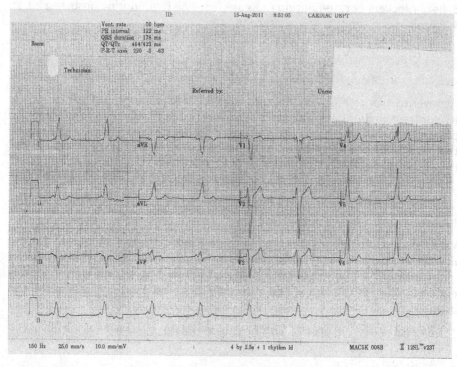

Figure 13.4 Wolff-Parkinson-White syndrome type A

How do you manage AVRT?

The specific management of orthodromic AVRT is:

1 Vagal manoeuvres
2 Adenosine may cardiovert the rhythm
3 CCBs are first-line if adenosine unsuccessful
4 DCCV is necessary in the presence of adverse signs

Antidromic AVRT may be mistaken for VT. Haemodynamically stable patients may respond to amiodarone or procainamide; instability necessitates DCCV. If in doubt, it should be treated as VT.

When AF develops in a patient with WPW syndrome, the accessory pathway allows for rapid conduction directly to the ventricles, bypassing the AV node. The complexes are broad and the rate is well over 200 bpm (Figure 13.5). Treatment with AV nodal blocking drugs (e.g. adenosine, beta-blockers or CCBs) may increase conduction via the accessory pathway and cause degeneration into VT or ventricular fibrillation (VF). Procainamide or DCCV are preferred. Haemodynamic instability necessitates urgent synchronised DCCV.

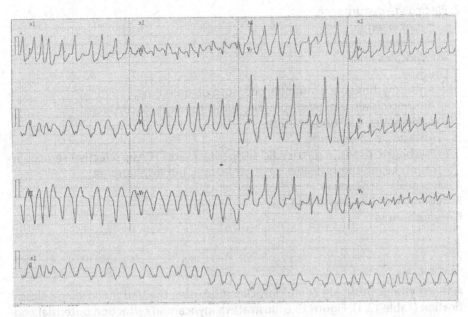

Figure 13.5 AF in Wolff-Parkinson-White syndrome

How do you differentiate VT from SVT with aberrancy?

A broad complex tachycardia is more likely to be ventricular tachycardia if there is:

1 AV dissociation (P waves may be seen superimposed on T waves or between QRS complexes)
2 Extreme axis deviation (lead I is positive, lead aVF is negative)
3 QRS >160 ms
4 *Fusion beats* (hybrid of sinus + ventricular complexes)
5 *Capture beats* (normal conduction of an atrial impulse through the AV node)
6 Concordance (either positive or negative) across the precordial leads
7 Notching seen near the top of the S wave – *Josephson's sign*
8 RSR' pattern with a taller R (right bundle branch block (RBBB) produces an RSR' pattern with a taller R')

What are the causes of a long QT interval?

1 Congenital
   - Romano-Ward syndrome (autosomal dominant)
   - Jervell-Lange-Neilson (autosomal recessive, associated with congenital deafness)

2 Electrolyte disturbance
 – Hypokalaemia
 – Hypomagnesaemia
 – Hypocalcaemia
3 Drugs
 – Antiarrhythmics, e.g. amiodarone, sotolol, quinidine
 – Antimicrobials, e.g. erythromycin, clarithromycin, fluconazole
 – Antiemetics, e.g. ondansetron
 – Antacids, e.g. cisapride
 – Psychiatric drugs, e.g. tricyclic antipepressants (TCAs), selective serotonin reuptake inhibitors (SSRIs), phenothiazines, butyrophenones
4 Myocardial ischaemia
5 Subarachnoid haemorrhage
6 Hypothermia

How are antiarrhythmic drugs classified?

Antiarrhythmic drugs are commonly classified using the Vaughn Williams classification (Table 13.1). Figure 13.6 illustrates a myocardial cell action potential and helps to explain the mechanisms of drug action. Antiarrhythmic drugs may also be classified according to which arrhythmias they are used to treat.

In addition to its class III activity, amiodarone also exhibits class I, II and IV activity.

Table 13.1 Vaughn-Williams classification of antiarrhythmic drugs

Class		Action	Drugs	Use
Class I		Na^+ channel blockers Reduce rate of rise of phase 0		
	Ia	Prolonged absolute refractory period (ARP)	Procainamide	SVT and VT
	Ib	Shortened ARP	Lignocaine Phenytoin	VT
	Ic	ARP unchanged	Flecainide Propafenone	SVT and VT
Class II		Beta-blockers Reduce AV node conduction, prolong phase 4, reduce contractility	Bisoprolol Metoprolol Esmolol	SVT
Class III		K^+ channel blockers Prolong phase 3, increase duration of action potential	Amiodarone Sotolol	SVT and VT
Class IV		Ca^{2+} channel blockers Reduce sinoatrial (SA) and AV node automatocity	Verapamil Diltiazem	SVT

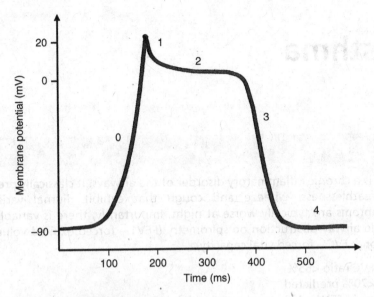

0 - Depolarisation (fast Na$^+$ influx)
1 - Repolarisation (K$^+$ efflux)
2 - Plateau phase (K$^+$ efflux balanced by Ca^{2+} influx through slow L-type Ca^{2+} channels)
3 - Repolarisation (L-type Ca^{2+} channels close)
4 - Resting membrane potential restored by Na$^+$/K$^+$ ATPase (Na$^+$ efflux, K$^+$ influx)

Figure 13.6 The myocardial action potential

Adenosine is an endogenous nucleoside with rapid onset and ultra-short duration of action. It acts on A$_1$ receptors, causing transient AV nodal block and is used in the diagnosis and treatment of SVT. It may cause severe bronchospasm and should be avoided in asthmatics.

Chapter 14

Asthma

What is asthma?

Asthma is a chronic inflammatory disorder of the airways. It classically presents with breathlessness, wheeze and cough that exhibit diurnal variation. The symptoms are typically worse at night. Importantly, there is variable but reversible airway obstruction on spirometry (FEV1 – forced expired volume in one second; FVC – forced vital capacity):

1 FEV1/FVC ratio <65%
2 FEV1 <70% predicted
3 Increase in FEV1 >12% from baseline following inhaled bronchodilator

There may be a history of atopy (eczema, allergic rhinitis) or exposure to occupational allergens. Asthma may be exacerbated by allergens, cold air, cigarette smoke or exposure to certain drugs, e.g. NSAIDs, aspirin, beta-blockers.

What is the pathophysiology of asthma?

Chronic airway inflammation results in smooth muscle hypertrophy and goblet cell hyperplasia. There is increased airway reactivity, mucosal and submucosal oedema and excessive secretion. This produces the typical symptoms of bronch-ospasm and mucus plugging, and eventually leads to scarring due to epithelial collagen deposition.

How do you diagnose life-threatening asthma?

The British Thoracic Society/Scottish Intercollegiate Guidelines Network (BTS/SIGN) guidelines describe four levels of severity in acute asthma (Table 14.1).

Table 14.1 The levels of severity of acute asthma

Moderate acute asthma	Increasing symptoms PEFR >50–75% best (within last 2 years) or predicted No features of acute severe asthma
Acute severe asthma	Any one of: i PEFR 33–50% best or predicted ii RR ≥25 per minute iii HR ≥110 bpm iv Inability to complete sentences
Life-threatening asthma	Any one of the following signs present in a patient with acute severe asthma

Clinical signs	Investigations
Altered conscious level Exhaustion Arrhythmia Hypotension Cyanosis Silent chest Poor respiratory effort	PEFR <33% best or predicted SpO_2 <92% PaO_2 <8 kPa 'Normal' $PaCO_2$ (4.6–6.0 kPa)

Near-fatal asthma	Raised $PaCO_2$ and/or requiring mechanical ventilation with raised inflation pressures

PEFR – peak expiratory flow rate

Reproduced from BTS/SIGN British Guideline on the management of asthma by kind permission of the British Thoracic Society

---

A 31-year-old man with brittle asthma is admitted to the Emergency Department (ED) with an acute attack following a short coryzal illness. He has been admitted three times within the last year, including one ICU admission during which he was intubated and ventilated. On your assessment he is drowsy, making poor respiratory effort and is unable to talk. He is cold, clammy and peripherally shut down. Auscultation reveals very quiet breath sounds with no audible wheeze.

His observations are:

SpO_2 91% on 15 l/min oxygen via a non-rebreathing mask

RR 37 per minute

HR 148 bpm

BP 94/59 mmHg

ABG on 15 l/min oxygen: pH 7.41, $PaCO_2$ 4.9 kPa, PaO_2 7.3 kPa, BE -7.4 mmol/l, HCO_3^- 16.1 mmol/l, lactate 4.8 mmol/l

What is your immediate management?

This patient has life-threatening asthma and is at high risk of deterioration. He is likely to require invasive ventilation. He should be managed with an ABCDE approach, treating abnormalities as they are found. Close liaison with the respiratory physicians is mandatory, and he should be admitted to critical care. Specific management involves:

1 **Airway assessment**
   – Administer oxygen titrated to SpO_2 94–98%
   – Indications for intubation in acute asthma include:
      i Poor or deteriorating respiratory effort
      ii Exhaustion
      iii Persistent or worsening hypoxia
      iv Drowsiness, confusion
      v Respiratory arrest
   – Hypercapnia is an indication of severity, but does not mandate intubation in itself
   – Consider ketamine (1–2 mg/kg) as induction agent
   – Avoid NMBAs that cause histamine release, e.g. atracurium

2 **Breathing**
   – Arterial blood gas (ABG) analysis will assist in categorising the severity of the asthma attack and help to guide intervention including intubation
   – Perform a CXR in patients with life-threatening asthma to look for pneumothorax/pneumomediastinum or consolidation
   – Concurrent administration of oxygen-driven **nebulised bronchodilators**
      i Salbutamol 2.5–5 mg (5–10 mg continuously over an hour if response is poor)
      ii Ipratropium bromide 250–500 mcg 4–6 hourly (produces significantly better bronchodilation than β_2-agonists alone)
   – Give **steroids** (prednisolone 40 mg orally od, or hydrocortisone 100 mg IV qds for five days total)
      – Steroids reduce mortality, relapses, subsequent hospital admission and requirement for β_2-agonist therapy
      – Early administration improves outcome
   – Administer **magnesium** ($MgSO_4$ 8 mmol (2 g) IV over 20 minutes) in patients who have had little or no response to nebulised bronchodilators – see page 282
      – May improve lung function and reduce intubation rates in patients with acute severe asthma
   – Consider **intravenous salbutamol** in patients where nebulisers cannot be administered reliably (monitor serum lactate)
   – Some patients with near-fatal or life-threatening asthma with a poor response to initial therapy may gain additional benefit from IV **aminophylline** (5 mg/kg loading dose over 20 minutes (omit if on maintenance oral therapy) then infusion of 0.5–0.7 mg/kg/hour)
   – Infective exacerbations are likely to be viral – antibiotics are not recommended routinely

- Leukotriene-receptor antagonists are not useful in acute asthma
- There is no evidence for the use of heliox, although it may reduce work of breathing as a bridge to resolution of bronchospasm

3 Circulation

- Patients are usually intravascularly deplete; CO is further decreased due to the impedance of venous return caused by airflow obstruction and high intrathoracic pressure
  - Careful fluid resuscitation should be performed
  - This is even more important in patients who require intubation as suppression of their sympathetic drive following induction of anaesthesia can cause cardiovascular collapse
- Pulsus paradoxus is an inadequate marker of severity and should not be used
- Electrolyte imbalance is common and should be monitored and corrected
  - Hypokalaemia is problematic with β_2-agonist therapy

> **Despite optimal medical therapy, the patient deteriorates further and requires intubation. What ventilatory strategies should be employed in patients with an acute asthma exacerbation?**

There is high airway resistance in asthma, which obstructs expiratory flow and can lead to breath stacking and air trapping (*dynamic hyperinflation*). This is associated with barotrauma and cardiovascular depression. Dynamic hyperinflation should be suspected when inspiratory flow is seen to commence before expiratory flow returns to baseline.

The aim is to minimise this with the following strategies:

1 Low PEEP (≤80% of intrinsic PEEP in spontaneously ventilating patients)
  - Intrinsic PEEP increases the magnitude of the drop in airway pressure that the patient must generate to trigger a breath, i.e. increases work of breathing
  - Careful application of extrinsic (i.e. ventilator) PEEP will reduce this gradient and the work of breathing
  - Intrinsic PEEP may be measured by performing an expiratory hold (aim <10 cmH_2O)
2 Prolonged expiratory time (I:E ratio of 1:2–1:4)
3 Controlled hypoventilation
  - Slow respiratory rate (10–14 breaths/minute)
  - Low tidal volumes (≤8 ml/kg)
  - Pressure limitation (P_{plat} <30 cmH_2O)
  - Permissive hypercapnia is generally well-tolerated with a pH >7.2, as long as adequate oxygenation is achieved

It may be necessary to temporarily disconnect the patient from the ventilator to manually decompress the hyperinflated lungs.

In the event of continued bronchospasm and difficulty in ventilating, are there any other adjunctive therapies that you are aware of?

1 Ketamine
   – Phencyclidine derivative that acts as an antagonist at the N-methyl-D-aspartate (NMDA) receptor and causes bronchodilation
   – Useful as an induction agent in acute asthma (1–2 mg/kg) – causes dissociative anaesthesia
   – Infusion may be used as an adjunct on the ICU
2 Volatile anaesthetic agents, particularly sevoflurane
   – Well-documented bronchodilating effects
   – May be added to the ventilator gas in intractable bronchospasm
3 VV ECMO
   – May be considered in patients with refractory status asthmaticus (i.e. who have not responded to aggressive medical therapy and mechanical ventilation)

Is there any evidence for the use of NIV in acute asthma?

A Cochrane Review of five trials (206 patients) in 2013 was inconclusive. There has been one small trial that showed improvement in hospitalisation rates, discharge from emergency departments and lung function. The use of NIV is not established in asthma, but its use could be considered on a trial basis on the ICU with a low threshold for intubation if reasonable improvement is not seen.

What are the risk factors for near-fatal asthma?

1 Previous ICU admission +/- mechanical ventilation
2 Oral steroid or theophylline use
3 Increasing use of β_2-agonists
4 Poor compliance with inhaled corticosteroids (including risk factors such as psychiatric history, drug and alcohol abuse, non-attendance at clinic appointments)
5 Altered perception of dyspnoea
6 Age >40 years
7 *Brittle asthma*
   i Type 1 – >40% diurnal variation in PEFR for >50% of the time despite intensive therapy
   ii Type 2 – sudden severe attacks on a background of 'well-controlled' asthma

Further Reading
British Thoracic Society (BTS)/Scottish Intercollegiate Guidelines Network (SIGN), 2016. British guideline on the management of asthma (QRG 153) [online]. Edinburgh: SIGN; 2016. Available at: www.brit-thoracic.org.uk/standards-of-care/guidelines/btssign-british-guideline-on-the-management-of-asthma/ (Accessed: 11 May 2017)

Lim W J, Mohammed Akram R, Carson K V, et al. Non-invasive positive pressure ventilation for treatment of respiratory failure due to severe acute exacerbations of asthma. *Cochrane Database Syst Rev* 2012; **12**: CD004360

Peck T, Hill S, Williams M. General anaesthetic agents. In: *Pharmacology for Anaesthesia and Intensive Care*. Cambridge University Press, 2014; 93–125

Chapter 15

Bronchopleural Fistulae

What is a bronchopleural fistula?

A bronchopleural fistula (BPF) is an abnormal communication between the bronchial tree and pleural space, which causes an air leak from the lung. It manifests clinically as a persistent air leak or a failure to re-inflate the lung despite chest tube drainage for 24 hours.

The size of the air leak is critical: small tears or punctures will heal quickly with conservative management, however larger structural damage to the lung or a major bronchus will not.

Significant morbidity and mortality is associated with bronchopleural fistulae and their diagnosis and management remains a therapeutic challenge.

What is an air leak and how are air leaks classified?

An air leak can be defined as any extrusion of air from a normally gas-filled cavity such as the upper airway, sinuses, tracheobronchial tree and GI tract.

Air leaks from the tracheobronchial tree can be classified into four functional types (Table 15.1).

Table 15.1 Robert David Cerfolio classification of air leaks

Type	Details
Continuous	Air leak is present throughout the respiratory cycle Seen in patients who are receiving mechanical ventilation or who have a BPF
Inspiratory	Air leak only during inspiration
Expiratory	Air leak only during expiration Most common post-pulmonary surgery
Forced expiration	Air leak only when patient performs forced expiration or coughs

What are the causes of a bronchopleural fistula?

The most common cause of a BPF is following pulmonary resection (4–10% post-pneumonectomy, 0.5% post-lobectomy).

Risk factors include:

1 Right-sided procedures
2 Uncontrolled pleural/pulmonary infection
3 Pre-operative steroids, radiation, diabetes
4 Malignancy
5 Mechanical ventilation for >24 hours

Other causes of BPF are as follows:

1 Trauma
2 ARDS
3 Infection, e.g. pneumonia, empyema, tuberculosis
4 Necrotising lung disease associated with chemotherapy or radiotherapy
5 Iatrogenic, e.g. line placement, lung biopsy
6 Persistent spontaneous pneumothorax
7 Complication of mechanical ventilation

What are the clinical features of a bronchopleural fistula?

The clinical features of a BPF can vary widely from a self-limiting condition to a life-threatening complication such as tension pneumothorax. Common presenting features include:

1 Dyspnoea
2 Hypotension
3 Subcutaneous emphysema
4 Cough with expectoration of purulent material
5 Shifting of the trachea and mediastinum
6 Persistent air leak in a mechanically ventilated patient
7 Persistent bubbling of intercostal drain

How is a bronchopleural fistula diagnosed?

Bronchopleural fistulae represent a diagnostic challenge. The following investigations are utilised:

1 CXR
   – Increase in intrapleural airspace
   – Appearance of a new air-fluid level
   – Development of a tension pneumothorax

2 Bronchoscopy
  – Can confirm and localise the BPF by visualisation of continuous return of bubbles on bronchial washing
  – Methylene blue test – selective instillation of methylene blue into segmental bronchi which then appears in chest drain
3 CT chest
  – Imaging technique of choice for visualising and characterising BPFs
  – Will demonstrate pneumothorax, pneumomediastinum and the underlying lung pathology
4 Others
  – Ventilation scintigraphy using radioactive gases, e.g. Xe-133 (accumulates in the pleural space and remains trapped in washout study)

How does a bronchopleural fistula differ from a pneumothorax?

A bronchopleural fistula is a direct communication between the central bronchial tree and the pleural cavity, causing an air leak from the lung. A pneumothorax involves a peripheral communication between a ruptured bleb or alveolar duct and the pleural cavity.

What are the potential physiological consequences of a bronchopleural fistula in a mechanically ventilated patient?

Mechanical ventilation of a lung with a BPF will lead to a continuous air leak, and will delay healing of fistulous tract. It also results in the following:

1 Inability to apply PEEP
2 Loss of effective tidal volume secondary to an inability to maintain adequate alveolar ventilation
3 Failure of lung re-expansion
4 Inappropriate cycling of the ventilator
5 Delayed weaning from the ventilator

How is a bronchopleural fistula managed?

Management options for a BPF include both medical and surgical treatments dependent on the condition of the patient and size of the air leak.

1 Resuscitation and initial management
  i Supportive care and monitoring
  ii Imaging as necessary: CXR, CT chest, bronchoscopy
  iii Treat life-threatening conditions:
    – Tension pneumothorax – needle decompression

- Major bronchial stump dehiscence – immediate re-suturing with reinforcement
- Pulmonary flooding – airway control, postural drain with affected side down

2 General conservative measures
   i Large bore chest drain insertion
      - All patients with low-flow BPF and empyema require chest drain insertion
      - Suction applied to the pleural space as necessary
      - The optimal amount of suction must be determined on an individual basis
   ii Control active infection
      - If empyema or infection are suspected, give appropriate antibiotics +/– drainage

3 Specific management in **ventilated patients**
   i Minimise alveolar distension and minute volume
      - Reduce PEEP, tidal volume, inspiratory time and respiratory rate
      - Tolerate permissive hypercapnia and lower SpO_2
   ii Encourage spontaneous ventilation
   iii Discontinue mechanical ventilation as soon as possible
      - Most air leaks will resolve spontaneously over a few days in the spontaneously ventilating patient who does not require the use of high levels of PEEP/CPAP

4 Management of **large or persistent leaks**
   Most BPFs close spontaneously once the underlying pathology improves and following discontinuation of mechanical ventilation. However, intervention is required in the case of continued air leak.
   i Other modes of ventilation
      - Use of high-frequency ventilation (HFV) and oscillation has been reported
   ii Independent lung ventilation using two ventilators or differential lung ventilation
      - Double lumen tube (DLT) insertion
      - Endobronchial occlusion/bronchial blocker
   iii Bronchoscopic repair
      - BPF >8 mm are not suitable for bronchoscopic repair
      - Bronchoscopy can be used to directly apply sealants (e.g. cyanoacrylate, fibrin agents, gelfoam)
   iv Surgery
      - Thoracoplasty
      - Bronchial stump stapling
      - Pleural abrasion and decortication
   v ECMO

What are the ICU-specific consequences of a large BPF?

1 Difficulty in weaning from mechanical ventilation
2 Hypoxia, hypercapnia
3 Inability to apply PEEP and expand remaining lung
4 Prolonged use of sedatives and muscle relaxants with associated risk of ICU-AW and delirium
5 Need for further operative procedures and ongoing imaging necessitating transfers away from the unit
6 Potential requirement for differential lung ventilation using DLT or HFV
7 High mortality and morbidity

Further Reading

Paramasivam E, Bodenham A. Air leaks, pneumothorax and chest drains. *Contin Educ Anaesth Crit Care Pain* 2008; 8(6): 204–209

Chapter 16

Burns

What is the pathophysiology of major burns?

Figure 16.1 illustrates the pathophysiology.

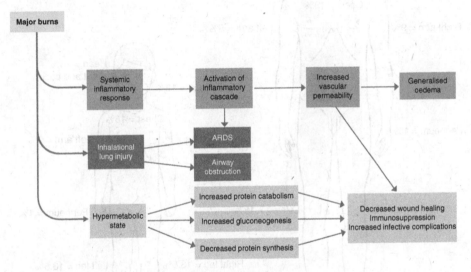

Figure 16.1 The pathophysiology of major burns

How is burn severity estimated?

1 Burn area
   Age-specific *Lund-Browder charts* provide an accurate assessment of burn injury as total body surface area (TBSA, %). Alternatively, the *Rule of Nines* may be used (Figure 16.2). The patient's palm and adducted fingers may also be used to represent 1% BSA, and an estimate of burn injury may be made on this basis.
2 Burn depth is assessed as follows:
   i *Superficial*
   - Involves epidermis only
   - Erythematous, painful and dry with no blistering

ii *Partial-thickness* (superficial or deep dermal, depending on degree of dermal injury)
  – Erythematous, painful and oedematous with blistering
iii *Full-thickness*
  – Destroys all layers of skin and may involve subcutaneous structures
  – Painless (nocioceptors destroyed) and white (no capillary return)

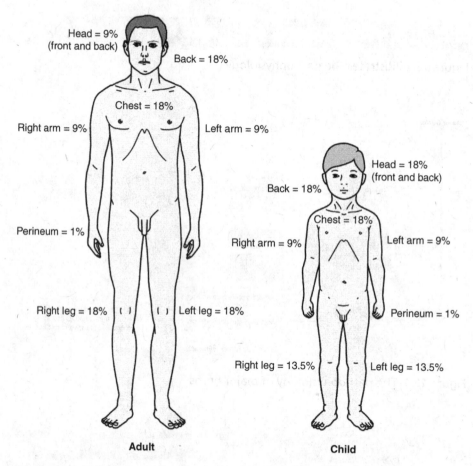

Figure 16.2 The Wallace Rule of Nines
Reproduced with permission from Hettiaratchy S, et al. (*Br Med J* 2004)

What are the management priorities in a patient presenting with major burns?

The management of the patient with major burns should follow an Advanced Trauma Life Support (ATLS) approach, treating life-threatening injuries as they are found. Particular care should be taken to assess for the presence of inhalation injury and to estimate the extent of the burns. Specific management involves:

1 **Airway (with C-spine control) and ventilatory management**
   - Features suggestive of potential inhalational injury include:
     i Facial burns
     ii Carbonaceous sputum
     iii Singeing of nasal/facial hair
     iv Oropharyngeal oedema
     v Stridor
     vi Voice change including hoarseness
   - Additional indications for endotracheal intubation:
     i Neck burns
     ii Respiratory failure
     iii Decreased conscious level
     iv To facilitate analgesia, imaging or other intervention in a multiply injured patient
   - Pre-emptive intubation is preferable and senior anaesthetic input is advisable
   - An uncut endotracheal tube (ETT) should be used to allow for evolving facial oedema (≥size 8.0 to facilitate bronchoscopy)
   - Institute LPV
   - Perform regular ABG analysis, consider carbon monoxide and cyanide poisoning

2 Establish large-bore IV access and commence **fluid resuscitation** with a warmed balanced crystalloid solution
   - The *Parkland Formula* is used to calculate fluid requirements in the first 24 hours following the burn injury:

   Volume of fluid required = 4ml × body weight (kg) × TBSA (%)

   - Half the volume is given in the first 8 hours, the remaining half over the following 16 hours
   - Monitor urine output and consider invasive BP and central venous pressure (CVP) monitoring

3 **Analgesia** is of the utmost importance
   - Full-thickness burns are painless, but partial-thickness burns can be very painful
   - Titrated opioid analgesia is first-line; ketamine may be useful

4 **Avoid hypothermia**
   - The hypothalamic set-point in patients with severe burns is reset to 38.5°C
   - Control the environmental temperature between 28-32°C with high humidity to reduce evaporative loss

5 **Early surgical management** may be indicated
   - Urgent escharotomy may be necessary in circumferential burns
   - Morbidity and mortality associated with deep burn injury is significantly reduced by surgical intervention

   – Debridement allows source control for the inflammatory response and reduces the hypermetabolic state

A thorough history should be taken of events surrounding the injury to help guide management:

1 What time did the fire start and did the patient self-extricate?
   – Assessment of duration of exposure
   – Whether there are likely to be any other injuries, e.g. jumping out of window to escape
2 What was the nature of the fire?
   – Were there any toxic chemicals?
3 Did it occur indoors or outside?
   – Risk of inhalation injury
4 Was there an explosion?
   – Blast injury
5 What was the patient's condition at the scene?
   – Including GCS, other obvious injuries and whether CPR was provided

What is inhalation injury and how is it managed?

Inhalation injury is suggested by prolonged smoke exposure in a confined space, particularly in the presence of neurological impairment affecting ability to escape (including intoxication). It includes:

1 *Upper airway thermal injury*
   – May cause significant oedema of the tongue, pharynx and larynx resulting in airway obstruction
   – Early prophylactic endotracheal intubation should be considered
2 *Chemical irritation throughout the respiratory tract*
   – Caused by direct injury to the respiratory epithelium and capillary endothelium by acidic or alkaline compounds released from burning material
   – Results in severe tracheobronchitis, impaired mucociliary clearance and loss of surfactant causing atelectasis
   – Early inflammation and capillary leak followed later by exudate formation produce an ARDS-type picture

The specific management of an inhalation injury involves:

1 **Early bronchoscopy** (within 24 hours)
   – Confirms diagnosis and allows grading of severity
2 **Bronchoalveolar lavage (BAL)/aggressive pulmonary toilet** (to remove foreign material and slough)
   – In patients with inhalation injury complicated by pneumonia there is a trend towards reduced duration of mechanical ventilation, mortality and ICU and hospital LOS in those who are bronchoscoped vs those who are not

3 **Triple nebuliser therapy** (conflicting evidence for efficacy)
    i Bronchodilators
    ii Heparin (to reduce fibrin deposition)
    iii NAC (mucolysis)
4 **Lung-protective ventilation** with consideration of $ECCO_2R$ or ECMO

Mortality in burns patients increases dramatically from 13.9% to 27.6% in the presence of inhalation injury.

What is 'burn shock'?

Burn shock is a term used to describe the combination of hypovolaemic, distributive and cardiogenic shock seen in a patient with major burns, which is refractory to massive fluid resuscitation.

When should infection be suspected/treated in these hypermetabolic patients?

Diagnosis of infection or sepsis is notoriously difficult in patients with major burns because they exhibit features of the systemic inflammatory response syndrome (SIRS) as a result of the burn insult. Regular microbiological surveillance is necessary, and three of the following criteria from the American Burn Association should be present in addition to documented infection before sepsis can be diagnosed in a patient with burns:

1 Temperature <36.5°C or >39°C
2 Respiratory rate (RR) >25 in a spontaneously breathing patient, or need for mechanical ventilation with minute volume >12 l/min
3 Heart rate (HR) >110 bpm
4 Glucose >12.8 mmol/l in a non-diabetic patient
5 Intolerance of enteral feed for >24 hours
6 Platelet count <100 x 10^9/l (≥3 days after resuscitation phase)

Short courses of targeted, narrow-spectrum antibiotic therapy can be used if there is *real* evidence of infection, and rigorous infection control measures are vital.

How does carbon monoxide/cyanide poisoning present? How is it diagnosed and what is the management?

Carbon monoxide and cyanide poisoning are outlined in Table 16.1.

Table 16.1 Carbon monoxide and cyanide poisoning

	Carbon monoxide poisoning	Cyanide poisoning
Pathophysiology	Carbon monoxide has an affinity for haemoglobin 250 times that of oxygen. There is impaired oxygen delivery to the tissues due to reduced oxygen carrying capacity and reduced dissociation once bound (left shift in the oxygen dissociation curve). Additionally, there is inhibition of cytochrome oxidase, resulting in impaired oxygen utilisation at the mitochondrial level	Cyanide inhibits mitochondrial cytochrome oxidase, blocking oxidative phosphorylation and resulting in anaerobic metabolism
Presentation	Nausea and vomiting, headache, hypotension. Neurological signs from mild confusion to coma and seizures. Cherry-red skin discolouration is infrequently seen	Breathlessness, hypotension, dizziness, vomiting and psychomotor agitation progressing rapidly to loss of consciousness (symptoms largely relate to hypoxia). Unexplained metabolic acidosis and high central venous saturation ($ScvO_2$) are also suggestive
Investigations	Carboxyhaemoglobin (HbCO) level on co-oximetry on ABG (normal HbCO <1%, in smokers may be <5%). SpO_2 will trend towards 100% (absorption spectra of HbCO similar to HbO_2) – SaO_2 should be measured by co-oximetry. PaO_2 will be normal	Lactic acidosis. High $ScvO_2$, i.e. low arterio-venous oxygen gradient. Cyanide levels take ≥3 hours to perform
Management	Administer 100% oxygen (reduces half-life from 4 hours in air to 1 hour). Intubate and ventilate if HbCO >25%. Hyperbaric oxygen therapy (HBOT) at 3 atm (reduces half-life to 15–20 minutes) indicated if: i HbCO >40% ii Pregnancy if HbCO >15% iii Coma	Supportive therapy directed at maximising oxygen delivery, i.e. 100% oxygen with intubation if necessary. Antidotes (chelators): i Hydroxycobalamin 5 g (2 doses) ii Dicobalt edetate iii Sodium thiosulphate, which converts cyanide to thiocyanate (renally excreted) may also be used

Table 16.1 (cont.)

	Carbon monoxide poisoning	Cyanide poisoning
Prognosis	Poor correlation between HbCO level and the presence or absence of symptoms at presentation, or with long-term outcomes HbCO >60% is likely to be fatal	Prognosis is reasonably good for patients with moderate symptoms if rapid supportive therapy and antidotes are provided Prognosis is poor in patients who suffer cardiac arrest secondary to cyanide toxicity, even if antidotes are administered promptly Patients who survive are at risk of neurological sequelae, e.g. anoxic encephalopathy Acute and delayed neurological manifestations (movement disorders, e.g. Parkinson-like syndrome, neuropsychiatric sequelae) have been reported

HbO_2 – oxyhaemoglobin; SaO_2 – arterial oxygen saturation

What are the criteria for referral to a burns centre?

The National Referral Network for Burn Care is now disbanded, but their recommendation of seeking specialist input from a burns centre (either referral to, or discussion with) in the following circumstances is very useful:

1 Age <5 or >60 years-old
2 The presence of comorbidities, especially those that affect healing:
  i Significant cardiorespiratory disease
  ii DM
  iii Pregnancy
  iv Immunosuppression
  v Liver disease, particularly cirrhosis
3 Site:
  i Face, hands, feet, perineum
  ii Any flexure, particularly neck or axilla
  iii Circumferential dermal or full-thickness burns of the torso, limbs or neck

4 Inhalational injury (excluding pure carbon monoxide poisoning)
5 Mechanism:
  i Chemical injury (>5% TBSA)
  ii Exposure to ionising radiation
  iii High pressure steam injury
  iv High tension electrical injury
  v Cold injury
  vi Hydrofluoric acid injury (>1% TBSA)
  vii Suspicion of non-accidental injury
6 Dermal or full-thickness burns TBSA >5% in under-16-year-olds or >10% if ≥16 years-old

What are the potential complications in a patient with major burns?

Secondary to over-resuscitation

- Generalised oedema
- Abdominal/limb compartment syndrome
- Pulmonary oedema
- Need for prolonged mechanical ventilation

Respiratory

- Airway obstruction or ARDS following inhalational injury

Cardiovascular

- Arrhythmias
- Myocardial ischaemia
- Cardiac failure
- Vasoplegia

Neurological

- Pain will be considerable in the short- and medium-term
- Patients may quickly become tolerant to opioids – adjunctive medications may be useful including ketamine, gabapentin and amitriptyline
- Fentanyl may be useful for dressing changes

Renal

- AKI due to under-resuscitation, abdominal compartment syndrome, rhabdomyolysis

Gastrointestinal

- Increased nutritional requirement due to hypermetabolism (peaks at 7–10 days, may last up to 2 years); there is increased protein catabolism, and early enteral feeding is associated with improved survival
- Stress ulceration

Haematological

- Venous thromboembolism

Infective

- Burn wound infection
- Pneumonia (aspiration, hospital- or ventilator-acquired)
- Sepsis related to indwelling lines and catheters

Metabolic

- Rhabdomyolysis due to muscle burns
- Compartment syndrome secondary to circumferential burns or following fluid resuscitation

Musculoskeletal

- Contractures
- Amputations

Importantly, the psychological impact of major burn injury may be significant.

Further Reading

Bishop S, Maguire S. Anaesthesia and intensive care for major burns. *Contin Educ Anaesth Crit Care Pain* 2012; **12**(3): 18–122

National Network for Burn Care, 2012. *National Burn Care Referral Guidance* [online]. Available at: www.britishburnassociation.org/downloads/National_Burn_Care_Referral_Guidance_-_5.2.12.pdf (Accessed 24 February 2017)

Chapter 17

Calcium

Calcium is the most abundant mineral found in the human body.

Table 17.1 Calcium homeostasis

Normal serum Ca^{2+}	2.2–2.6 mmol/l
Total body calcium	Around 1 kg, 99% of which is stored in the bones and teeth
Average daily requirement	0.1 mmol/kg/day
Absorption	Kidneys Small intestine Bone
Homeostasis	Calcium enters the plasma by absorption from the gut and by reabsorption from the bones. Regulated by: i Parathyroid hormone ii Vitamin D
Excretion	Secretion into the GI tract Renal excretion (calcitonin inhibits tubular reabsorption of calcium, increasing renal loss) Deposition in the bone
Roles	Essential in bone mineralisation Neuronal function Coagulation Cofactor for many enzymes (e.g. lipase) and proteins Essential in endocrine, exocrine and neurocrine function Calcium ions are amongst the most important second messengers used in signal transduction Mediates muscle contraction Calcium can bind to several different calcium-modulated proteins such as troponin-C and calmodulin which are necessary for promoting contraction in muscle

What do you understand about calcium homeostasis?

Calcium homeostasis is the mechanism by which plasma concentration of calcium is maintained between the narrow limits of 2.2–2.6 mmol/l. The kidneys are the organs primarily responsible for this control. Calcium in plasma exists in three forms:

1 Free ions (~1.2 mmol/l)
2 Ions bound to plasma proteins, primarily albumin (40–50%, reduced by metabolic acidosis, increased by respiratory alkalosis)
3 Diffusible complexes (<10%)

The amount of total calcium in the plasma varies with the level of plasma albumin; however, the biological effect of calcium is determined by the amount of ionised calcium.

Parathyroid hormone (PTH) is important in ensuring the tight plasma control of ionised calcium. Its actions are:

1 Calcium release from bone (increased osteoclast activity)
2 Increased reabsorption from distal convoluted tubule (DCT)
3 Reduced phosphate reabsorption, leading to increased ionised calcium levels (less phosphate available to complex with calcium)
4 Vitamin D3 conversion into 1,25-dihydroxy-vitamin D3, which causes increased GI calcium absorption

Calcitonin is released from the C-cells of the thyroid in response to hypercalcaemia and opposes the action of PTH:

1 Inhibition of calcium absorption from the GI tract
2 Inhibition of osteoclast activity
3 Stimulation of osteoblast activity
4 Inhibition of tubular reabsorption leading to increased excretion
   – BUT it also *inhibits* reabsorption of phosphate in the DCT

Hypercalcaemia

Define hypercalcaemia

Serum calcium >2.6 mmol/l.

How does hypercalcaemia present?

The features of hypercalcaemia are classically described by the phrase: *groans* (constipation), *bones* (bony pain), *moans* (psychosis) and *stones* (kidney stones).

Cardiac arrhythmias can occur with ECG abnormalities including a short QT interval (QTc) and broad T-waves. Cardiac arrest may result if the calcium concentration is >3.75 mmol/l.

See Table 17.2 for a summary of the symptoms and signs of hyper- and hypocalcaemia.

Table 17.2 Symptoms and signs of hyper- and hypocalcaemia

	Hypercalcaemia	Hypocalcaemia
Symptoms	**Bones** (osteolysis, bony pain, fractures) **Stones** (renal colic) **Psychic moans** (depression, hallucinations, confusion that may progress to coma) **Abdominal groans** (anorexia, nausea and vomiting, constipation, pancreatitis, peptic ulceration) **Others:** General malaise, weakness and hyporeflexia Nephrogenic diabetes insipidus (DI)	Mental status changes
Signs	Dehydration Calcification in skin, cornea	Neuromuscular excitability: – Tetany – *Chvostek sign* (contracture of facial muscles produced by tapping ipsilateral facial nerve) – *Trousseau sign* (carpopedal spasm with contraction of fingers elicited by inflating a blood pressure cuff) – Seizures
ECG features	Short QTc Prolonged PR interval Widened QRS Wide T-waves May progress to high grade AV block and arrest	Prolonged QTc AV block Torsades de pointe *may* occur

What causes hypercalcaemia?

Hypercalcaemia is associated with a number of disease processes (see Table 17.3).

How do you treat hypercalcaemia?

The management of hypercalcaemia should follow an ABCDE approach, treating abnormalities as you find them. The ultimate treatment is directed at the underlying cause, but specific management of hypercalcaemia involves:

1 IV hydration with 0.9% saline
   – This forces a diuresis – monitor K^+ and Mg^{2+}
2 Bisphosphonate therapy
   – Pamidronate 60–90 mg IV over 2–4 hours

Table 17.3 Causes of hypercalcaemia

Malignancy	Secondary deposits in bone, myeloma, ectopic PTH & 1,25-(OH)D
Endocrine	Primary hyperparathyroidism (including adenoma and multiple endocrine neoplasia), hyperthyroidism, familial hypocalcuric hypercalcaemia, tertiary hyperparathyroidism
Granulomatous diseases	Sarcoidosis, TB
Drugs	Thiazide diuretics, lithium, aminophylline, vitamin D
Miscellaneous	Rhabdomyolysis, milk-alkali syndrome, renal failure

3 Diuretics
  - Furosemide can be used (although this promotes bony uptake of calcium)
4 Stop medications that contribute to hypercalcaemia
  - Calcium, vitamin D, thiazide diuretics
5. Additional therapies
  - Calcitonin, mobilisation, RRT

Hypocalcaemia

Define hypocalcaemia

Hypocalaemia is defined as a serum calcium level of <2.2 mmol/l. It is severe if Ca^{2+} <1.9 mmol/l.

What are the causes of hypocalcaemia?

The causes of hypocalcaemia in critical care are multifactorial. The more common causes include hypoalbuminaemia, hyperventilation or the transfusion of citrated blood.

Other causes are listed in Table 17.4.

What ECG changes would you see in a patient with low calcium?

The predominant change is prolongation of the QT interval, which may progress to polymorphic VT, although less commonly than with hypokalaemia and hypomagnesaemia. Arrhythmias are uncommon.

Hypocalcaemia is treated with calcium supplementation (oral or parenteral, depending on severity). Of note, calcium chloride contains three times as many calcium ions as calcium gluconate (6.8 mmol vs 2.2 mmol in 10 ml 10% solution).

Table 17.4 Causes of hypocalcaemia

Endocrine	Primary hypoparathyroidism Congenital deficiency (DiGeorge syndrome) Pseudohypoparathyroidism (resistance to PTH) Vitamin D deficiency
Malnutrition	Decreased dietary intake Intestinal malabsorption Vitamin D-dependent rickets Osteomalacia
Drugs	Furosemide Calcitonin Bisphosphonates Phenytoin Aminoglycosides Amphotericin B
Miscellaneous	Acute hyperphosphataemia Tumour lysis syndrome Rhabdomyolysis Acute renal failure Acute pancreatitis

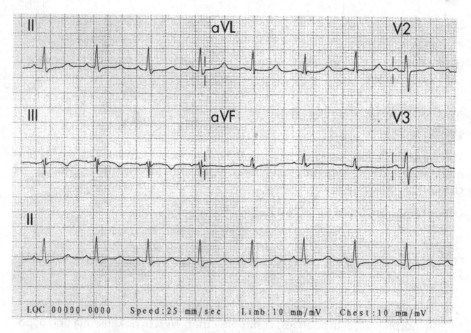

Figure 17.1 Prolonged QTc in a patient with DiGeorge syndrome and a Ca^{2+} of 1.32 mmol/l
Reproduced with permission from Kar PS, et al. (*J Clin Pathol* 2005)

Further Reading

Parikh M, Webb S. Cations: potassium, calcium and magnesium. *Contin educ anaesth crit care pain* 2012; **2**(4): 195–198

Aguillera I M, Vaughan R S. Calcium and the Anaesthetist. *Anaesthesia* 2000; **55**: 779–790

Chapter 18

Cardiac Output Monitoring

What is fluid responsiveness?

Fluid responsiveness is a term applied to a situation in which a patient's cardio-vascular system (CVS) is challenged with a bolus of IV fluid and the response assessed. Patients fit into one of two groups:

1 Non-responder
   - No response to a fluid challenge
   - This may mean that the patient is intravascularly replete and that another cause of shock should be sought (e.g. obstructive, cardiogenic) *or* they are so hypovolaemic that not enough fluid has been given to result in improvement (e.g. active haemorrhage)
2 Responder
   - Patient responds to a fluid challenge with improvement in clinical and/or haemodynamic parameters (response may be sustained or short-lived)
   - This may imply that the patient is volume deplete and requires further fluid

What methods can we use to determine whether someone might be fluid responsive?

There are several indications that a patient may benefit from a fluid challenge:

1 Clinical signs
   - Tachypnoea
   - Tachycardia +/– hypotension
   - Peripheral-core temperature difference
   - Evidence of end organ dysfunction (oliguria, confusion/low GCS, high lactate)
   - Observing a *swing* in the arterial line or SpO_2 trace
2 Administering a fluid challenge (i.e. a straight-leg raise or administering 250 ml of fluid over 5 minutes) and reviewing the following parameters:
   - HR
   - BP
   - CVP
3 Cardiac output monitoring
4 Echocardiography
   - LV *kissing* walls
   - RV volume status

– IVC collapsibility/distensibility index (in spontaneously ventilating and mechanically ventilated patients respectively)

Classify types of cardiac output monitoring and give examples of each

Cardiac output monitoring (COM) can be classified as non-invasive, minimally invasive and invasive (see Table 18.1).

Table 18.1: Classification of types of CO monitoring

Classification	Method	Principle
Non-invasive	Transthoracic impedence	Bioimpedence (changes in electrical current produced by fluid shifts in thorax)
	Transthoracic echo	LV and RV volume status, IVC collapsibility index
Minimally invasive	PiCCO	Pulse contour analysis, calibrated using transpulmonary thermodilution, needs CVC
	LiDCO	Pulse power analysis, calibrated with transpulmonary lithium dilution, CVC or venflon
	FloTrac	Pulse contour analysis, non-calibrated
	Oesophageal Doppler probe	Doppler principle, aortic cross-sectional area
	TOE	LV and RV volume status
Invasive	Pulmonary artery catheter	Area under thermodilution curve (CO calculated using Stewart-Hamilton equation)

CVC – central venous catheter

Describe the pulmonary artery catheter

The pulmonary artery catheter (PAC, also known as the Swan-Ganz catheter) is usually 8 French in calibre and 110 cm in length. It has the following components:

1 Distal lumen that is used to measure the PCWP and for sampling mixed venous blood
2 Proximal lumen that opens about 30 cm from the tip that is used to monitor CVP and may be used to administer cold injectate to permit measurement of CO by thermodilution
3 There may be another proximal lumen 26 cm proximal to the tip that can be used for fluids or drugs

4 Thermistor located 3.7 cm proximal to the tip of the PAC, which is transduced by the cardiac output monitor

5 10 cm long thermal filament, enabling calculation of CO using thermodilution without the need for a cold saline bolus

6 A further lumen with a built-in clamp is connected to a balloon that is located at the catheter tip: this is used to inject up to 1.5 ml of air into the balloon to facilitate floatation.

A diagram of the PAC is shown in Figure 18.1.

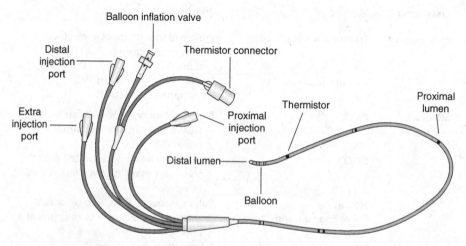

Figure 18.1 A pulmonary artery catheter

Describe the normal pressures and waveforms that you encounter as the PAC is advanced

The balloon is inflated once the PAC is within the RA, allowing the catheter to *float* through the heart into the PA. Right atrial pressure (RAP) is similar to CVP (usually 3–8 mmHg in a non-ventilated patient). Once the PAC advances into the RV the pressure trace develops a systolic component (~25 mmHg) and a low diastolic component (0–10 mmHg). As the catheter floats into the pulmonary artery (PA), the diastolic pressure increases (10–20 mmHg, due to pulmonary vascular resistance) and a dicrotic notch can be seen (due to closure of the pulmonary valve). The balloon then carries the catheter into a branch of the PA into which it *wedges*. This trace is similar to the CVP waveform (PCWP, 4–12 mmHg) and reflects left atrial pressure (LAP). The trace is shown in Figure 18.2.

It is important that the PAC tip sits in West zone 3, so that there is a continuous column of blood between the PAC and the LA.

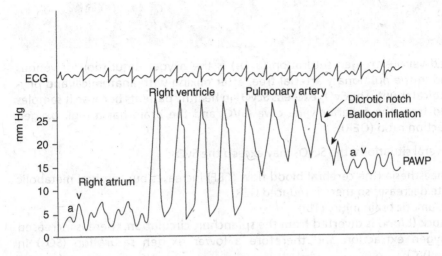

Figure 18.2 Normal pressures and waveforms seen as a pulmonary artery catheter is advanced

If the PAC is inserted via the right internal jugular vein (IJV), the RA is located at approximately 15–20 cm, the RV is at 25–30 cm and the PA is a further 10 cm distally.

It is important to deflate the balloon once the PCWP has been taken, otherwise the lung supplied by the artery in which the PAC is wedged will become ischaemic and risk infarction.

What information is measured and what is derived?

This is summarised in Table 18.2.

Table 18.2 Measured and derived variables obtained from the pulmonary artery catheter

Measured	Derived (using CO = [MAP-CVP]/SVR)	
Cardiac output	Cardiac index	(CO/BSA, l/min/m^2)
CVP	SV	(CO/HR, ml/beat)
RAP	SVI	(SV/BSA, ml/beat/m^2)
RVP	SVR	(dynes.sec/m^5)
PAP	SVRI	(dynes.sec/m^5)
PCWP	PVR	(dynes.sec/m^5)
SvO$_2$	PVRI	(dynes.sec/m^5)
Core temperature		

RVP – right ventricular pressure; PAP – pulmonary artery pressure; BSA – body surface area; SV – stroke volume; SVI – stroke volume index; SVRI – systemic vascular resistance index; PVR – pulmonary vascular resistance; PVRI – pulmonary vascular resistance index

Tell me about SvO$_2$. How does it compare to central venous saturation (ScvO$_2$)?

Mixed venous oxygen saturation (SvO$_2$) is the oxygen saturation of venous blood in the pulmonary arterial tree, after mixing with anatomical and physiological shunt. The SvO$_2$ exceeds ScvO$_2$ in healthy patients because it samples blood from the superior vena cava (SVC) and the brain has a high oxygen extraction ratio (OER).

In several situations, the ScvO$_2$ may *exceed* the SvO$_2$:

1 Anaesthesia (the cerebral blood flow (CBF) increases but cerebral metabolic rate decreases so there is reduced OER)
2 Traumatic brain injury (TBI)
3 Shock (blood is diverted from the splanchnic circulation, there is increased oxygen extraction and therefore a lower oxygen saturation (SO$_2$) in the IVC)

What are the complications associated with use of pulmonary artery catheters?

Complications associated with obtaining central venous access:

1 Bleeding / haematoma
2 Air embolism
3 Vascular injury
4 Arterial puncture
5 Pneumothorax
6 Tamponade

Complications associated with floating the catheter:

1 Arrhythmias
2 Tamponade
3 Valvular trauma
4 Misplacement (incorrect West zone, unable to pass through the heart)
5 Knotting of catheter

Complications associated with the PAC being in situ:

1 Venous thromboembolism
2 Pulmonary infarction
3 Pulmonary arterial rupture

Do you know of any evidence for or against the use of PAC?

The **PAC-man** trial (2005) was a pragmatic RCT that showed no difference in in-hospital, ICU or 28-day mortality, or ICU or hospital LOS. There was a 10% complication rate associated with PAC use. The authors concluded that whilst there was no clear evidence of benefit or of harm, the PAC is potentially useful in undifferentiated shock, right ventricular failure (RVF) and pulmonary hypertension (although the study was underpowered for this).

Tell me about the oesophageal doppler as a CO monitor

The Doppler effect states that when a sound wave is reflected off a moving object, the frequency shift is proportional to the velocity of the object. This principle is utilised in the oesophageal Doppler probe, which emits ultrasound waves that are reflected off red blood cells (RBCs) travelling in the descending aorta, producing a velocity-time curve of blood flow. The stroke distance (the distance travelled by the blood in one heartbeat) is then calculated. The aortic cross-sectional area (CSA) is determined from a nomogram based on the patient's height and weight, and multiplied by the stroke distance to give stroke volume.

The probe is 90 cm long, with markers at 35, 40 and 45 cm to aid placement. The descending aortic Doppler trace is normally obtained between 35–40 cm when the probe is placed orally. The probe must be directed posteriorly, pointing towards the descending aorta. Audible and visual signals are used to aid focussing, but the oesophageal Doppler monitor (ODM) is significantly operator dependent.

Several assumptions are made when using the ODM:

1 That the angle of the probe to the direction of blood flow is constant
2 That the aortic CSA is constant throughout the cardiac cycle
3 That there is laminar flow within the aorta
4 That 70% of the cardiac output enters the descending aorta

Draw a typical trace and tell me what each part means

A typical ODM trace is shown in Figure 18.3.

Stroke distance (SD) is the distance in cm that a column of blood moves along the aorta with each contraction of the LV. It is the area under the velocity-time curve. This is converted into stroke volume by multiplying by aortic CSA.

Mean acceleration (MA) and *peak velocity (PV)* may be used as markers of LV contractility. The peak velocity decreases with age (90–120 cm/s for a 20-year-old; 70–100 cm/s for a 50-year-old; and 50–80 cm/s for a 70-year-old).

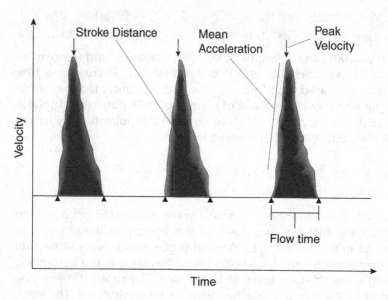

Figure 18.3 The oesophageal Doppler trace

Flow time corrected (FTc) is the time in milliseconds that the heart spends in systole, corrected for heart rate. Typical values in a healthy adult are 330–360 ms. A low value indicates high afterload (often due to hypovolaemia) and a high value indicates low afterload, e.g. vasoplegia in sepsis.

Are there any guidelines for the use of ODM? What are they based on?

The concept of goal-directed therapy came from the introduction of protocolised care for patients with sepsis by **Rivers** in his trial in 2001, which produced compelling results. However, the recent **ARISE, ProCESS** and **ProMISe** trials all concluded that protocolised care is no better than usual care. These trials are discussed in the 'Sepsis' topic (see page 414).

There are several studies that have demonstrated reduced complication rates and shorter LOS in hospital when the ODM is used perioperatively to guide fluid therapy. NICE advises that the oesophageal Doppler should be considered for use in patients undergoing high risk or major surgery (MTG3).

Tell me about the differences between PiCCO and LiDCO™

The differences are summarised in Table 18.3.

Table 18.3 The differences between PiCCO and LIDCO™

	PiCCO	LiDCO™
Arterial line	Thermistor-tipped, femoral	Standard
Central line	Yes	Not needed
Calibration	Transpulmonary thermodilution	Transpulmonary lithium dilution (0.5–2 ml Li$^+$) (LiDCO *rapid* does not require calibration)
Waveform analysis	Pulse contour analysis algorithm Assumes area under systolic portion of arterial pressure trace is proportional to SV	Pulse power analysis algorithm Assumes that fluctuations of arterial pressure around the mean (pulsatility) are proportional to SV Baseline voltage due to Na$^+$ measured Change in voltage due to Li$^+$ is converted to [Li$^+$] and a [Li$^+$]/time curve is produced This is used to calculate plasma flow Blood flow = plasma flow/(1-Hct)
Special measurements	Global end-diastolic volume (GEDV, reliable predictor of fluid responsiveness) Extravascular lung water (EVLW, measurement of pulmonary oedema, useful in limiting fluid resuscitation and weaning from mechanical ventilation)	
Problems		Affected by use of non-depolarising NMBAs

Hct – haematocrit

Further Reading

Harvey S, Harrison D A, Singer M, et al. Assessment of the clinical effectiveness of pulmonary artery catheters in management of patients in intensive care (PAC-Man): a randomised controlled trial. *Lancet* 2005; **366**(9484): 472–477

Invasive Monitoring. In: Al-Shaikh B, Stacey S. *Essentials of Anaesthetic Equipment*, 4th ed. Philadelphia, PA: Churchill Livingstone Elsevier, 2013; 177–199

National Institute for Health and Care Excellence, 2011. CardioQ-ODM oesophageal Doppler monitor. Medical Technologies Guidance 3. Available at: www.nice.org.uk/guidance/mtg3 (Accessed: 15 May 2017)

Oesophageal Doppler Monitoring using the CardioQ & CardioQ-ODM Workbook for Operating Department Practitioners & Theatre Staff. Datex Medical, Chichester, West Sussex. 9051–5402 Issue 2, 2009

Chapter 19

Cardiogenic Shock

What is cardiogenic shock?

Cardiogenic shock is defined as the evidence of tissue hypoperfusion secondary to primary cardiac failure after correction of preload. It represents the extreme end of the spectrum of acute decompensated cardiac failure (<2% of cases).

It is characterised by:

1 SBP <90 mmHg or a decrease in MAP by >30 mmHg
2 HR >60 bpm
3 Oliguria
4 With or without evidence of organ congestion

Describe the pathophysiology of cardiogenic shock

The pathophysiology is illustrated in Figure 19.1.

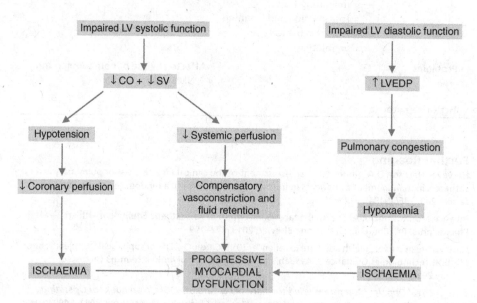

Figure 19.1 The pathophysiology of cardiogenic shock

What are the causes of cardiogenic shock?

The most common cause of cardiogenic shock is acute decompensation of established cardiac failure. Decompensation can be triggered by non-compliance with medication, an acute ischaemic event, arrhythmia, hypertensive crisis, brain injury, sepsis, drug abuse or volume overload. Less frequently it can present de novo in a patient with previously normal cardiac function.

The causes of acute cardiac failure are outlined in Table 19.1.

Table 19.1 Causes of acute cardiac failure

Acute coronary syndromes (ACS)		
Arrhythmias		
Valvular pathology	Acute valvular regurgitation, e.g. rupture of chordae tendinae, endocarditis	
	Decompensation of severe aortic stenosis	
Viral myocarditis	*Coxsackievirus*	
	Adenovirus	
Tamponade	Trauma	
	Aortic dissection	
	Pericardial effusion / pericarditis	
High output cardiac failure	Thyroid storm	
	Severe anaemia	
Decompensation of chronic cardiac failure	**Hypertensive heart disease**	i.e. diastolic heart failure
	Dilated cardiomyopathy	Alcohol
		Toxins, e.g. heavy metals
		Drugs, e.g. doxorubicin, MDMA, cocaine
		Peripartum cardiomyopathy
	Restrictive cardiomyopathy	Infiltration, e.g. sarcoidosis, amyloidosis, haemochromatosis, connective tissue disorders
		Radiation
	Congenital	Hypertrophic cardiomyopathy

MDMA – 3,4-methylenedioxy-methamphetamine

How does it present?

Cardiovascular

- Cool peripheries with prolonged capillary refill time (CRT) due to peripheral vasoconstriction
- Tachy- or bradycardia
- Arrhythmias
- BP may be high due to high SVR or low if decompensated
- Myocardial ischaemia
- Signs of RVF including peripheral oedema, raised jugular venous pressure (JVP) and hepatomegaly with right upper quadrant (RUQ) tenderness

Respiratory

- Tachypnoea with evidence of pulmonary oedema
- Hypoxaemia

Neurological

- Low GCS
- Confusion/altered mental state

Renal

- Oliguria

How do you manage patients with cardiogenic shock?

Cardiogenic shock should be managed with an ABCDE approach, treating abnormalities as they are found. Specific management involves:

1 Administer 100% oxygen
  Consider NIV or invasive ventilation if necessary
2 Obtain large bore IV access and take bloods for FBC, U+Es, LFTs, cardiac enzymes, brain natriuretic peptide (BNP), clotting screen, viral serology if indicated clinically
3 Perform 12 lead ECG, CXR and echocardiography
4 Administer 250 ml warm fluid bolus – use caution, ideally guided by cardiac output monitoring, CVP and/or echocardiography
5 Have a low threshold for inotropic support
  i **Adrenaline**
    - Low dose: β_1 and β_2 effects (tachycardia, positive inotropy, vasodilatation)
    - High dose: α_1 effects (vasoconstriction)
  ii **Dobutamine**
    - Predominantly β_1 effects (tachycardia, positive inotropy, vasodilatation – often used in combination with noradrenaline for this reason)

- Some β_2 activity (vasodilatation)
6 Consider vasodilators to reduce preload and afterload and reduce myocardial work
    i **Milrinone / enoximone**
        - Phosphodiesterase-3 (PDE$_3$) inhibitor (increases cyclic adenosine monophosphate (cAMP): reduces PVR and SVR, positive inotropy and lusitropy)
        - Useful in diastolic heart failure
    ii **GTN**
        - Nitric oxide donor – predominantly causes venodilatation
7 Start a vasopressor if BP is low to maintain coronary perfusion
    i **Noradrenaline** – first line
        - α_1-mediated vasoconstriction
    ii **Vasopressin**
        - V$_1$ receptor-mediated vasoconstriction (located in vascular smooth muscle)
        - V$_2$ receptor-mediated water retention (located in collecting ducts)
8 Consider **levosimendan**
    - Sensitises troponin C to calcium (positive inotropy)
    - Opens adenosine triphosphate (ATP)-dependent potassium channels (increased coronary perfusion, reduced preload, reduced afterload)
    - Overall effect: increased contractility without increasing myocardial oxygen consumption (VO$_2$)
    - Evidence that short-term IV levosimendan improves short- and long-term survival in patients with cardiac failure
9 Mechanical support
    i Intra-aortic balloon pump (IABP)
    ii Ventricular assist device (VAD) as bridge to recovery or to transplant

A summary of the physiological basis of the approach to acute decompensated cardiac failure is shown in Table 19.2.

Table 19.2 The physiological approach to decompensated cardiac failure

Aim	Mechanism	Method
Reduce myocardial oxygen demand	Reduce HR	Ensure adequate preload Beta-blockade if diastolic dysfunction Sedation
	Reduce afterload	Vasodilators Diuretics if volume overload Sedation
Improve myocardial oxygen delivery	Increase myocardial perfusion	Vasodilators Inotropes (caution as may increase VO$_2$)
	Increase oxygen carrying capacity	Increase FiO$_2$ *Consider* blood transfusion

How does an IABP work?

The IABP is inserted via the femoral artery, usually following primary coronary intervention (PCI). The balloon lies within the descending aorta just distal to the origin of the left subclavian artery (CXR confirms correct positioning).

– Low density helium is pushed into the balloon during diastole, producing an augmented DBP to *improve coronary perfusion*
– The balloon is deflated during systole (as the aortic valve opens) to *reduce myocardial afterload*
– The overall effect is to improve myocardial oxygen delivery and reduce myocardial oxygen demand

Balloon pump cycling is coordinated via the ECG or via the invasive blood pressure (IBP) trace:

– Inflation occurs in the middle of the T wave/at the dicrotic notch
– Deflation occurs at the peak of the R wave/just before the systolic upstroke on the IBP trace.

The augmented arterial trace is shown in Figure 19.2.

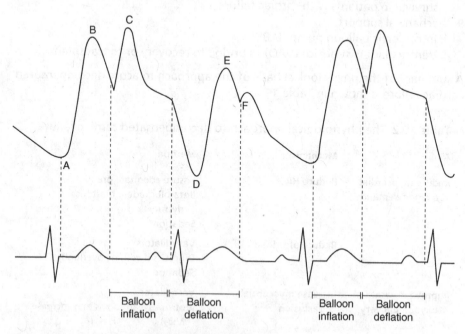

Figure 19.2 The arterial trace in a patient with a balloon pump in situ
A - unassisted DBP; B - unassisted SBP; C - diastolic augmentation; D - augmented DBP; E - unassisted beat; F - natural dicrotic notch

What are the contraindications to IABP insertion?

There are three absolute contraindications to placement of a balloon pump:

1 Aortic regurgitation
2 Aortic dissection/aneurysm
3 Severe peripheral vascular disease

Relative contraindications:

1 Arterial tortuosity
2 Left ventricular outflow tract obstruction
3 Sepsis
4 Contraindications to anticoagulation including coagulopathy and HIT

What are the complications of IABP placement?

Complications may be divided into those related to the vascular access necessary for insertion, and those related to the presence of the IABP within the lumen of the aorta.

Vascular

1 Bleeding
2 Haematoma, pseudoaneurysm
3 Dissection
4 Perforation

Balloon-related

1 Mesenteric/renal ischaemia (balloon position too low)
2 Left upper limb/cerebral ischaemia (balloon position too high)
3 Helium embolus
4 Haemolysis
5 Thrombocytopenia

What is a ventricular assist device? What are the indications for their use? Are there any complications?

A VAD is a surgically placed mechanical device that can support either the left (LVAD), right (RVAD), or both (BiVAD) ventricles. BiVAD implantation is uncommon as RV failure often results from pulmonary hypertension secondary to LV failure and will improve after LVAD insertion.

They reduce myocardial work, allowing the ventricles to rest whilst ensuring forward flow and organ perfusion. Third generation devices use an impellar and provide continuous centrifugal flow. They can be used as a bridge to recovery instead of VA ECMO in acute heart failure or as a bridge to transplantation in chronic cardiac failure. They may also be used as a long-term treatment modality for patients with end-stage heart failure who are unsuitable transplant candidates.

Complications include:

1 Bleeding
   - Most common complication post-VAD insertion
   - Blood product transfusion should be guided by near-patient testing, and early re-exploration may be required
2 Cardiac tamponade
   - This results in decreased VAD flows, increasing CVP, reduced MAP/escalation of inotropic support, metabolic acidosis, oliguria
   - The treatment is immediate surgical decompression to evacuate the blood clot
3 Haemodynamic disturbance
   - If a patient is hypovolaemic post-LVAD insertion, the interventricular septum is entrained leftwards towards the inflow cannula
   - TOE is helpful
4 RV failure
   - This leads to RV dilatation, high atrial pressures (>20 mmHg), reduced RV contractility and severe tricuspid regurgitation
   - This may be managed medically but occasionally may necessitate a short-term RVAD
5 Fluid overload
   - May occur as fluid is mobilised as a result of the higher cardiac output achieved with the VAD
6 Infection
   - Antibiotic prophylaxis is used
7 Intra-cardiac thrombosis
   - Due to decreased VAD flows
   - Produces altered sound on auscultation

Further Reading

Brookes L, 2016. REVIVE II and SURVIVE: Use of levosimendan for the treatment of acute decompensated heart failure [online]. London: Medscape. Available at: www.medscape.org/view article/523043 (Accessed 27 November 2016)

Harris P, Kuppurao L. Ventricular assist devices. *Contin Educ Anaesth Crit Care Pain* 2012; 12(3): 145–151

Krishna M, Zacharowski K. Principles of intra-aortic balloon pump counterpulsation. *Contin Educ Anaesth Crit Care Pain* 2009; 9(1): 24–28

Summers R L, Sterling S. Early emergency management of acute decompensated heart failure. *Curr Opin Crit Care* 2012; 18: 301–307

Chapter 20

Care of the Heart Beating Organ Donor

Summarise the pathophysiological changes associated with brain stem death

Brainstem death causes widespread cardiovascular, respiratory, endocrine, metabolic and haematological changes.

Cardiovascular

1 An increase in BP initially occurs in an attempt to maintain cerebral perfusion in the face of rising ICP
   - Cerebral herniation with pontine ischaemia will occur as ICP continues to increase resulting in a catecholamine storm
   - This hyperadrenergic state results in marked sympathetic stimulation with intense vasoconstriction, raised SVR and tachycardia
   - The resultant increase in afterload to both ventricles causes acute myocardial ischaemia
2 The classic *Cushing's reflex* (hypertension with bradycardia) may occur, secondary to reflex baroreceptor activity and/or central midbrain activation of the parasympathetic nervous system
3 Eventual foramen magnum herniation results in loss of sympathetic tone, leading to peripheral vasodilatation, hypotension and haemodynamic instability necessitating vasopressor treatment

Respiratory

1 Raised pulmonary hydrostatic pressure aggravated by capillary endothelial damage results in pulmonary oedema
2 Apnoea and cardiac arrest result if ventilation is not supported

Endocrine

1 Pituitary ischaemia leads to cranial DI, which results in fluid loss and further electrolyte abnormalities
2 Hypothalamic dysfunction leads to hypothermia and functional hypothyroidism

Coagulation

Coagulation abnormalities can occur secondary to the effects of catecholamines on platelet function alongside the impact of damaged brain tissue on plasminogen activator and thromboplastin release.

How is the cardiovascular system managed and what cardiovascular parameters should be targeted in a heart beating brain-dead donor?

The NHS Blood and Transplant (NHSBT) group have produced a donation after brain death (DBD) donor optimisation care bundle that advocates the following cardiovascular goals in the management of the brain-dead donor (see Table 20.1).

Table 20.1 Cardiovascular targets for heart beating organ donors

Cardiovascular parameter	Target range
HR	60-120 bpm
SBP	> 100 mmHg
MAP	60–80 mmHg
PCWP	10–15 mmHg
Cardiac index (CI)	> 2.1 l/min/m^2
SvO$_2$	> 60%
CVP	6–10 mmHg
SVRI	1800–2400 dynes.sec/cm^5/m^2

Restoring an effective circulating volume should be the first priority; COM is important to guide such treatment. Fluid overload should be avoided and following restoration of circulating volume, fluids should be restricted. With hypotension in the context of vasodilation, vasopressin is recommended (infusion of up to 4 units/hour). If the cardiac index does not respond to restoration of volume status and vascular tone, inotropic support is required (dopamine is the preferred inotrope as per the NHSBT DBD care bundle).

What are the goals of ventilatory management?

1 Perform lung recruitment manoeuvres
2 Lung protective ventilation
   - Tidal volumes 4–8 ml/kg ideal body weight
   - Optimum PEEP (5–10 cmH$_2$O)
   - Peak inspiratory pressures limited to <30 cmH$_2$O
3 Regular chest physiotherapy

4 Head up 30-45°
5 Primary respiratory/arterial blood gas targets as per Table 20.2

Table 20.2 Ventilatory parameters in the brain dead organ donor

Parameter	Target range
pH	7.35–7.45
PaO_2	> 10 kPa
$PaCO_2$	4.5–6 kPa
SpO_2	> 94% for the lowest FiO_2 (ideally <0.4)

What are the principles of managing metabolic, endocrine and haematological issues?

Metabolic

1 Administering 15 mg/kg methylprednisolone has been shown to attenuate the increase in extravascular lung water index and improve oxygenation
   – Methylprednisolone use is associated with increased organ retrieval and it should be given as soon as possible
2 Active warming may be required to ensure the patient's temperature is 36–37.5°C

Endocrine

1 An insulin infusion is usually necessary to maintain a blood glucose of 4–10 mmol/l
2 Early vasopressin (vs noradrenaline) may prevent the need for additional treatment in DI
3 Levels of all anterior pituitary hormones can decrease and hypothyroidism can occur
   – T_3 replacement was previously given empirically to brainstem dead donors, although its use is associated with adverse effects such as arrhythmias and so is no longer routine
4 Hypernatraemia in the donor is associated with poor liver graft function
   – If Na^+ >155 mmol/l, water can be given enterally or a low sodium IV fluid (5% dextrose) used judiciously

Haematological

1 Blood and blood products are transfused as indicated clinically to optimise oxygen delivery
   – Transfusion triggers should be those used locally
   – There is emerging evidence that blood transfusions may adversely affect organ function post transplantation

2 Coagulation derangement should be corrected only if there is significant ongoing bleeding

What is cranial diabetes insipidus and how is it treated?

Cranial DI results from primary deficiency of anti-diuretic hormone (ADH) due to pituitary ischaemia/dysfunction. It is characterised by:

1 Urine output >4 ml/kg/hour
2 Serum sodium >145 mmol/l
3 Serum osmolality >300 mosmol/kg
4 Urine osmolality <200 mosmol/kg

Diabetes insipidus should be treated at an early stage. If there is a dramatic and unexpected rise in urine output, treatment should be commenced even before confirmation with plasma and urinary electrolytes. Fluid replacement with solutions containing minimal sodium should be instigated. Desmopressin (DDAVP 0.5–4 mcg IV) is the drug of choice if the DI is not effectively treated by the vasopressin used for cardiovascular management.

Further Reading

Gordon J, McKinlay J. Physiological changes after brainstem death and management of the heart-beating donor. *Contin Educ Anaesth Crit Care Pain* 2012; **12**(5): 225–229.

NHS Blood and Transplant, 2016. Donor optimisation [online]. Available from www.odt.nhs.uk/donation/deceased-donation/donor-optimisation/ (Accessed 5 February 2017)

NHS Blood and Transplant, 2016. Donation after circulatory death [online]. Available from www.odt.nhs.uk/donation/deceased-donation/donation-after-circulatory-death/ (Accessed 5 February 2017)

Chapter 21

Chronic Liver Disease in the ICU

What are the causes of cirrhotic liver disease?

The main causes of cirrhosis are listed in Table 21.1.

Table 21.1 Causes of cirrhosis

Toxins	Alcohol
Infective	Hepatitis B and C
Drugs	Methotrexate Methyldopa Amiodarone
Cholestatic conditions	Primary biliary cirrhosis Primary sclerosing cholangitis
Autoimmune	Autoimmune hepatitis
Hereditary	Wilson's disease Haemochromatosis Alpha-1 antitrypsin deficiency Type IV glycogen storage disease
Vascular	Budd-Chiari syndrome Veno-occlusive disease
Other	Non-alcoholic fatty liver disease (NAFLD)

What scoring systems are commonly used for prognostication in chronic liver disease?

Two scores are mainly used in clinical practice for patient counselling, clinical decision making and stratifying risk in therapeutic trials: The *Child-Turcotte-Pugh score* (CPS) and the *Model for End-stage Liver Disease* (MELD).

The CPS (Table 21.2) was originally proposed in 1964 to predict prognosis and is well established, but it has several drawbacks, which led to the development of MELD.

Table 21.2 Child-Turcotte-Pugh score

Parameter	Points assigned 1	2	3
Encephalopathy	None	Grade I-II	Grade III-IV (or chronic)
Ascites	None	Mild-moderate (diuretic-controlled)	Severe (diuretic-refractory)
Bilirubin (μmol/l)	< 34	34 – 50	> 50
Albumin (g/l)	> 35	28 – 35	< 28
INR	< 1.7	1.7 – 2.3	> 2.3
Class		% survival at 1 year	% survival at 2 years
A	5–6 points	100	85
B	7–9 points	81	57
C	10–15 points	45	35

The MELD score is used to predict mortality in hospitalised patients with cirrhosis, and is calculated by the following formula:

MELD = (3.78 × ln[serum bilirubin(mg/dl)]) + (11.2 × ln[INR]) + (9.57 × ln[serum creatinine(mg/dl)]) + 6.43

The UK Model for End-Stage Liver Disease (UKELD) was developed in 2008 to aid in the selection of liver transplant patients in the UK.

SOFA scoring can also help discriminate the survivors from the non-survivors.

List some common reasons for ICU admission in patients with cirrhosis

1 Bleeding – commonly due to varices
2 Hepatic encephalopathy and low GCS
3 Alcoholic hepatitis
4 Acute kidney injury
5 Severe sepsis

In the UK, hospital mortality for cirrhotic patients is >50% with little change in recent times. Patients with cirrhosis and severe sepsis requiring organ support have a mortality of 65–90% (dependent on the number of organs failing), compared with 33–39% in non-cirrhotic patients.

What is portal hypertension?

Portal hypertension (portal pressure >10 mmHg) is associated with the development of a porto-systemic collateral venous circulation, ascites and splenomegaly. It is diagnosed clinically as portal pressures can only be measured directly e.g. during transjugular intrahepatic portosystemic shunt (TIPSS) insertion.

The main complication of portal hypertension is massive upper GI haemorrhage secondary to gastroesophageal varices.

What is the treatment of massive variceal haemorrhage?

Massive upper gastrointestinal (UGI) bleeding secondary to varices should be managed with an ABCDE approach, treating abnormalities as they are found. Specific management involves:

1 **Volume resuscitation**
   Transfusion of blood and blood products according to local protocols for major haemorrhage
2 **Administration of vasoconstrictors**
   e.g. terlipressin or somatostatin
3 **Endoscopic therapy** performed within 24 hours of presentation to control haemorrhage
   Variceal band ligation is the preferred endoscopic method
4 **Prevention of complications**
   Antibiotics are recommended for all patients with suspected or confirmed variceal bleeding

If there is failure to control active bleeding:

- **Balloon tamponade** with Sengstaken-Blakemore tube until further endoscopy, TIPSS or surgery can be performed
- Consider transfer to a centre with liver transplant service for uncontrolled bleeding from portal hypertension

The following procedures should be considered for the prevention of rebleeding when pharmacologic and/or endoscopic therapy have failed:

1 TIPSS
2 Orthotopic liver transplantation

What is a transjugular intrahepatic portosystemic stent shunt?

A TIPSS is an endovascular procedure that establishes communication between the inflow portal vein and the outflow hepatic vein, using a stent. It is performed to reduce portal pressures in patients with complications related to portal hypertension (variceal bleeding, diuretic-resistant ascites). The goal is to divert blood into the hepatic vein so as to reduce the pressure gradient between portal and systemic circulations. Importantly, hepatic encephalopathy may then develop because blood from the portal vein will then bypass the liver and its metabolic processes.

What is hepatorenal syndrome?

Hepatorenal syndrome (HRS) is a particular type of renal failure affecting patients with cirrhosis or fulminant liver failure. It is a pre-renal AKI that is not responsive to fluid therapy. There is abnormal autoregulation with renal vasoconstriction (due to sympathetic stimulation despite reduced renal prostaglandin synthesis) and dilatation of splanchnic vessels.

Hepatorenal syndrome is characterised by a low fractional excretion of sodium and a progressive rise in the plasma creatinine concentration in a patient with chronic liver disease.

The diagnostic criteria are:

1 Cirrhosis with ascites
2 Creatinine >133 μmol/l
3 No improvement in creatinine after two days of diuretic withdrawal and volume expansion with albumin
4 Absence of shock
5. Absence of nephrotoxins
6 Absence of renal parenchymal disease

There are two types of HRS:

Type I: Rapidly progressive decline in kidney function and carries a mortality of >50%
Type II: More indolent course, associated with diuretic-resistant ascites

A trial of treatment with terlipressin and plasma expansion with albumin should be considered. TIPSS has been shown to improve renal function in patients with HRS. The definitive treatment is liver transplantation.

What is spontaneous bacterial peritonitis and how is a diagnosis established?

Spontaneous bacterial peritonitis is defined as an ascitic fluid infection without an evident intra-abdominal, surgically treatable source. It almost always occurs in patients with cirrhosis and ascites. A high index of suspicion is required for its presence, as signs and symptoms can be non-specific. Presenting features include fever, hypotension, abdominal pain and altered mental status.

A peritoneal fluid neutrophil count >250 cells/mm^3 is the accepted criterion for the diagnosis of spontaneous bacterial peritonitis and/or positive peritoneal fluid culture.

Patients should receive empiric antibiotic therapy based on local susceptibility testing.

A single-centre RCT in 2016 demonstrated that terlipressin improved haemodynamics and had a mortality benefit when compared to noradrenaline in patients with cirrhosis and septic shock of all causes. Further work is required before this becomes standard practice.

What are the clinical features of hepatopulmonary syndrome?

Hepatopulmonary syndrome is a poorly understood condition that presents with intrapulmonary shunting and hypoxia in patients with cirrhosis. Classically, dyspnoea and hypoxaemia are worse in the upright position (referred to as *platypnoea* and *orthodeoxia*, respectively). The syndrome carries a very poor prognosis, and is an indication for orthotopic liver transplantation in suitable candidates.

What is alcoholic hepatitis and what is the treatment?

Alcoholic hepatitis is a syndrome of progressive inflammatory liver injury associated with long-term heavy intake of ethanol. Patients with severe acute alcoholic hepatitis have a mortality of 50% or greater within 30 days.

The diagnosis is made in a patient with history of significant alcohol intake, fever and worsening LFTs (including elevated bilirubin and aminotransferases). Patients do not necessarily have cirrhosis.

The treatment is supportive with steroids given for more severe cases to reduce inflammation. Transfer to a tertiary referral centre may be required in severe cases. Pentoxyphylline has been shown to reduce the incidence of HRS in alcoholic hepatitis. Ultimately, alcohol abstinence is necessary in the long term.

Further Reading
Elsayed I A S, Battu P K, Irving S. Management of acute upper GI bleeding. *BJA Educ* 2017; **17**(4): 117–123

Kamath P S, Wiesner R H, Malinchoc M et al. A model to predict survival in patients with end-stage liver disease. *Hepatology* 2001; **33**(2): 464–70

O'Brien A J, Welch C A, Singer M, Harrison D A. Prevalence and outcome of cirrhosis patients admitted to UK intensive care: a comparison against dialysis-dependent chronic renal failure patients. *Intensive Care Med* 2012; **38**(6): 991–1000

Tripathi D, Stanley A J, Hayes P C et al. UK guidelines on the management of variceal haemorrhage in cirrhotic patients. *Gut* 2015; **64**: 1680–1704

Chapter 22

Chronic Obstructive Pulmonary Disease

What is chronic obstructive pulmonary disease?

Chronic obstructive pulmonary disease (COPD) is a progressive inflammatory condition affecting peripheral and central airways, lung parenchyma and pulmonary vasculature. The Global Initiative for Chronic Obstructive Lung Disease (GOLD, 2017) defines COPD as:

> A common, preventable and treatable disease characterised by persistent respiratory symptoms and airflow limitation that is due to airway and/or alveolar abnormalities usually caused by exposure to noxious particles and gases.

Expiratory airflow limitation is the result of a combination of small airway inflammation (obstructive bronchiolitis) and parenchymal destruction (emphysema).

Whilst cigarette smoking is the key noxious stimulus resulting in the development of COPD, other risk factors exist including air pollution, occupational exposure and genetic factors such as α_1-antitrypsin deficiency.

How is COPD diagnosed and severity ascertained?

The diagnosis of COPD should be considered in anyone with dyspnoea, a chronic cough or regular sputum production. Both NICE and GOLD have published guidelines for the diagnosis of COPD.

The diagnosis and assessment of severity of COPD is multi-faceted; it is based on symptoms, spirometry, functional assessment and the presence of complications:

1 *Symptoms*
   A diagnosis of COPD should be considered in smokers over the age of 35 presenting with exertional breathlessness, a chronic cough, regular sputum production and frequent winter bronchitis or wheeze
2 *Spirometry*
   Requires demonstrable airway obstruction, with a post-bronchodilator FEV1/FVC of <0.7

3 *Severity*

No single measure correlates exactly with true severity in an individual patient

Severe COPD is characterised by:

i Dyspnoea on minimal exertion that severely restricts daily activities (see Table 22.1 for the modified British Medical Research Council (MRC) breathlessness scale)

ii Spirometry (Table 22.2)

iii Presence of severe hypoxaemia, hypercapnia, pulmonary hypertension, heart failure or polycythaemia

Table 22.1 Modified MRC dyspnoea scale

Grade 1	Not troubled by breathlessness except on strenuous exercise
Grade 2	Short of breath when hurrying on the level or walking up a slight hill
Grade 3	Walks slower than most people on the level Stops after 15 mins of walking at own pace
Grade 4	Stops for breath after walking about 100 yards or after a few minutes at own pace
Grade 5	Too breathless to leave the house, or breathless when dressing or undressing

Table 22.2 GOLD classification of airflow limitation severity in COPD (based on post-bronchodilator FEV1)

In patients with FEV1/FVC < 0.7		
GOLD 1	Mild	FEV1 ≥ 80% predicted
GOLD 2	Moderate	FEV1 50 – 79% predicted
GOLD 3	Severe	FEV1 30 – 49% predicted
GOLD 4	Very severe	FEV1 < 30% predicted

Reproduced with kind permission from www.goldcopd.org

What is the pathophysiology of COPD and what are the consequences?

The pathophysiology of COPD involves (GOLD, 2017):

1 *Airflow limitation and gas trapping*

Peripheral airway limitation traps gas during expiration, resulting in hyperinflation. Static hyperinflation reduces inspiratory capacity and is commonly associated with dynamic hyperinflation during exercise leading to increased dyspnoea and limitation of exercise capacity.

2 *Gas exchange abnormalities*

Gas transfer for oxygen and carbon dioxide worsens as the disease progresses. Reduced ventilatory drive and increased dead space lead to reduced ventilation, which in turn leads to carbon dioxide retention. Abnormalities in alveolar ventilation and a reduced pulmonary capillary bed further worsen V/Q abnormalities.

3 *Mucous hypersecretion*

Mucus hypersecretion results in a chronic cough and is due to chronic airway irritation by cigarette smoke and other noxious agents. This leads to an increased number of goblet cells and enlarged submucosal glands.

4 *Pulmonary hypertension*

Hypoxic vasoconstriction of the small pulmonary arteries results in structural changes including intimal and smooth muscle hyperplasia, causing pulmonary hypertension. This usually occurs late in the course of COPD.

5 *Exacerbations*

During exacerbations (secondary to a number of factors including bacterial and viral infections and environmental pollutants) there is increased hyperinflation and gas trapping with reduced expiratory flow, leading to increased dyspnoea.

6 *Systemic features*

Coexisting diseases are common. Hyperinflation and airflow limitation affect cardiac function and gas exchange. Skeletal muscle wasting and cachexia result, which in turn may initiate or worsen comorbidities.

What are the indications for intensive care admission in patients with COPD?

1 Persistent or worsening hypoxaemia and/or severe or worsening respiratory acidosis (pH <7.25) despite supplemental oxygen and NIV
2 Need for invasive mechanical ventilation
3 Need for vasopressors/inotropes
4 Changes in mental state/consciousness
5 Severe dyspnoea responding poorly to initial treatment

What is the management of an exacerbation of COPD?

The patient with an acute exacerbation of COPD (AECOPD) should be managed with an ABCDE approach, treating abnormalities as they are found. Specific management principles include:

1 **Investigations**
   i Blood tests to look for evidence of infection and organ dysfunction (FBC, CRP, cultures, U+Es, LFTs, clotting screen)
   ii Sputum MC+S
   iii Arterial blood gas analysis required at regular intervals
   iv CXR to identify focal consolidation/pneumonia
   v Consider TTE to identify right heart dysfunction and pulmonary hypertension
2 **Pharmacological therapies**
   i β_2-agonists
      – Short-acting β_2-agonists, e.g. nebulised salbutamol 2.5 mg
      – Short-acting anticholinergics, e.g. nebulised ipratropium bromide 250–500 mcg

ii Steroids
  – Systemic steroids can improve FEV1, oxygenation and shorten recovery
iii Antibiotics when indicated, e.g. pyrexia, systemic features of infection, raised inflammatory markers, CXR changes
iv Oral mucolytics in patients with productive cough, e.g. carbocysteine 750 mg tds
v Methylxanthines (e.g. aminophylline) are *not* recommended due to their increased side effect profile

3 **Respiratory support**
  i Oxygen to target saturations 88–92%
    – This targeted approach is associated with less respiratory acidosis and decreased mortality in COPD patients
    – Hypercapnic respiratory failure secondary to excessive oxygen administration can result primarily from increased V/Q mismatching
  ii Controlled oxygen delivery via fixed performance (Venturi) devices
  iii Non-invasive ventilation
    – Should be the first mode of ventilation used in patients with COPD
    – The use of NIV in patients with moderate or moderate-severe COPD respiratory acidosis has been shown to prevent endotracheal intubation and improve survival
    – NIV facilitates weaning and improves the success of extubation in patients with COPD
  iv Invasive ventilation
4 Measures for **prevention** of further exacerbations
  i Optimise bronchodilators and mucolytics
  ii Pneumococcal and annual influenza vaccines
  iii Assess need for continuing oxygen therapy long term (see below)

What are the specific indications for NIV in a COPD exacerbation?

NIV has resulted in a reduction in mortality of around 50% in the management of acute type 2 respiratory failure in COPD over the last decade. The BTS recommends that NIV should be considered in:

1 Patients with a persisting or worsening respiratory acidosis (PaCO$_2$ >6.5 kPa, pH <7.35) despite optimal medical therapy
2 Patients with severe acidosis (i.e. pH <7.25)
  – Such patients may benefit from NIV but have a higher risk of treatment failure, and should be managed in a HDU/ICU setting with the intention to proceed to invasive ventilation if NIV fails
3 As the ceiling of treatment for patients who, for whatever valid reason, are not candidates for intubation

Worsening physiological parameters, particularly pH and RR, indicate the need to change the management strategy (i.e. clinical review, change of NIV interface, adjustment of ventilator settings and consideration of intubation)

What other key interventions have shown benefit in the management of COPD?

1 Smoking cessation
 i Smoking cessation is a key intervention for all patients who continue to smoke
 ii Counselling and many different forms of pharmacotherapy exist to facilitate smoking cessation
2 Long term oxygen therapy (LTOT) confers survival benefit in COPD and improves pulmonary haemodynamics. The BTS recommends that LTOT should be considered in:
 i Patients with stable, chronic COPD and a resting PaO_2 ≤7.3 kPa
 ii Patients with a resting PaO_2 ≤8 kPa *and* evidence of peripheral oedema, polycythaemia (haematocrit >55%) or pulmonary hypertension

What are the indications for intubation and invasive ventilation in AECOPD?

The BTS guidelines advise invasive ventilation in:

1 Imminent respiratory arrest
2 Severe respiratory distress
3 Failure of, or contraindications to, NIV
4 Persisting pH <7.15 or deterioration in pH despite NIV
5 GCS <8

What are the principles of invasive ventilation for a patient with COPD?

Limited expiratory flow rates in COPD patients (as a result of airway narrowing) lead to breath-stacking and the development of intrinsic PEEP, as in asthmatics (see page 83).

Intrinsic PEEP has the following physiological consequences:

1 Decreased venous return and consequent hypotension
2 Increased PVR and right heart strain
3 Pulmonary barotrauma, volutrauma, hypercapnia and acidosis

Ventilating patients with COPD therefore involves a compromise between achieving normocapnia, oxygenation and cardiovascular stability. Ventilatory principles include:

1 Reduced respiratory rate or I:E ratio
 – Produces prolonged expiratory time, reducing the risk of breath-stacking
 – Reduced minute volume will consequently lead to hypercapnia, acidosis, increased PVR and potential haemodynamic instability

2 Application of extrinsic PEEP
  - Keeps small airways open during expiration
  - If values are kept below intrinsic PEEP, there should be no significant increases in alveolar pressure and no worsening of cardiovascular effects
3 Treatment of bronchospasm
  - Optimise gas flow

Is there any evidence for the use of acetazolamide in mechanically ventilated patients with COPD?

The **DIABOLO** trial (JAMA, 2016) was a double-blinded multi-centre RCT that investigated this. Patients with a history of COPD who had been invasively ventilated for <24 hours and had a metabolic alkalosis were randomised to receive acetazolamide or placebo for up to 28 days. There was no difference in duration of mechanical ventilation.

Is it appropriate to admit patients with an exacerbation of severe COPD to critical care?

As a group, critically ill patients with severe COPD have a high mortality: one recent retrospective review showed that those who are intubated and mechanically ventilated have an in-hospital mortality of 25%. However, the BTS advises that clinicians are likely to underestimate survival in AECOPD: duration of ICU stay and survival is better than most other medical reasons for invasive ventilation.

The appropriateness of invasive ventilation in the critically ill patient with severe COPD should be addressed on a case-by-case basis. It is generally agreed that functional status in the prior period of stability and FEV1 before ICU admission can be helpful in decision making. Forward planning and patient consultation regarding escalation of care is important and certainly a management plan in the event of NIV failure should be made early in the admission.

Patients should be stratified into management groups depending on their pre-morbid state, reversibility of acute illness, relative contraindications to ventilatory support and their wishes.

Further Reading
Davidson A C, Banham S, Elliott M, et al. BTS/ICS guideline for the ventilatory management of acute hypercapnic respiratory failure in adults. *Thorax* 2016; **71**: ii1–ii35

GOLD, 2017. Global Strategy for the Diagnosis, Management and Prevention of COPD [online]. Available at: http://goldcopd.org/gold-2017-global-strategy-diagnosis-management-prevention-copd/ (Accessed: 1 May 2017)

Hardinge M, Annandale J, Bourne S, et al. The BTS guideline for home oxygen use in adults. *Thorax* 2015; **70**: i1–i43

Lumb A, Biercamp C. Chronic obstructive pulmonary disease and anaesthesia. *Contin Educ Anaesth Crit Care Pain* 2014; **14** (1): 1–5.

National Institute for Health and Care Excellence, 2010. Chronic obstructive pulmonary disease in over 16s: diagnosis and management. Clinical guideline 101 [online]. Available at: www.nice.org.uk/guidance/CG101 (Accessed: 16 May 2017)

Chapter 23

Colloids

Define the term *colloid*

A colloid is a fluid containing large molecules that exert an oncotic pressure at the capillary membrane. These molecules are effectively suspended in a crystalloid solution.

What colloids are you aware of?

Colloids may be classified into natural and synthetic. Natural colloids include blood and its constituents, and albumin. Synthetic colloids include gelatins and hydroxyethyl starches (HES). See Table 23.1 for a summary of the synthetic colloids.

Table 23.1 Comparison of synthetic colloids

Colloid	Average Molecular Weight	Advantages	Disadvantages
Gelatins Modified bovine collagen suspensions	35 kDa	Long shelf life	Rapidly excreted by the kidneys (most molecules much smaller than 35 kDa), so actual effect ~1.5 hours Potential anaphylaxis
Hydroxyethyl starches Corn / potato starch suspensions Large ethylated, polymerised amylopectin molecules	Several available Different average MW: – Low MW (70–130 kDa) – Medium MW (200 kDa) – High MW (450 kDa)	Longer plasma half-life than other synthetic colloids (>6 hours)	Higher MW solutions, e.g. 450 kDa (especially those with high substitution ratios, e.g. 450/0.7) impair factor VIII and vWF, causing coagulopathy Increased incidence of renal failure and mortality in critically ill

vWF – von-Willebrand Factor

What is albumin? In what form do we use it?

Albumin is a globular, single polypeptide with a molecular weight (MW) of 69 kDa. It is highly negatively charged and is repelled by the negatively charged glycocalyx of the endothelium. This property extends its intravascular half-life to 5–10 days when given as a volume expander (assuming intact capillary endothelium).

Human albumin solution (HAS) is a solution containing protein derived from plasma, serum and normal placentas. It is available in two concentrations in the UK: isotonic (4.5%) or concentrated (20%). It is prepared from thousands of pooled donations, and therefore carries a theoretical risk of transmission of new variant Creutzvelt-Jacob disease (CJD).

Where is albumin produced?

Albumin is produced in the liver at a rate of 0.2 g/kg/day under the influence of neuroendocrine systems and the plasma oncotic pressure. It is synthesised quickly, and released into the blood without being stored. Albumin accounts for approximately 50% of plasma proteins and the normal range is 35–50 g/l. It is a negative acute phase protein, with its production being suppressed in physiological stress. Hence hypoalbuminaemia is almost universal in the critically ill.

What are the functions of native albumin?

The functions of albumin are:

1 Transport molecule
   - Cations (calcium, sodium, potassium)
   - Hormones, e.g. T_4, steroids
   - Unconjugated bilirubin
   - Bile salts
   - Acidic drugs, e.g. barbiturates, warfarin, NSAIDs (drugs may compete for binding sites)
2 Maintenance of oncotic pressure
   - Albumin contributes ~80% of colloid oncotic pressure in healthy patients
3 Acid base balance (acts as a buffer)

When do we use albumin?

1 Fluid resuscitation
   - The *Surviving Sepsis* guidelines recommend the use of albumin in fluid resuscitation once large volumes of crystalloid have been given

- HAS is not often used for this purpose in the UK
2 Prophylaxis and management of HRS
3 To facilitate large volume paracentesis in cirrhosis
4 As a replacement fluid in plasmapheresis

Do you know of any evidence surrounding the use of albumin in critically ill patients?

In 1998, a Cochrane review based on a meta-analysis of 32 trials demonstrated no difference in mortality between hypovolaemic patients (following surgery or trauma) who received albumin volume expansion when compared to those treated with crystalloids. Interestingly, there was an increased mortality rate in patients with burns who were treated with albumin as compared to those treated with crystalloids. Overall, albumin administration appeared to be associated with an increased overall mortality rate when compared to patients treated with other forms of fluid therapy. This meta-analysis resulted in a drastic reduction in the use of HAS in intensive care. However, two further meta-analyses appeared to contradict these findings.

The **SAFE** trial (NEJM, 2004) was a double-blinded multi-centre Australian RCT comparing the use of 4% HAS compared with normal saline for fluid resuscitation in ICU patients. There was equivalent mortality in the two groups. Additionally, there was a non-significant trend favouring the use of normal saline in trauma, and albumin in sepsis. Subgroup analysis revealed a significant increase in mortality in patients with traumatic brain injury who received albumin.

The **ALBIOS** trial (NEJM, 2014) was a non-blinded multi-centre Italian RCT comparing the use of 20% HAS (to maintain serum albumin ≥30 g/l) with crystalloid fluids alone, in adults with severe sepsis or septic shock. Despite the fact that the study was not blinded, there was no difference in mortality between the groups implying that routine albumin replacement in critically ill patients with sepsis confers no survival advantage.

Are there any disadvantages to using albumin?

1 The use of HAS as a resuscitative fluid worsens 28-day mortality and long term outcomes in patients with TBI
2 Albumin is more expensive to produce and to buy than crystalloids
3 In patients with endothelial dysfunction and capillary leak, the use of albumin may worsen third space loss (protein molecules leak into the interstitial space, drawing water with them)
4 There is a theoretical risk of new variant CJD transmission with albumin use

In non-septic critically ill patients there is no mortality benefit to the use of albumin versus crystalloids.

What is the evidence surrounding the use of starches in critically ill patients?

Following the introduction of HES on to the global market, reports began to emerge of significant adverse effects including deterioration in renal function in critically ill patients.

The **VISEP** (Efficacy of Volume Substitution and Insulin Therapy in Severe Sepsis) trial (NEJM, 2008) was a German multi-centre RCT that focused on the safety and efficacy of HES versus lactated Ringer's solution in patients with severe sepsis and septic shock. It was stopped early for safety reasons. They demonstrated that HES increases risk of AKI and need for RRT; however, the trial used high doses of hyperoncotic HES and may not be relevant to usual practice. This trial also addressed the role of intensive glycaemic control in these patients, and found a significant increase in adverse events related to hypoglycaemia (a finding echoed in the NICE-SUGAR trial in 2008).

The Scandinavian **6S** trial (NEJM, 2012) was a double-blinded multi-centre RCT comparing the use of HES (130/0.42) with Ringer's lactate. There was no difference in 28-day mortality, but a significant increase in 90-day mortality and use of RRT in the intervention group. Patients in the HES group were more likely to receive blood products, with a trend towards more severe bleeding.

In 2012, Myburgh et al. conducted the **CHEST** trial (NEJM), a double-blinded multi-centre Antipodean RCT comparing the use of 6% HES (130/0.4) with normal saline for fluid resuscitation in critically ill patients. There was no difference in 90-day mortality, but the use of RRT was greater in the patients receiving HES (by RIFLE criteria the saline group had more *risk* and *injury* AKI, but less *failure*). Additionally, patients in the intervention group received more blood products.

Several studies reporting benefits of HES were retracted on the grounds of ethical and scientific misconduct in 2011, and following publication of the CHEST trial in 2013, HES was withdrawn from the British market.

Further Reading
Vincent J L, Russell J A, Jacob M, et al. Albumin administration in the acutely ill: what is new and where next? *Crit Care* 2014; **18**: 231–241

Chapter 24

Critical Incidents in the ICU

What is a patient safety incident?

A patient safety incident refers to any healthcare event that is:

- Unexpected
- Unintended
- Undesired
- Associated with actual/potential harm

Why are critically ill patients at particular risk of a patient safety incident?

Patients on the ICU are:

1 Undergoing highly invasive treatments with concomitant complications
2 Receiving frequent parenteral drugs/fluids
3 Undergoing intensive interventions
4 Lacking capacity/autonomy
5 Lacking physiological reserve
6 More likely to be sedated or unable to communicate concerns

What are the stages involved in patients receiving medications and at which stage do most errors occur?

The broad stages involved in the process of delivering medication to patients are:

1 Prescription
2 Transcription
3 Preparation
4 Dispensing
5 Administration

The majority of errors occur in the administration phase.

What are medication errors and adverse drug events? How common are they?

Medication errors are any mistake in the prescription, preparation or administration of a drug that does not necessarily cause harm. A recent systematic review revealed rates of medication errors varied widely from 8.1 to 2344 per 1000 patient days.

Adverse drug events (ADEs) are medication errors where harm occurs. The overall incidence of ADEs again vary widely from 5.1 to 87.5 per 1000 patient days.

Why are medication errors more common on the ICU?

There are many risk factors for medication errors specific to the ICU. These factors can be divided into patient-, environmental- and medication-specific factors (Table 24.1).

Table 24.1 Risk factors for medication errors in critical care

Patient factors	Environment and human factors	Medication specific
Severity of illness	High turnover of patients and providers	Number of medications (risk of medication interactions)
Extremes of age	Difficult working conditions, high stress	Types of medications – Use of infusions and boluses – Pump programming – Use of estimated weights
Prolonged hospitalisation (increased exposure and susceptibility to ADEs)	Emergency admissions	
Sedation, lack of capacity	Knowledge and performance deficits	
Altered pharmacodynamics	Communication problems, inadequate information technology	

Are there any measures that have been shown to reduce medication errors in the ICU?

A multifaceted approach is required to reduce medication errors on the ICU:

1 Eliminate environmental and situational risk factors
   i Avoid excessive working hours
   ii Minimise interruptions/distractions
   iii Trainee supervision
2 Optimise the medication process
   i Computerised physician prescription systems and intravenous infusion devices
   ii Medication standardisation
3 Prevention of oversights
   i Adequate staffing
   ii Pharmacist involvement
   iii Education and quality assurance

What is a never event?

NHS England define Never Events as:

Serious incidents that are wholly preventable, as guidance or safety recommendations that provide strong systemic protective barriers are available at a national level and should have been implemented by all healthcare providers.

Can you name the never events that may relate to intensive care?

All organisations providing NHS care should use the Never Events list in Table 24.2 (NHS England 2015/16).

Table 24.2 The Never Events list (2016)

Surgical	Wrong site surgery * Wrong implant/prosthesis Retained foreign object post-procedure *
Medication	Mis-selection of a strong potassium-containing solution * Wrong route of administration of medication * Overdose of insulin due to abbreviations or incorrect device * Overdose of methotrexate for non-cancer treatment Mis-selection of high strength midazolam for conscious sedation
Mental Health	Failure to install functional or collapsible shower or curtain rails
General	Falls from poorly restricted windows Chest or neck entrapment in bed rails Transfusion or transplantation of ABO-incompatible blood products or organs * Misplaced nasogastric or orogastric tubes * Scalding of patients

* represents those applicable to ICU

What is the correct procedure for confirming the position of a nasogastric tube?

Between September 2011 and March 2016, 95 incidents relating to the use of misplaced NG tubes were reported to the National Reporting and Learning System (NRLS), prompting a further Patient Safety Alert to be issued in July 2016 as a result of the risk of severe harm and death.

The National Patient Safety Agency (NPSA) 2011 guidelines state:

1 *Nothing* should be introduced down an NG tube until the position is confirmed
2 *1st line test method: pH testing*
   - A pH of between 1 and 5.5 is the safe range
   - Tube position must be checked using pH indicator strips that are CE marked, intended by the manufacturer to test human gastric aspirate and have a clear definition between pH 5–6
   - Each pH result must be documented on the nasogastric monitoring form kept at the patient's bedside
3 *2nd line test method: chest X-ray*
   - Used when no aspirate is obtained or pH indicator paper fails to confirm a pH in the safe range
   - Documentation following X-ray should include:
     i Who authorised the X-ray
     ii Who confirmed the position of the NG tube; the person must be evidenced as competent to do so
     iii Confirmation that the X-ray viewed was the most current X-ray for the correct patient
     iv The rationale for confirmation of position of the NG tube
4 Checking the external tube markings for displacement remains vital

Due to the use of gastric acid suppressing agents and the particular risk of NG misplacement in the unconscious critically ill patient, many ICUs are now advocating X-ray confirmation for each NG tube that is inserted.

Waiting for X-ray confirmation can cause delays in time-critical administration of enteral medicine or optimal nutritional practices. It is possible that new technologies such as electromagnetic NG tube placement may allow faster/ equally safe practices.

What processes are in place to help minimise the risk of a never event?

The following processes are commonly employed to minimise the occurrence of never events:

1 Two person checking of drugs/blood
2 Barcode scanners
3 Checklists (e.g. the World Health Organisation (WHO) surgical safety checklist)
4 Debriefs
5 Standardisation of processes
6 Team training in communication and awareness of human factors
7 Mandatory learning modules and competency-based training for staff
8 Growing culture of open communication to enable learning from mistakes

What you would you do if you were involved in a never event?

Failure to report a never event is unacceptable and a potential sign of cultural and safety failings in an organisation.

Following a single never event, immediate steps should be taken to ensure that patient safety systems and procedures are reviewed. The following points summarise the requirements when a Never Event is identified:

1 Patient safety is paramount
   - Ensure the patient is stable, and any complications are treated immediately
2 Inform the consultant(s) responsible for patient care and departmental lead that a Never Event has occurred
3 Inform the patient/family/carer as soon as possible
   - Ensure details of the conversation are documented in the patient notes
4 Complete an incident report as per local policy
   - Never Events should also be reported on the Strategic Executive Information System within two days
5 Never Events must be highlighted to the relevant commissioner within two working days as per the Serious Incidents Framework
6 Never Events must be investigated in line with the Serious Incidents Framework (e.g. root cause analysis)

Further Reading

NHS England Patient Safety Domain, 2015. *Never Events List 2015/16* [online]. Available at: www.england.nhs.uk/wp-content/uploads/2015/03/never-evnts-list-15-16.pdf (Accessed: 18 February 2017)

NHS Improvement, 2016. *Resource Set Initial Placement Checks for Nasogastric and Orogastric Tubes* [online]. Available at: https://improvement.nhs.uk/resources/resource-set-initial-placement-checks-nasogastric-and-orogastric-tubes/ (Accessed: 25 February 2017)

Wilmer A, Louie K, Dodek P, et al. Incidence of medication errors and adverse drug events in the ICU: a systematic review [online]. *Qual Saf Health Care* 2010; **19** (5): e7. Available at: http://qualitysafety.bmj.com/content/19/5/e7.long (Accessed: 25 February 2017)

Chapter 25

Delirium

Define delirium

Delirium is an acute change in consciousness and awareness that fluctuates over time. Patients may have:

1 Disordered thinking
2 Reduced attention
3 Abnormal sleep/wake cycle
4 Abnormal psychomotor activity
5 Abnormal perceptions
6 Abnormal emotional behaviour

The criteria from the *DSM IV* (1994) requires four diagnostic criteria be present to diagnose delirium:

a) Disturbance of consciousness (i.e. reduced clarity of awareness of the environment) with reduced ability to focus, sustain, or shift attention
b) A change in cognition (such as memory deficit, disorientation, language disturbance) or the development of a perceptual disturbance that is not better accounted for by a pre-existing, established, or evolving dementia
c) The disturbance develops over a short period of time (usually hours to days) and tends to fluctuate during the course of the day
d) There is evidence from the history, physical examination and laboratory findings that:
  i The disturbance is caused by the direct physiological consequences of a general medical condition
  ii The symptoms in criterion i. developed during substance intoxication, or during or shortly after, a withdrawal syndrome, or
  iii The delirium has more than one aetiology.

The *ICD-10* (1992) definition is similar:

a) Clouding of consciousness, i.e. reduced clarity of awareness of the environment, with reduced ability to focus, sustain, or shift attention
b) Disturbance of cognition, manifested by both:
  i Impairment of immediate recall and recent memory, with relatively intact remote memory
  ii Disorientation in time, place or person

c) At least one of the following psychomotor disturbances:
   i Rapid, unpredictable shifts from hypo-activity to hyper-activity
   ii Increased reaction time
   iii Increased or decreased flow of speech
   iv Enhanced startle reaction
d) Disturbance of sleep or the sleep-wake cycle, manifested by at least one of the following:
   i Insomnia, which in severe cases may involve total sleep loss, with or without drowsiness, or reversal of the sleep-wake cycle
   ii Nocturnal worsening of symptoms
   iii Disturbing dreams and nightmares which may continue as hallucinations after awakening
e) Rapid onset and fluctuations of the symptoms over the course of the day
f) Objective evidence from history, physical and neurological examination or underlying cerebral or systemic disease (other than psychoactive substance-related) that can be presumed to be responsible for the clinical manifestations in a-d.

What is the pathophysiology of delirium?

It is thought to be due to neurotransmitter imbalance, with reduced acetylcholine and increased dopamine resulting in neuronal excitability. Additionally, there may be cerebral microvascular dysfunction following exposure to inflammatory mediators, or global failure of oxidative metabolism resulting in cerebral insufficiency.

How common is it?

Very common. The prevalence is higher in the more severely unwell patients, with up to 70–80% of mechanically ventilated patients affected and 50% of less unwell patients.

How does it present?

There are three main subtypes of delirium:

1 Hyperactive delirium (~1%)
   – Confused
   – Agitated
   – Combative, aggressive
   – Paranoid
2 Hypoactive delirium (35%)
   – Inattentive
   – Stuporous
   – Withdrawn
   – Often mistaken for depression
3 Mixed (64%)

What are the risk factors for the development of delirium?

Patient factors:

1 Age
2 Comorbidities
3 Baseline cognitive impairment or psychiatric history
4 Alcohol or substance abuse

Factors relating to acute illness:

1 High APACHE II score
2 Sepsis
3 Hypoxaemia
4 Metabolic derangement, e.g. acidaemia, hypo/hypernatraemia, hypo/hyper-calcaemia
5 Surgery, particularly use of CPB

Iatrogenic:

1 Disturbed sleep/wake cycle
2 Sedative medications (in particular benzodiazepines)
3 Anticholinergic medication

Are there any consequences of delirium? Why is delirium important?

Delirium is associated with:

1 Short term complications:
   – Risk of adverse events including accidental extubation / line removal
2 Medium term complications:
   – Increased LOS on ICU and in hospital
   – Increased duration of mechanical ventilation
   – Increased mortality (independent risk factor for three-fold increase in mortality at 90 days)
3 Long term complications:
   – Risk of post-traumatic stress disorder (PTSD)
   – Risk of long term cognitive impairment

How do you diagnose delirium in the ICU?

Several bedside scoring systems have been developed to assess ICU delirium. The two most widely accepted tools are the Confusion Assessment Method-ICU (CAM-ICU, see Figure 25.1) and Intensive Care Delirium Screening Checklist (ICDSC, see Table 25.1).

CAM-ICU Worksheet

Feature 1: Acute Onset or Fluctuating Course	Score	Check here if Present
Is the patient different than his/her baseline mental status? OR Has the patient had any fluctuation in mental status in the past 24 hours as evidenced by fluctuation on a sedation/level of consciousness scale (i.e., RASS/SASA), GCS, or previous delirium assessment?	Either question Yes →	☐

Feature 2: Inattention		
Letters Attention Test (See training manual for alternate Pictures) Directions: Say to the patient "*I am going to read you a series of 10 letters. Whenever you hear the letter 'A,' indicate by squeezing my hand.*" Read letters from the following letter list in a normal tone 3 seconds apart. S A V E A H A A R T or C A S A B L A N C A or A B A D B A D A A Y Errors are counted when patient fails to squeeze on the letter "A" and when the patient squeeze on any other than "A."	Number of Errors >2 →	☐

Feature 2: Altered Level of Consciousness		
Present if the Actual RASS score is anything other than alert and calm (zero)	RASS anything other than zero →	☐

Feature 4:Disorganized Thinking		
Yes/No Questions (See training manual for alternate set of questions) 1. Will a stone float on water? 2. Are there fish in the sea? 3. Does one pound weigh more than two pounds? 4. Can you use a hammer to pound a nail? **Errors are counted when the patient incorrectly answers a question.** Command Say to patient: "Hold up this many fingers" (Hold 2 fingers in front of patient) "Now do the same thing with the other hand" (Do not repeat number of fingers) * If the patient is unable to move both arms. for 2nd part of command ask patient to "Add one more finger" **An error is counted if patient is unable to complete the entire command.**	Combined number of errors >1→	☐

OVerall CAM-ICU Feature 1 plus 2 and either 3 or 4 present = CAM-ICU po itive	Criteria Met →	☐ **CAM-ICU Positive** (Delirium Present)
	Criteria Not Met →	☐ **CAM-ICU Negative** (No Delirium)

Figure 25.1 CAM-ICU checklist
Reproduced with kind permission from Professor EW Ely

Table 25.1 ICDSC checklist

Altered level of consciousness	Exaggerated response to normal stimulation	RASS +1 to +4	1 point
	Normal wakefulness	RASS 0	0 points
	Response to mild or moderate stimulation (follows commands)	RASS –1 to –3	1 point
	Response only to intense and repeated stimulation	RASS –4	Delirium assessment cannot be completed in patients who are stuporous or comatose
	No response	RASS –5	
Inattention Score 1 point if any of these present	Difficulty in following commands Easily distracted by external stimuli Difficulty in shifting focus		
Disorientation	Any obvious mistake in time, place or person scores 1 point		
Hallucination, delusion, psychosis Score 1 point if any of these present	Unequivocal clinical manifestation of hallucinations or of behaviour probably due to hallucinations or delusions Gross impairment in reality testing		
Psychomotor agitation or retardation Score 1 point if either present	Hyperactivity requiring the use of additional sedative drugs or restraints in order to control potential danger to self or others Hypoactivity or clinically noticeable psychomotor slowing		
Inappropriate speech or mood Score 1 point if either present	Inappropriate, disorganised or incoherent speech Inappropriate display of emotion related to events or situation		
Sleep/wake cycle disturbance Score 1 point if any of these present	Sleeping less than 4 hours at night Waking frequently at night (not including wakefulness initiated by medical staff or loud environment) Sleeping during most of the day		
Symptom fluctuation	Fluctuation of the manifestation of any item or symptom over 24 hours scores 1 point		

Reproduced with permission from Bergeron N, et al. (*Intensive Care Med* 2001)

What can be done to reduce the risk of delirium?

1 The *ABCDE bundle* (**Vasilevskis, et al,** Chest, 2010) can be used
   - *Awake and Breathing* (daily sedation holds +/– spontaneous breathing trials (SBTs) to reduce the amount of sedation given and total days of mechanical ventilation)
   - *Choice of sedation* (minimising the use of medications that can provoke delirium, e.g. benzodiazepines)
   - *Coordination* (regular orientation and ensuring patients have their glasses and hearing aids)
   - *Delirium monitoring* (with CAM-ICU or similar)
   - *Early mobilisation* has been shown to reduce acute cognitive and physical dysfunction in ICU patients
2 Sleep hygiene
3 Removing invasive devices when no longer required

How is delirium managed?

The non-pharmacological methods are outlined above. Pharmacological methods include:

1 Antipsychotics are the drugs of choice in patients posing a risk to themselves or others (e.g. haloperidol, olanzepine, quetiapine)
2 Recent evidence supports the use of dexmedetomidine (α_2 agonist) over propofol and benzodiazepines for sedation

The **DahLIA trial** (JAMA, 2016) was a double-blind multi-centre RCT (although underpowered) comparing dexmedetomidine infusion with placebo in patients who were neurologically inappropriate for extubation. It showed a statistically significant reduction in median ventilator-free hours at day seven and a significant reduction in the use of antipsychotics, as well as a non-significant reduction in ICU LOS in patients treated with dexmedetomidine.

The **Midex-Prodex trial** (JAMA, 2012) was a double-blind multi centre parallel trial design (depending on the usual practice in the recruiting ICU) that showed non-inferiority of dexmedetomidine when compared to midazolam or propofol sedation (i.e. time at target sedation without rescue medication). Duration of sedation was significantly shorter with dexmedetomidine compared to midazolam; the slightly shorter duration for dexmedetomidine against propofol was not statistically significant. There was also a non-significant reduction in ICU LOS in the dexmedetomidine group compared to the other two groups.

Further Reading

Bergeron N, Dubois M J, Dumont M, Dial S, Skrobik Y. Intensive Care Delirium Screening Checklist: evaluation of a new screening tool. *Intensive Care Med* 2001; **27**: 859–64

Ely E W, Margolin R, Francis J, et al. Evaluation of delirium in critically ill patients: Validation of the Confusion Assessment Method for the Intensive Care Unit (CAM-ICU). *Crit Care Med* 2001; **29**: 1370–1379

King J. Delirium in intensive care. *Contin Educ Anaesth Crit Care Pain* 2009; **9**(5): 144–147

Chapter 26

Diabetic Emergencies

Diabetic Ketoacidosis

What is diabetic ketoacidosis?

Diabetic ketoacidosis (DKA) is a potentially life-threatening metabolic complication of diabetes defined by the biochemical triad of ketonaemia, hyperglycaemia and acidaemia.

What is the pathophysiology of DKA?

Diabetic ketoacidosis usually occurs as the result of absolute or relative insulin deficiency which, when combined with increases in glucagon, catecholamines and cortisol stimulates lipolysis, free fatty acid production and ketogenesis. Accumulation of the ketoacids (3-β-hydroxybutyrate, acetone and acetoacetate) then results in a metabolic acidosis. Hyperglycaemia results from increased hepatic gluconeogenesis and glycolysis in addition to reduced glucose uptake peripherally due to insulin deficiency.

The marked fluid depletion characteristic of DKA is the result of several processes:

1 Osmotic diuresis secondary to hyperglycaemia
2 Vomiting (commonly seen in DKA)
3 Reduced oral intake secondary to reduced consciousness

What are the causes of DKA?

Common precipitating factors include surgery, intercurrent infection, myocardial infarction and non-compliance with drug therapy.

What are the clinical features of DKA?

The clinical features of DKA include thirst, polyuria, nausea, vomiting, abdominal pain, dehydration, smell of ketones on the breath, Kussmaul breathing (deep, laboured and gasping breathing pattern secondary to severe metabolic acidosis), confusion and coma.

What are the diagnostic criteria for DKA?

As stated by the Joint British Diabetes Societies, all three of the following must be present:

1 Capillary blood glucose >11 mmol/l
2 Ketonaemia >3 mmol/l or urine ketones >2+ on urine dipsticks
3 Venous bicarbonate <15 mmol/l and/or venous pH <7.3

What are the indications for consideration of admission to HDU/ICU?

The presence of one or more of the following may indicate severe DKA, and therefore a higher level of care should be considered:

1 Blood ketones >6 mmol/l
2 Bicarbonate <5 mmol/l
3 Venous/arterial pH <7.1
4 Hypokalaemia on admission <3.5 mmol/l
5 GCS <12
6 SpO_2 <92% (assuming normal baseline function)
7 Systolic BP <90 mmHg
8 Heart rate <60 or >100 bpm
9 Anion gap >16

$$\text{Anion gap} = (Na^+ + K^+) - (Cl^- + HCO_3^-)$$

What is the treatment of DKA?

Most hospitals have clear guidelines/protocols for the management of DKA.

The patient with DKA should be managed with an ABCDE approach, treating abnormalities as they are found. Specific management focuses on the following principles:

1 **Fluid and electrolyte replacement**
   – Aims:
      i Restore circulating volume
      ii Clear ketones
      iii Correct electrolyte imbalance
   – Crystalloid fluid replacement should be used and 0.9% sodium chloride is the fluid of choice (although debate over this persists)
   – Initial hypotension (SBP <90 mmHg) should be treated with 500 ml boluses of 0.9% sodium chloride
   – Fluid replacement should be continued with 1 litre over the first hour, a further litre over 2 hours, followed by another litre over 4 hours
   – Modify rate and volume of fluid in young and elderly patients, and those with renal and heart failure (increased risk of cerebral oedema)

- The potassium debt is typically 3–5 mmol/kg: Each bag of 0.9% sodium chloride should be supplemented with potassium when the plasma potassium is <5.5 mmol/l

2 **Insulin therapy and metabolic treatment targets**

Role of insulin: Suppression of ketogenesis, reduction of blood glucose, correction of electrolyte disturbance

- A fixed rate insulin infusion should be commenced (0.1 units/kg/hour)
- *Do not* give an initial insulin bolus
- If the patient normally takes a long-acting insulin analogue this should be continued
- Close monitoring of venous blood gases and urinary/blood ketones is essential to closely monitor treatment efficacy
- Overall targets for treatment:
    i Decrease blood ketone level by 0.5 mmol/l per hour
    ii Increase venous bicarbonate by 3 mmol/l per hour
    iii Decrease capillary blood glucose by 3 mmol/l per hour
    iv Maintain potassium 4.0–5.5 mmol/l
- If these targets are not achieved, then the fixed rate insulin infusion rate should be increased
- 10% glucose infusion may be necessary to avoid hypoglycaemia and allow the continuation of the insulin infusion to suppress ketogenesis

3 **Treatment of the underlying cause**
4 **Other supportive treatments**
    i Thromboprophylaxis (mechanical and pharmacological)
    ii Stress ulcer prophylaxis
    iii Consider enteral feeding as necessary

What is the commonest cause of death in DKA?

Cerebral oedema (more so in children and young adults).

How does the management of DKA differ in children?

The markedly increased risk of cerebral oedema in the paediatric population necessitates judicious use of fluid.

1 A 10 ml/kg bolus of 0.9% sodium chloride be given *only* if the child is shocked (poor peripheral pulses, prolonged capillary refill with tachycardia and/or hypotension)
2 Fluid requirement = deficit + maintenance – volume used in resuscitation
This volume of fluid is given over 48 hours in the paediatric population (rather than 24 hours)

Fluid deficit (ml) = Body weight × % dehydration × 10

3 Maintenance fluid volumes are lower than standard and it is important not to over-estimate fluid requirement
4 Insulin therapy is delayed for one hour

Hyperglycaemic Hyperosmolar State

What is hyperglycaemic hyperosmolar state?

The characteristic features of a hyperglycaemic hyperosmolar state (HHS) are severe hyperglycaemia and fluid depletion with no or mild ketosis. It is usually seen in elderly patients with uncontrolled type 2 DM and often other significant comorbidity.

What is the mortality associated with HHS?

Hyperglycaemic hyperosmolar state is associated with significant morbidity and a higher mortality than DKA (15–30%).

What are the clinical features of HHS?

The characteristic features of HHS include:

1 **Hypovolaemia**
   Significant fluid losses are evident, estimated to be between 100–220 ml/kg
2 Marked **hyperglycaemia** (>30 mmol/l)
   Without significant hyperketonaemia (<3 mmol/l)
   Without significant acidosis (pH >7.3, bicarbonate >15 mmol/l)
3 Serum **hyperosmolarity**
   Osmolality >320 mosmol/kg

The presenting signs and symptoms are generally non-specific: anorexia, malaise and weakness, which progresses to severe dehydration, renal impairment and coma.

Whilst DKA tends to present within hours of onset, HHS develops over many days and consequently dehydration and metabolic disturbance may be very severe.

What are the goals of treatment of HHS?

A hyperglycaemic hyperosmolar state should be managed with an ABCDE approach, treating abnormalities as they are found. Specific treatment involves:

1 **Treatment of the underlying cause**
2 **Normalisation of osmolality**
   – It is very important to calculate osmolality regularly to monitor the response to treatment

$$\text{Osmolality} = (2Na^+ + glucose + urea)$$

3 **Replacement of fluid and electrolyte losses**
   – Debate persists around the speed and type of fluid required; however, the Joint British Diabetes Societies suggests:

- 0.9% sodium chloride (+/- potassium as necessary) is generally advocated, as the majority of losses are sodium, chloride and potassium
- 0.45% sodium chloride is only used if osmolality is no longer declining despite adequate fluid resuscitation
- Replace potassium if <5.5 mmol/l
- Targets for treatment:
  i K⁺ 4.0–5.5 mmol/l
  ii Na⁺ reduction by ≤10 mmol/l in 24 hours
  iii Glucose reduction by ≤5 mmol/l per hour

4 **Normalisation of blood glucose**
  - Fluid replacement alone will result in a falling blood glucose (there is a risk however of precipitously dropping the osmolality)
  - Start a low dose insulin infusion (0.05 units/kg/hour) *only once glucose values are no longer decreasing with fluid resuscitation* (unless ketonaemia is identified)

5 **Prevention of complications**
  - Thrombotic events (including myocardial infarction (MI) and ischaemic stroke) are more common than in DKA
  - Care of pressure areas is mandatory in this group of patients

What are the indications for potential admission to HDU/ICU?

1 Osmolality >350 mosmol/kg
2 Sodium >160 mmol/l
3 pH <7.1
4 K⁺ <3.5 or >6 mmol/l
5 GCS <12
6 SpO₂ <92% on room air
7 SBP <90 mmHg
8 Heart rate <60 and >100 bpm
9 Urine output <0.5 ml/kg/hour
10 Creatinine >200 μmol/l
11 Hypothermia
12 MI, stroke or other serious comorbidity

Further Reading

British Society for Paediatric Endocrinology and Diabetes, 2015. *BSPED Recommended Guideline for the Management of Children and Young People under the Age of 18 Years with Diabetic Ketoacidosis* [online]. Available at: www.bsped.org.uk/clinical/docs/DKAguideline.pdf (Accessed: 16 November 2016)

Joint British Diabetes Societies Inpatient Care Group, 2013. *The Management of Diabetic Ketoacidosis in Adults* [online]. Available at: www.diabetologists-abcd.org.uk/jbds/JBDS_IP_DKA_Adults_Revised.pdf (Accessed: 16 November 2016)

Joint British Diabetes Societies Inpatient Care Group, 2012. The management of the hyperosmolar hyperglycaemic state (HHS) in adults with diabetes [online]. Available at: www.diabetologists-abcd.org.uk/jbds/jbds_ip_hhs_adults.pdf (Accessed: 16 November 2016)

Chapter 27

Diagnosing Brainstem Death

What is the definition of brain death?

Death is defined as the simultaneous and irreversible loss of both the capacity for consciousness and the capacity to breathe.

Brain death is a complete and irreversible loss of brain and brainstem function as a result of neurological injury. The heart is still beating but respiratory function is dependent on a ventilator.

The Academy of the Medical Royal Colleges UK (AoMRC) code for the diagnosis of death by neurological criteria outlines three essential components:

1 Fulfilment of essential preconditions
2 Exclusion of potentially reversible causes of coma
3 Formal demonstration of coma and apnoea

What are the pre-conditions for brainstem testing?

1 The patient should be deeply unconscious, apnoeic and mechanically ventilated
2 Irreversible brain damage of known aetiology
   – On the rare occasions where this is uncertain, an extended period of observation and support may be required to confirm the pathology is indeed irreversible

What are the exclusion criteria?

It is essential to ensure that coma is not secondary to reversible factors such as CNS depressant drugs, biochemical/metabolic abnormalities or hypothermia. The AoMRC code of practice sets out guidelines on such causes (Table 27.1).

Approaches to possible drug intoxication as the cause of coma include:

1 A period of observation 2–3 times the elimination half-life of the drug in question
2 Administration of specific antagonists
3 Plasma analysis (Table 27.2)
4 Confirmatory test to confirm absence of cerebral blood flow/perfusion

Table 27.1 AoMRC potentially reversible causes for coma

System	Factor	Lower limit	Upper limit	Notes
Circulatory	MAP	> 60 mmHg		
Respiratory	pH	7.35	7.45	
	pCO_2		<6.0 kPa	
	pO_2	>10 kPa		
Metabolic	Temperature	34 °C		
Biochemical	Sodium	115 mmol/l	160 mmol/l	Derangements as
	Potassium	>2 mmol/l	3 mmol/l	a result of the
	Magnesium	0.5 mmol/l	3 mmol/l	process of
	Phosphate	0.5 mmol/l		brainstem
				death (i.e.
				diabetes
				insipidus) may
				not require
				correction
				before testing
	Glucose	3 mmol/l	20 mmol/l	Check immediately before brainstem testing

Table 27.2 Plasma analysis of agents with long or unpredictable half lives

Midazolam	Brainstem testing should not be undertaken if midazolam level is >10 µg/l
Thiopentone	Brainstem testing should not be undertaken if thiopentone level is >5 mg/l

Who can perform a brain death examination?

Two competent clinicians who have held General Medical Council (GMC) registration for more than 5 years, one of whom must be a consultant.

How is brainstem testing performed?

Formal brainstem testing consists of two components: An examination of the integrity of the sensory and motor pathways of cranial nerve (CN) reflexes (Table 27.3) and the apnoea test.

Table 27.3 Cranial nerve tests

Test	Afferent	Efferent	Procedure
Pupillary reflex	II	III	A bright light is shone into each eye in turn to look for direct and consensual reflexes
Corneal reflex	V	VII	The cornea is brushed lightly with a swab
Response to painful stimulus	V	VII	A painful stimulus is applied to the supraorbital ridge
Vestibulo-ocular reflex	VIII	III, IV, VI	Visualise the tympanic membrane prior to beginning the test. Instil 50 ml ice cold saline into each external auditory meatus in turn, looking for eye movement/nystagmus
Gag reflex	IX	X	The pharynx is stimulated with a spatula/similar device
Cough reflex	X	X	A bronchial catheter is passed down the endotracheal tube to stimulate the carina

Apnoea test procedure:

1 Increase the FiO_2 to 1.0
2 Perform an ABG to confirm that the measured $PaCO_2$ and SaO_2 correlate with the monitored values
3 Decrease the minute volume by lowering the respiratory rate until end-tidal CO_2 is at above 6.0 kPa
   Check an ABG to ensure $PaCO_2$ >6.0 kPa and the pH is less than 7.4
4 Maintain apnoeic oxygenation by either instilling 5 l/min oxygen via suction catheter or by using CPAP (and possibly a prior recruitment manoeuvre)
5 Five-minute observation period to look for the presence of spontaneous respiratory activity
   Ensure haemodynamic stability throughout the test
6 Perform a final ABG to confirm an increase in $PaCO_2$ of >0.5 kPa.

Following completion, the ventilator should be reconnected and any acid-base abnormality must be corrected before performing the second set of tests. There is no defined time interval between both sets of tests.

When is the legal time of death?

The time at which the first set of tests was completed.

What auxiliary tests are available?

There are several circumstances where brain death cannot be confirmed according to clinical testing alone. These include:

1 Inability to exclude the influence of residual sedative drugs
2 High cervical cord injury
3 Severe maxillofacial injury

Confirmatory tests can be performed to establish diagnosis of brainstem death in these circumstances. Testing can be divided into flow studies and studies of brain electrical activity (Table 27.4).

Table 27.4 Auxiliary tests to aid confirmation of brain death

Measures of brain electrical activity	EEG	Most popular and validated test worldwide. Little value in hypothermia or drug intoxication as these factors can suppress neuronal activity.
	Somatosensory evoked potential (SSEP)	A peripheral stimulus given (i.e. median nerve) and a response is measured at the contralateral primary sensory cortex
Flow studies	Cerebral angiography	A confirmatory test reveals absence of intracerebral filling beyond the entry of the carotid and vertebral arteries into the skull
	Transcranial Doppler	Useful only if a reliable waveform is found. Complete absence of flow may not be reliable if inadequate windows exist.

Further Reading

Academy of the Medical Royal Colleges, 2008. A Code of pactice for the diagnosis and confirmation of death. Available at: www.aomrc.org.uk/publications/reports-guidance/ukdec-reports-and-guidance/code-practice-diagnosis-confirmation-death/ (Accessed: 5 February 2017)

NHS Blood and Transplant. Donation after brain-stem death [online]. Available at: https://www.odt.nhs.uk/deceased-donation/best-practice-guidance/donation-after-brain-stem-death/ (Accessed: 5 February 2017)

Oram J, Murphy P. Diagnosis of death. *Contin Educ Anaesth Crit Care Pain* 2011; **11**(3): 77–81

Chapter 28

Diarrhoea

What is the definition of the term *diarrhoea*?

There are no universally accepted definitions of diarrhoea. WHO define it as *the passage of three or more loose or liquid stools per day*. The British Society of Gastroenterology's definition is similar, but provides an alternative quantitative definition as *the passage of greater than 200 g of stool per day*. Other definitions include the passage of more stool than is normal for an individual person, or the passage of watery stool. The Bristol Stool Chart classes type 6 or 7 stool as diarrhoea.

What is the incidence of diarrhoea in intensive care?

Approximately 25–50% of patients will have diarrhoea during their intensive care admission.

What is the pathophysiology of diarrhoea?

Diarrhoea is essentially due to an imbalance of water and solute transport in the gastrointestinal tract and may result from one or more of four different patho-physiological mechanisms (Table 28.1).

What are the causes of diarrhoea on the intensive care unit?

The causes of diarrhoea can be divided into infective and non-infective.

Infective causes:

1 Bacterial, e.g. *E. coli, Salmonella, Campylobacter jejuni, Clostridium difficile, Shigella*
2 Viral, e.g. *Norovirus, Rotavirus*
3 Fungal, e.g. *Candida*
4 Protozoal, e.g. *Cryptosporidia, Giardia lamblia*

Non-infective causes:

1 Inflammatory bowel disease (IBD), e.g. Ulcerative colitis, Crohn's
2 Drug-related, e.g. enteral feeds (the commonest cause of non-infective diarrhoea in ICU), antibiotics including beta lactams and macrolides, oral magnesium salts, laxatives, chemotherapy agents, NSAIDs, alcohol, antacids

Table 28.1 Different types of diarrhoea

Type	Pathophysiology	Example
Osmotic	There is failure of the GI tract to absorb osmotically active solutes, meaning that water is retained within the gut lumen Improves with starvation	Enteral feed-associated diarrhoea
Secretory	There is increased secretion or reduced reabsorption of salt and water across the gut mucosa Large volume diarrhoea often results Does not improve with starvation	Enterotoxin production, e.g. *Vibrio cholerae* causes sodium secretion into bowel Laxative use
Inflammatory	There is loss of integrity of the GI mucosa due to inflammation, impaired absorption of bowel contents and exudative fluid loss Bloody diarrhoea may result if the process affects the colon	Inflammatory bowel disease
Dysmotility	There may be rapid transit time through the GI tract and the water and electrolyte load from the small bowel overwhelms the absorptive capacity of the colon	Following recovery from ileus

3 Mesenteric ischaemia
4 Bacterial overgrowth causing bile salt malabsorption
5 Short gut syndrome
6 Post-ileus recovery or overflow diarrhoea in impaction or pseudo-obstruction
7 Food intolerance, e.g. Coeliac disease, lactose intolerance
8 Others e.g. anxiety, irritable bowel syndrome

What are the problems with ongoing diarrhoea in an ICU patient?

Diarrhoea causes patient-related problems and organisational problems.

Patient-related:

1 Increased risk of pressure sores
2 Increased risk of infection

Organisational:

1 Significant workload for nursing staff
2 Infection control risk to other patients on the ICU: barrier precautions and meticulous hand hygiene are essential

How would you manage a patient with diarrhoea?

The patient with diarrhoea should be managed with an ABCDE approach, treating abnormalities as they are found. Specific management includes:

1 History and examination
   - Travel and exposure to potential sources of infection
   - Onset, duration and characteristics of the diarrhoea
   - Presence of systemic symptoms
   - Drug history including immunosuppressants and any medication that was recently stopped
   - Determine whether the patient is dehydrated
   - Abdominal tenderness and localised peritonism should raise concern – seek a surgical opinion
   - Rectal examination will exclude impaction and overflow diarrhoea as a differential

2 Investigation should initially be directed towards excluding infective causes and includes:
   i Blood tests (FBC, U+E, CRP, LFTs, coagulation screen, blood cultures)
   ii Stool samples should be sent for:
      - Microscopy, culture and sensitivity (MC+S)
      - *C. difficile* toxin
      - Virology
      - Cysts, ova and parasites
   iii Radiological investigation should be tailored to clinical findings
      - Plain abdominal X-ray should be performed in any patient with abdominal tenderness or with confirmed *C. difficile* infection
      - Erect CXR if perforation is suspected
      - CT abdomen and pelvis with or without contrast to further delineate pathology e.g. in mesenteric ischaemia
   iv Flexible sigmoidoscopy/colonoscopy
      - If diarrhoea persists and no cause has been found, consider performing a flexible sigmoidoscopy or colonoscopy
      - Caution should be exercised in patients with acute colitis, who are at high risk of perforation with this procedure

3 Specific points to remember:
   i Early and regular surgical review is indicated in immunosuppressed patients and those with significant abdominal tenderness, elevated white cell count (WCC) or associated organ dysfunction

ii Treatment for diarrhoea is largely supportive, aimed at maintaining hydration, monitoring and correcting electrolytes and acid-base balance, and avoiding complications

iii Infection should be treated with appropriate antimicrobial agents

iv In the case of enteral feed-associated diarrhoea, changing the feed or enriching the feed with fibre may help
 – Once infection and overflow have been excluded, an anti-motility drug may be given, e.g. loperamide 2 mg up to 4 hourly

v A bowel management system may be employed to reduce nursing workload and mitigate the increased risk of pressure sores

vi Meticulous infection control measures should be employed

What is *Clostridium difficile*?

Clostridium difficile is an anaerobic, spore-forming gram positive bacillus. It produces two toxins: Toxin A (an enterotoxin, which causes fluid sequestration in the bowel) and Toxin B (a cytotoxin, which is detected with the CDT test). It is a common and serious nosocomial infection often arising in situations where the patient's normal gut flora have been eradicated, such as following broad spectrum antibiotic therapy. *C. difficile* infection produces copious, offensive, watery stools with a characteristic odour. The spores are not killed by alcohol gel, so handwashing with soap and water is mandatory.

What are the risk factors for *C. difficile* infection?

Risk factors for *C. difficile* infection include:

1 Age >60
2 Broad spectrum antibiotic therapy
3 Underlying malignancy
4 Albumin <25 g/l
5 Renal disease
6 Pulmonary disease
7 Proton pump inhibitor therapy

Tell me specifically how you would approach a patient with confirmed *C. difficile* infection

The patient should be investigated as previously discussed, isolated, and the infection control team informed. Full barrier precautions should be employed and handwashing with soap and water should be carried out before and after every contact with the patient or their environment.

The treatment of *C. difficile* infection is with oral or parenteral metronidazole or oral vancomycin.

C. difficile diarrhoea will progress to fulminant pseudomembranous colitis in approximately 20%, and mortality in this group of patients approaches 20%. The patient is at risk of developing toxic megacolon and perforation.

Further Reading

Thibault R, Graf S, Clerc A, et al. Diarrhoea in the ICU: respective contribution of feeding and antibiotics. *Crit Care* 2013; 17(4): R153

Tirlapur N, Puthucheary Z A, Cooper J A, et al. Diarrhoea in the critically ill is common, associated with poor outcome, and rarely due to Clostridium difficile [online]. Available at: www.nature.com/articles/srep24691 (Accessed: 8 March 2017)

Chapter 29

Disorders of Consciousness

What are the main disorders of consciousness? What are the features of each?

Consciousness encompasses two main components: arousal and awareness. A disrupted relationship between these two components characterise disorders of consciousness.

The main disorders of consciousness (DOC) as defined by the Royal College of Physicians working party guideline (2013) are:

1 **Coma** (absent wakefulness and absent awareness)
   - A state of unrousable unresponsiveness, lasting more than 6 hours in which a person:
     i Cannot be awakened
     ii Fails to respond normally to painful stimuli, light or sound
     iii Lacks a normal sleep-wake cycle *and*
     iv Does not initiate voluntary actions
2 **Vegetative state** (VS) (wakefulness with absent awareness)
   - Severe cortical damage with preservation of some brainstem activity
   - Preserved capacity for spontaneous or stimulus-induced arousal, evidenced by:
     i Sleep-wake cycles
     ii Range of reflexive and spontaneous behaviours
   - Complete absence of environmental awareness and awareness of self
3 **Minimally conscious state** (MCS) (wakefulness with minimal awareness)
   - A state of severely altered consciousness in which minimal but clearly discernible behavioural evidence of self or environmental awareness is demonstrated
   - MCS is characterised by inconsistent but reproducible responses above the level of spontaneous or reflexive behaviour, indicating some degree of interaction with their surroundings.

Following acute brain injury, many patients will progress through stages of coma, VS and MCS as they emerge into a state of full awareness (Figure 29.1). Some will remain in a vegetative or minimally conscious state for the rest of their lives.

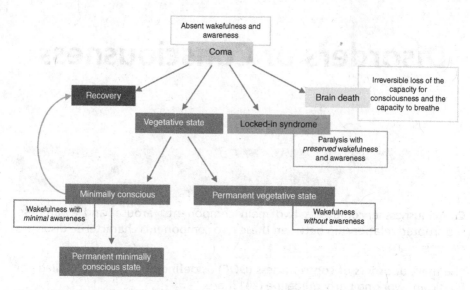

Figure 29.1 States of consciousness following acute brain injury

What are the causes of disordered consciousness?

A brain injury giving rise to disordered consciousness may result from one of many causes. The major causes are listed in Table 29.1.

Table 29.1 Common causes of brain injury resulting in disorders of consciousness

Aetiology	Examples
Traumatic brain injury	Direct impact head injury Diffuse axonal injury (DAI) resulting from deceleration
Vascular event	Intracerebral haemorrhage (ICH) Subarachnoid haemorrhage (SAH) Ischaemic stroke
Toxic / metabolic	Alcohol Drugs in overdose or poisons Anaesthetics, benzodiazepines, opioids Severe hypoglycaemia, hyper- or hypo-osmolar states
Infection / inflammation	Encephalitis Abscess Vasculitis Sepsis (including tropical diseases)
Hypoxia / hypoperfusion	Cardiorespiratory arrest Profound hypovolaemia Drowning
Systemic illness	Liver failure Renal failure Endocrine causes e.g. myxoedema

How would you manage a patient presenting with disordered consciousness?

The management of a patient with disordered consciousness should follow an ABCDE approach, treating abnormalities as they are found. A GCS ≤8 necessitates intubation to protect the airway, prevent secondary brain injury and facilitate imaging. Other specific management includes:

1 **History, examination and investigation**
   - Identify the cause of brain injury and potential complications
   - Exclude other conditions that may impair consciousness (metabolic/infective disorders, hydrocephalus etc.)
   - Blood tests including glucose, haematology, full biochemistry, TFTs, ammonia (if hepatic encephalopathy suspected), ABG
   - Specimens for culture
   - Blood alcohol values, toxicology screen
   - Consider lumbar puncture (LP) if no signs of raised ICP
   - Imaging (CT or MRI) – Exclude structural, operable reasons for DOC (e.g. hydrocephalus, haemorrhage)
2 **Maintain normal physiology**
   - Rapidly correct hypoxaemia and hypotension
   - Correct hypoglycaemia with 50 ml 50% glucose
   - Correct hypo- and hyperthermia
   - Correct electrolyte abnormalities and ensure adequate hydration
3 **Review medication**
   - Review and withdraw any medications that may affect arousal
   - Consider specific antagonists
4 **Electroengephalogram (EEG) or trial of an anticonvulsant** (if subclinical seizure activity is suspected)
5 **Detailed neurological assessment**
   - Confirm sensory, visual and auditory pathways are intact
6 **ICP management**
   - If raised ICP is present, consider insertion of an ICP monitor and initiate therapy to reduce raised ICP
7 **Further investigations**
   - Electrophysiological tests e.g. visual, auditory or somatosensory evoked potentials (SSEPs)

How can you prognosticate in disordered consciousness?

A careful neurological examination is the foundation for prognostication in DOC. The prognosis for coma, VS and MCS is difficult to establish at an individual level, but certain factors point toward a better outcome. These factors include young age, traumatic aetiology and short duration of the state.

Adequate time must be allowed for the metabolism of sedative drugs and NMBAs (at least 72 hours post-return of spontaneous circulation (ROSC)). Hypothermia invalidates standard guidelines and makes prognosticating patients in a coma after cardiac arrest particularly problematic. The 2014 European Resuscitation Council (ERC) consensus guidelines recommend waiting 72 hours *after* return of normothermia.

Multiple predictors should be utilised to prognosticate (see Table 29.2), hence the process is dependent on locally available tests and expertise. Ultimately, an uncertain observation outcome should equate to a prolonged period of observation. Absence of clinical improvement over time suggests a worse outcome.

Figure 29.2 illustrates the prognostication algorithm suggested by the ERC following a cardiac arrest, which should be applied ≥72 hours post-ROSC if after the exclusion of confounding factors, the patient remains unconscious with a GCS motor score of 1 or 2.

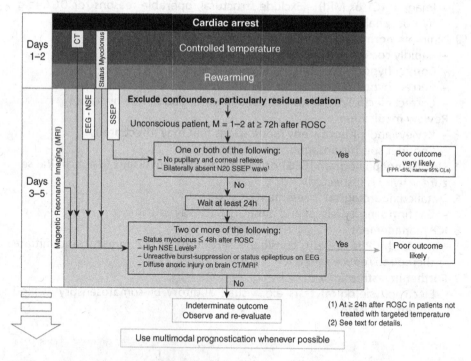

Figure 29.2 ERC prognostication algorithm
Reproduced with kind permission from Sandroni C, et al. (*Intensive Care Med* 2014)
FPR – false positive rate; CIs – confidence intervals

Table 29.2 Tools to prognosticate in adult comatose survivors of cardiac arrest

Predictor	Detail	Advantages	Disadvantages
SSEPs (Somatosensory evoked potentials)	Bilateral absence of SSEP N20 wave at ≥72 hours post-ROSC is used to predict poor outcome	Reliable test to predict poor outcome Not influenced by sedatives, analgesics, NMBAs or metabolic insults	Requires appropriate skill and expertise Avoid electrical interference Affected by hypothermia
EEG	The following features are used at ≥72 hours post-ROSC to predict poor outcome: i Absence of EEG reactivity to external stimuli ii Presence of burst-suppression iii Status epilepticus	Non-invasive Of prognostic significance alongside aiding in assessing level of consciousness which may be masked by sedation etc. Detects non-convulsive status epilepticus	Operator-dependent Non-quantitative Lacking standardisation Interpretation requires considerable expertise
Biomarkers	Neuron-specific enolase (NSE) S-100B Released following injury to neurons, hence likely to correlate with the severity of neurological injury	Quantitative results Likely independence from the effects of sedatives	Difficult to find a consistent threshold for identifying patients with poor outcome Haemolysis creates false positives, hence sampling at multiple time points is ideal Need for standardisation of the measuring techniques
Imaging	MRI CT Useful in excluding further causes of coma such as SAH Brain CT and MRI should only be used for prognosticating poor outcome after cardiac arrest only combination with other predictors	Advantages of MRI over brain CT: i Better spatial definition ii High sensitivity for identifying ischaemic brain injury	Performing an MRI is problematic in clinically unstable patients Limited evidence for the role of MRI and CT in prognostication

What is locked-in syndrome and how does it differ from DOC?

Locked-in syndrome usually results from brainstem pathology that disrupts the voluntary control of movement without abolishing either wakefulness or awareness. Patients who are locked-in are paralysed but conscious and can usually communicate by blinking their eyes.

Further Reading

Gossaries O, et al. Disorders of Consciousness: Coma, Vegetative and Minimally Conscious State. In: Cvetkovic D, et al. *States of Consciousness*, The Frontiers Collection. Springer-Verlag Berlin Heidelberg 2011; 29–55

Patel S, Hirsch N. Coma. *Contin Educ Anaesth Crit Care Pain* 2014; **14**(5): 220–223

Royal College of Physicians, 2013. Prolonged disorders of consciousness national clinical guidelines. Report of a working party [online]. www.rcplondon.ac.uk/guidelines-policy/prolonged-disorders-consciousness-national-clinical-guidelines (Accessed: 27 November 2016)

Sandroni C, Cariou A, Cavallaro F, et al. Prognostication in comatose survivors of cardiac arrest: An advisory statement from the European Resuscitation Council and the European Society of Intensive Care Medicine. *Intensive Care Med* 2014; **40**(12): 1816–1831

Chapter 30

Donation after Circulatory Death

What are the ethical principles that govern the management of a donation after circulatory death (DCD) donor prior to withdrawal of life-sustaining support?

No treatment specifically aimed at organ donation should be started prior to the decision to withdraw treatment being made.

Legal Guidance in the UK stipulates that maintenance of life-sustaining treatment can be considered to be in the best interests of a patient who wanted to be a donor if it facilitates donation and does not cause them harm or distress (this can include increases in FiO_2 and ventilatory support, changing the rate of fluid administration or inserting venous cannulae). Agents can be used to maintain arterial pressure (in accordance with local policy).

It is not appropriate to initiate treatment against the wishes of the family.

What is the process of controlled organ donation after circulatory death?

Once the retrieval team is prepared in the operating theatre, and when the family is ready, life-sustaining treatment is withdrawn.

Following cessation of cardio-respiratory function, there is a five-minute period to confirm monitored asystole prior to certification of death by a doctor independent of the retrieval team. After certification of death, the relatives may spend up to five minutes with the patient before transfer to the operating theatre (if longer is required, the donation process will require review).

In cases of lung donation, reintubation will be required (if the patient has been extubated) following confirmation of death. The lungs should be recruited with a single breath on instruction of the retrieval team and CPAP maintained with 100% O_2. Ventilation is not reinstated until after the chest has been opened and the aorta clamped.

What is functional warm ischaemia and how does this vary for different organs?

Functional warm ischaemia (FWI) starts when the systolic blood pressure falls <50 mmHg or SpO_2 <70%. Stand-down times from the onset of FWI vary by organ and by receiving centre. Approximate timings are as follows and will vary with each case:

Liver	30 minutes
Pancreas	30 minutes
Lungs	60 minutes (from onset of FWI to mechanical re-inflation of lungs)
Kidney	120 minutes

Tell me about the Maastricht classification for donation after circulatory death

Donation after circulatory death refers to the retrieval of organs for the purpose of transplantation from patients whose death is diagnosed and confirmed using cardio-respiratory criteria.

There are two principle types of DCD: controlled and uncontrolled. Uncontrolled DCD occurs after a cardiac arrest that is unexpected, whereas controlled DCD occurs after planned withdrawal of life-sustaining treatments. The Maastricht criteria describe the clinical circumstances in which DCD can occur (see Table 30.1).

Table 30.1 The Maastricht classification for donation after circulatory death

Category	Type	Circumstances	Typical location
1	Uncontrolled	Dead on arrival	ED
2	Uncontrolled	Unsuccessful resuscitation	ED
3	Controlled	Cardiac arrest follows planned withdrawal of life-sustaining treatment	ICU
4	Either	Cardiac arrest in a patient who is brain dead	ICU
5	Uncontrolled	Cardiac arrest in hospital inpatient	Hospital

What are the absolute contraindications to organ donation?

The only absolute contraindications to referral as a potential organ donor are:

1 Variant CJD
2 HIV disease (but not HIV infection)

Patients with one or more of the following conditions are unlikely to be accepted as potential donors, as per NHS Blood and Transplant:

1 Active invasive cancer in the last 3 years excluding non-melanoma skin cancer and primary brain tumour
2 Primary intracerebral lymphoma
3 All secondary intracerebral tumours
4 Haematological malignancy
5 Melanoma (except completely excised stage 1 cancers)
6 Untreated systemic infection
7 Active and untreated TB
8 West Nile virus
9 History of Ebola infection

There is no longer an upper or lower age limit for potential donors.

Further Reading

Dunne K, Doherty P. Donation after circulatory death. *Contin Educ Anaesth Crit Care Pain* 2011; **11**(3): 82–86

Intensive Care Society/NHS Blood and Transplant/British Transplantation Society, 2010. *Organ Donation after Circulatory Death. Report of a Consensus Meeting* [online]. Available at: www.odt.nhs.uk/pdf/DCD_Consensus_2010.pdf (Accessed: 5 February 2017)

NHS Blood and Transplant, 2016. *Donation after Circulatory Death* [online]. Available at: www.odt.nhs.uk/deceased-donation/best-practice-guidance/donation-after-circulatory-death/ (Accessed: February 2017)

Chapter 31

Drowning

Define *drowning*

Drowning is defined as primary respiratory impairment following submersion or immersion in a liquid medium, whatever the outcome. The terms *near-drowning* (used to describe survivors of drowning) and *dry drowning* (used to describe drowning victims without aspiration that are now thought to have died from another cause prior to submersion) were abandoned in 2002. Drowning may be classified according to clinical findings at the scene (Table 31.1).

Table 31.1 Classification of drowning

Class 1	No evidence of aspiration
Class 2	Evidence of aspiration but with adequate ventilation
Class 3	Evidence of aspiration with inadequate ventilation
Class 4	Absent ventilation and circulation

What are the pathophysiological changes that occur during drowning?

The pathophysiology of drowning is outlined in Figure 31.1. Other effects include:

Cardiovascular

i The *diving reflex* (aims to conserve oxygen)
  - Stimulated by the application of cold water to the face
  - Mediated by CN V_1
  - Results in apnoea, bradycardia and vasoconstriction
ii A massive catecholamine surge follows the diving reflex, causing:
  - Profound vasoconstriction
  - Arrhythmias
  - Pulmonary oedema
iii Progressive hypoxaemia and hypothermia leading to bradycardia, pulmonary hypertension and cardiac failure

iv In patients with cardiac arrest due to drowning, an initial shockable rhythm is
present in approximately 5% of cases only

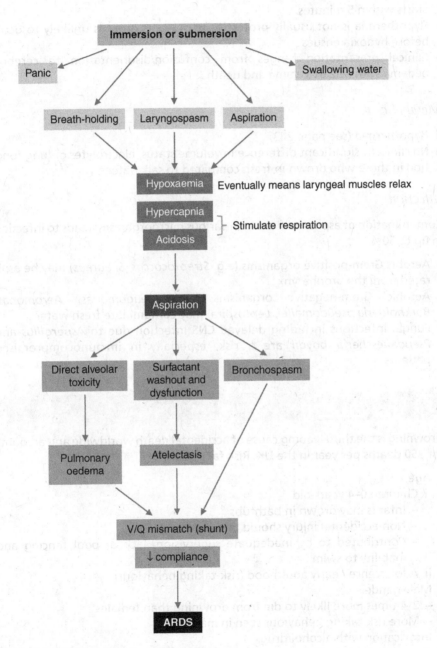

Figure 31.1 Pathophysiology of drowning

Neurological

Hypoxic brain injury

- Leading cause of morbidity and mortality in drowning
- Starts within 5 minutes
- Hypothermia is not usually protective because its onset is unlikely to occur before hypoxia ensues
- Clinical presentation ranges from confusion/disorientation to cerebral oedema with seizures, coma and death

Metabolic

i Hypothermia (see page 243)
ii No clinically significant difference in volume status, electrolytes or lung function in those who drown in fresh compared to salt water

Infection

Contamination of aspirated fluid with various microorganisms leads to infection in up to 50%

- Aerobic Gram-positive organisms (e.g. *Streptococcus, S. aureus*) may be aspirated from the oropharynx
- Aerobic Gram-negative organisms (e.g. *Pseudomonas, Aeromonas, Burkholderia pseudomallei, Leptospira*) may contaminate fresh water
- Fungal infections including delayed CNS infection due to *Aspergillus* and *Pseudallescheria boydii* are a risk, especially in immunocompromised patients

What are the risk factors for drowning?

Drowning is the third leading cause of accidental death worldwide and accounts for 350 deaths per year in the UK. Risk factors are:

1 Age:
  i Children 0–4 years-old
    - Infants may drown in bathtubs
    - Non-accidental injury should be considered
    - Contributed to by inadequate supervision, lack of pool fencing and inability to swim
  ii Adolescence / early adulthood (risk-taking behaviour)
2 Male gender
  - 2–4 times more likely to die from drowning than females
  - More risk-taking behaviour seen in males
3 Intoxication with alcohol/drugs
4 Occupation and hobbies
  i Scuba diving

   ii Farming
   iii Fishing
5 Medical conditions
   i Cardiac: ischaemic heart disease (IHD), cardiomyopathies, arrhythmias (especially channelopathies and long QT syndrome)
   ii Neurological: epilepsy, cerebrovascular disease
   iii Diabetes
   iv Depression
6 Conditions increasing the risk of drowning in open water
   i Currents
   ii Rip tides
   iii Waves
   · iv Cold water

What is the immediate management of a drowning victim?

The victim should be removed from the water promptly. The chances of a spinal injury in a drowning victim are very low. Spinal precautions are only necessary if there is a history of diving in shallow water or signs of severe injury after recreational activity such as kitesurfing.

Cardiac arrest and neurological injury in drowned patients are primarily due to hypoxia, and so the Advanced Life Support (ALS) priorities are different as compared with typical adult arrest scenarios (when the primary cause is more likely to be cardiac). Important points are:

1 Administer *five rescue breaths* (with oxygen if available)
2 If there is no response, begin compressions
3 Compression only CPR is not appropriate in drowning
4 The effects of hypothermia should be taken into consideration (see page 243)

On arrival to hospital, the management priorities are:

1 Initial management should follow an **ATLS approach**:
   – Secure the airway with an ETT if indicated
   – Respiratory examination may reveal signs of aspiration (dyspnoea, wheeze, crackles)
   – Record the GCS on scene and on arrival (has prognostic significance)
   – Treat any life-threatening injuries
2 **Optimise oxygenation**
   – Lung protective ventilatory strategy
   – No evidence to support the use of steroids
   – Bronchoscopy may be useful to remove aspirated debris
3 **Optimise cardiac output**
   – Significant hypovolaemia is common, especially in prolonged submersion and hypothermia – prompt fluid resuscitation is key
   – Inotropes/vasopressors should be considered in the presence of haemodynamic instability

4 **Neuroprotective measures** (see page 480)
   – No evidence to support the routine use of barbiturates or ICP monitoring
5 **Temperature control** to ~34°C
6 There is no evidence to support the routine use of prophylactic **antibiotics**, but empirical antibiotics may be considered in:
   i Patients who drown in grossly contaminated water
   ii Patients who develop signs of pneumonia

Is there any evidence for the use of ECMO in drowning?

A retrospective review of the ECLS international registry by **Burke, et al** (Resuscitation, 2016) revealed 247 patients who received ECLS following drowning between 1986 and 2015. Cardiac arrest with ROSC prior to ECLS occurred in 34.8%, ECLS was initiated during cardiac arrest (ECPR) in 31.2%, and 34.0% did not arrest prior to ECLS. Overall survival was 51.4%, with a statistically significant increase in survival across all three categories of patient. Interestingly, the use of veno-venous ECLS, a surrogate for predominantly respiratory failure, was associated with better survival than the use of veno-arterial ECLS in patients with cardiopulmonary failure. The presence of AKI and need for CPR during ECLS were associated with increased mortality.

What are the indicators for a poor prognosis in drowning victims?

1 Submersion >5–10 minutes
2 Resuscitation not attempted for >10 minutes after rescue
3 >25 minutes of resuscitation
4 GCS <5 or unreactive pupils on arrival to hospital
5 Pulseless and apnoeic on arrival to hospital
6 pH <7.10 on initial arterial blood gas

Further Reading

Burke C R, et al. Extracorporeal life support for victims of drowning. *Resuscitation* 2016; **104**: 19–23

Deakin C, et al. on behalf of the Resuscitation Council (UK), 2015. Prehospital resuscitation [online]. Available at: www.resus.org.uk/resuscitation-guidelines/prehospital-resuscitation/ (Accessed: 19 March 2017)

Martinez F E, Hooper A J. Drowning and immersion injury. *Anaesth Int Care Med* 2014; **15**(9): 420–423

Chapter 32

Encephalitis

Define *encephalitis* and tell me how it presents

Encephalitis is inflammation of the brain parenchyma. Most pathogens are viral and gain access to the CSF via haematogenous spread; some pathogens invade directly via neuronal transport.

Acute encephalitis usually develops over a number of days and a prodromal illness may be absent. Patients may present with:

1 Personality change
2 Headaches
3 Confusion
4 Seizures including status epilepticus
5 Focal neurology
6 Coma

What are the causes of encephalitis?

Encephalitis may be caused by viruses (most common), bacteria, fungi and TB. It may also occur as the result of an autoimmune process such as anti-NMDA receptor or anti-gamma-aminobutyric acid (GABA)-B receptor encephalitis.

Specifically, which viruses cause encephalitis?

The most common causative viral pathogens are:

1 HSV-1
2 Enterovirus
3 VZV
4 EBV
5 Rabies
6 CMV

How would you attempt to diagnose encephalitis?

1 History and examination:
   - Full history from the patient

– Collateral history important, as patient may be confused
– Particular focus on neurological examination

2 Blood tests:
  – FBC (WCC and differential may help to differentiate bacterial meningitis from viral meningo-encephalitis)
  – CRP
  – U+E, LFTs, TFTs (to exclude other causes of confusion)
  – Clotting to assess coagulopathy as a lumbar puncture may be necessary
  – Blood cultures
  – Autoimmune serology
  – Consider HIV testing

3 Imaging:
  – CT brain +/- contrast
  – MRI (more sensitive and is the investigation of choice if available)

4 EEG

5 LP (if not contraindicated, i.e. signs of raised ICP or coagulopathy):
  – Urgent cell count and gram stain
  – Cytology
  – Viral polymerase chain reaction (PCR)
  – Biochemistry (glucose, protein)
  – Culture (bacteria and fungi)
  – Autoantibodies

What are the differential diagnoses of encephalitis?

1 Infection
  – Meningitis
  – Cerebral abscess
  – Sepsis causing confusion/altered mental state
  – HIV

2 Vascular
  – Ischaemic stroke/TIA
  – Intracranial haemorrhage
  – Posterior reversible encephalopathy syndrome (PRES) – usually in hypertensive patients

3 Malignancy
  – Primary including lymphoma
  – Metastases

4 Toxins/metabolic encephalopathy
  – Hepatic encephalopathy
  – Uraemia
  – Thyroid crisis
  – Electrolyte disturbance, particularly sodium (but also magnesium and calcium)
  – Illicit drugs, e.g. cocaine, MDMA, amphetamines, lysergic acid diethylamide (LSD)

- Overdose, e.g. TCAs, SSRIs
- Serotonin syndrome or neuroleptic malignant syndrome

5 Automimmune
- Anti-NMDA or anti-GABA-B receptor encephalitis
- Vasculitis,
- Cerebral lupus
- Acute disseminated encephalomyelitis (ADEM), e.g. secondary to viral infection or following vaccination to rabies

6 Other
- Non-convulsive status epilepticus

What is the treatment?

The patient with encephalitis should be managed with an ABCDE approach, treating abnormalities as they are found. Specific management involves:

1 Antiviral therapy with aciclovir 10 mg/kg tds, continued for at least 14 days
2 A third generation cephalosporin, e.g. ceftriaxone 2 g tds, may be added to cover bacterial meningitis
3 The role of steroids in HSV encephalitis is controversial

What is the prognosis?

When treated the mortality of HSV encephalitis is approximately 10%. If untreated, the mortality approaches 80%.

Of those who survive, the complication rate is high. Patients most commonly suffer memory loss, but may also suffer behavioural and personality changes, speech problems or epilepsy.

How would your treatment differ in patients with immunocompromise?

Consideration should be given to testing for HIV if status unknown, as well as for opportunistic infections such as fungal encephalitis (*Cryptococcus neoformans*).

What are the CSF findings in viral meningitis/encephalitis?

Typical CSF findings in various pathologies are outlined in Table 32.1.

Table 32.1 CSF findings in meningoencephalitis

	Normal	Bacterial	Viral	Fungal	TB
Opening pressure (cmH$_2$O)	10–20	High	Normal/high	Very high	High
Appearance	Clear	Turbid	Gin clear	Fibrin web	Turbid
CSF:plasma glucose ratio	50–66%	Low (<50%)	Normal	Low/normal	Very low (<30%)
Protein (g/l)	<0.45	High (>1)	Normal	High (0.2–5)	High (1–5)
Cell Count (per mm^3)	<5	>1000	<500	100–500	50–1500
WCC differential	Lymphocytes	Polymorphs	Lymphocytes	Lymphocytes	Lymphocytes

Further Reading

Johnstone C, Hall A, Hart I J. Common viral illnesses in intensive care: presentation, diagnosis, and management. *Contin Educ Anaesth Crit Care Pain* 2014; **14** (5): 213–219

Solomon T, Michael B D, Smith P E, et al. Management of suspected viral encephalitis in adults – Association of British Neurologists and British Infection Association National Guidelines. *J Infect* 2012; **64**: 347–373

Chapter 33

Fire in the ICU

What key components are required for a fire to start?

The *fire triad* requires the presence of three components:

1 An oxidiser
2 An ignition source
3 Fuel

How should a medical gas cylinder be set-up to minimise patient risk with regard to fire safety?

1 Set up the cylinder for use prior to placing it close to the patient
   - The valve should be opened and flow selected away from the patient, as these are the stages most likely to be associated with ignition
2 Place the cylinder in a specific holder
   - Cylinders should be placed in holders designed to be fitted at the bottom of the bed or the back of wheelchairs
3 Avoid placing the cylinder on the bed next to the patient
   - If placing the cylinder on the bed is unavoidable, set it up and turn it on before putting it on the bed

How can fire be prevented on the ICU?

Open breathing systems are frequently used on ICU, hence prevention focuses on minimisation of ignition sources and safe use of fuel:

1 Safe use of electronic equipment with regular maintenance and safety checks
2 Cylinder explosions may result from oil or grease coming into contact with oxygen under pressure and training for the safe use of pressurised oxygen cylinders should be available in every hospital
3 The orderly stacking of waste and other flammable products in designated areas helps reduces fire risk
4 Ensure adequate fire doors, ventilation and escape routes when designing a new facility.

In 2011, a CD oxygen cylinder caught fire on the ICU at the Royal United Hospital, Bath. Subsequently the Safe Anaesthesia Liaison Group (SALG) of the Royal

College of Anaesthetists and AAGBI have produced a safety alert regarding fire safety (Figure 33.1).

SALG RECOMMENDATIONS

1 Although oxygen is a safe product to administer and handle, at high concentrations and under pressure it is potentially dangerous and should be treated with respect.
2 Oxygen cylinders should be handled with care, and where possible, positioned in specially designed holders, rather than being laid on a patient's bed.
3 All staff should undergo regular training in fire prevention and fire procedures, which should include training in situ in the clinical areas in which they work. Special attention should be given to the location of fire call points, fire extinguishers and medical gas shut off valves.
4 Every hospital should have a fire evacuation policy specifically for its Intensive Care Unit (ICU) and theatre suite.
5 Any problems with oxygen cylinders and associated equipment must be reported immediately to the medical gas supplier and the MHRA.

Figure 33.1 Safe Anaesthesia Liaison Group (SALG) recommendations to promote fire safety on ICU
Reproduced with permission from the Royal College of Anaesthetists (originally published in Fire Safety on Intensive Care and in Theatre, 2013)

How should a fire in critical care be managed?

There are three key goals:

1 Patient and staff safety
2 Manage the fire
3 Identify the cause and address future prevention

In the event of a fire in a critical care setting, the acronym **RACER** can be used:

Rescue

 i Remove patients and staff from immediate danger
 ii Caution with safe disconnection of lines and tubing
 iii Hand ventilation of patients will be necessary

Alert others

 i Raise the alarm as soon as possible
 ii Call 5555 and state location, type and size of fire
 iii Notify co-workers

Contain

 i Close all doors and windows
 ii Turn-off oxygen/flammable gases

Extinguish

i   Department of Health advice is to leave the fire, evacuate the area, close fire doors and await fire services

ii   Only attempt to extinguish a fire if it is small (the size of a waste paper basket)

iii   Select an appropriate fire extinguisher (Table 33.1)

iv   **PASS** is another acronym to guide the fire extinguisher user:
   - **P**ull the lock pin from its place
   - **A**im the nozzle at the base of the flames
   - **S**queeze the handles together; and
   - **S**weep from side to side at the base of the flames

Table 33.1 BS EN3 fire extinguisher colour coding

Type	Water	Water mist	Foam	Powder	CO$_2$
BS EN3 Colour code	Signal red	White with red print	Red with cream panel above instructions	Red with French blue panel above instructions	Red with black panel above instructions
Use	Organic solids, e.g. wood, paper	Organic solids Fats	Organic solids Flammable liquids	Organic solids Flammable liquids Flammable gases Electrical fires	Electrical fires

Relocate

i   Evacuate via fire exits:
   - Visitors first
   - Stable patients
   - Unstable patients
   - Staff

ii   Horizontal evacuation should be utilised (people moved to next lateral fire compartment) +/– vertical evacuation

iii   Stay in the evacuation area until ordered to move by the fire marshal

iv   Assembly points should be adhered to

Once the fire is extinguished, any patients/staff involved should be assessed for smoke inhalation and airway burns and a plan made for ongoing care.

Further Reading

Miles L F, Scheinkestel C D, Downey G O. Environmental emergencies in theatre and critical care areas: power failure, fire, and explosion. *Contin Educ Anaesth Crit Care Pain* 2015; **15**(2): 78–83.

Safe Anaesthesia Liaison Group (SALG). Promoting fire safety on intensive care and in theatre [online]. London: SALG. Available at: www.rcoa.ac.uk/document-store/fire-safety-intensive-care-and-theatre (Accessed: 28 December 2016)

Chapter 34

Fungal Infection and Antifungal Therapy

Why is fungal infection important in critically ill patients?

The incidence of invasive fungal infection is increasing in intensive care patients. There are a number of factors responsible for this:

1 Increasing numbers of immunosuppressed patients, e.g. cancer, chemotherapy, transplant recipients, HIV infection
2 Increasing use of invasive devices
3 Broad-spectrum antibiotic therapy
4 Increasingly aggressive medical and surgical interventions

What do we mean by the term *invasive fungal infection*?

A disseminated or invasive fungal infection is either the presence of a fungus in the blood (i.e. fungaemia) or a deep-seated infection that has occurred as a result of haematogenous spread. The term distinguishes systemic infection from colonisation of a non-sterile site (with no evidence of infection) and superficial infection, e.g. dermatitis, oesophagitis.

Which fungal pathogens are important in critically ill patients?

Candida is the 6-10th most common pathogen isolated in European ICUs. *C. albicans* accounts for approximately 50% of cases of fungal infection, whilst non-albicans candida species account for the majority of the remainder. The incidence of non-albicans *Candida* species is increasing, possibly due to increased use of fluconazole to which several of these species are resistant. *Aspergillus* rates are steadily rising and represent up to 15% of all cases.

What are the risk factors for the development of fungal infection?

1 ICU admission
   - There are high rates of fungal colonisation and transmission in patients admitted to the ICU

2 High APACHE II score
3 The presence of comorbidities, especially pulmonary disease including COPD and bronchiectasis, liver failure and DM
4 AKI requiring RRT
5 Immunosuppression
6 Broad-spectrum antibiotic therapy
7 Parenteral nutrition
8 Any breach of normal defences, e.g. vascular and urinary catheters, surgical wounds, burns, ETT
9 General surgery, especially abdominal surgery and perforated hollow viscus
10 *Candida* colonisation of multiple sites

What are the criteria used to diagnose fungal infection?

There are definitive and suggestive criteria. They are positive in only 30–50%, so a high index of suspicion should be maintained.

Definitive criteria:

1 Single positive blood culture – should *never* be mistaken for a contaminant
2 Positive culture from a biopsy specimen
3 Endophthalmitis
4 Burn wound invasion
5 Positive culture from ascitic fluid or CSF

Invasive fungal infection is suggested by the presence of three colonised sites.

What would lead you to suspect disseminated fungal infection in a patient on the ICU?

A high index of suspicion should be maintained as fungal infection may not produce any outwardly apparent clinical features, especially in immunocompromised patients. Signs include a non-specific inflammatory response and evidence of organ dysfunction. Treatment for fungal infection should be considered (especially in high risk patients) if there is:

1 Persistent fever despite antibiotic therapy and negative microbiology
2 High grade fungiuria in an *uncatheterised* patient
3 Fungiuria that persists after catheter removal
4 Fungus cultured from ≥2 sites
5 Confirmed visceral fungal lesions

How should a patient be investigated for suspected fungal infection?

1 Perform blood cultures (usually positive in only 50% of cases)
2 Examine the retinas for endophthalmitis (may be clinically silent)

3 Catheter urine sample for culture
4 Consider echocardiography if endocarditis is suspected
5 Take biopsies of any tissue suspected of potential fungal infection, e.g. bone, skin

How would you manage a patient with suspected fungal infection?

Patients with suspected fungal infection should be managed with an ABCDE approach, treating abnormalities as they are found. Importantly, antifungal therapy should be initiated immediately: one should not wait for microbiological confirmation and as such there should be close liaison with the microbiologist regarding appropriate antifungal agent and duration of treatment. Specific management for the following cases includes:

1 *Candida* isolate
   - Often isolated from respiratory secretions; however, true infection of the lower respiratory tract is rare
   - Isolated growth of *Candida* from respiratory specimens should not prompt the use of antifungal therapy in most patients
2 Asymptomatic candiduria
   - Change the catheter
   - Treat if candiduria persists or in high risk patients
   - The presence of pyuria is unhelpful as may represent concomitant bacterial infection in 25% of cases
3 Candidaemia
   - Change the line, send tip for MC+S
   - In non-neutropenic patients there is evidence for improved outcomes with early line removal
   - Consider rewiring the CVC in patients with difficult venous access, sending the tip of the old line for culture, and removing/replacing the new line only if the tip is found to be colonised with the same species
   - *C. parapsilosis* forms biofilms, so if this organism is isolated then the line should be removed

What is the prognosis of candidaemia?

Candidaemia has an overall mortality rate of 40–63%, and an attributable mortality rate of 20–40%. Early treatment with antifungals confers a better prognosis.

Tell me about *Aspergillus*

Aspergillus species are spore-forming moulds found in the soil. Only a few *Aspergillus* species are potentially pathogenic to humans: *Aspergillus fumigatus* is the most common, followed by *Aspergillus niger*. The most common site of infection with *Aspergillus* is the lung. An aspergilloma (fungal ball) is considered to be a saprophytic condition, whilst various types of invasive aspergillosis are considered true infections. *Aspergillus* pneumonia typically presents with non-specific symptoms such as fever, cough, dyspnoea, pleuritic pain or haemoptysis. Microbiological diagnosis is often difficult, but PCR can be used to detect fungal DNA, and galactomannan (present in the cell wall of *Aspergillus*) can be detected in blood and BAL specimens.

What classes of antifungal drugs are you aware of?

These are summarised in Table 34.1.

Table 34.1 The commonly used antifungal agents.

Class of Drug	Examples	Notes
Polyenes	Amphotericin B	Fungicidal (bind ergosterol in fungal cell wall, causing cell death)
		Broad spectrum of activity
		Fevers, chills and rigors common (reduced by premedication with antihistamines)
		Dose-limiting nephrotoxicity (liposomal preparations, e.g. AmBisome®, associated with reduced incidence)
Azoles		Fungistatic (inhibit ergosterol synthesis)
	Fluconazole	Active against *Candida* (non-albicans species may be resistant), not *Aspergillus* 100% oral bioavailability CyP450 inhibition (rifampicin reduces fluconazole levels) Prolonged QT interval
	Itraconazole	Increased spectrum of activity against yeasts and *Aspergillus*
	Voriconazole	Active against all *Candida* species First line treatment for invasive aspergillosis
Echinocandins	Caspofungin Anidulafungin	Inhibit cell wall glucan synthesis: fungicidal against *Candida*, fungistatic against *Aspergillus*
		Exhibit synergy with polyenes
		Low oral bioavailability (IV only)
		Good side effect profile, few interactions

Table 34.2 provides a broad guide to appropriate therapy for the more common fungi.

Table 34.2 Antifungal therapy guide according to causative organism

Condition	Antifungal
Candidiasis Non-albicans *Candida* (may be resistant to fluconazole)	Fluconazole Amphotericin / Echinocandin
Aspergillosis	Voriconazole / amphotericin (or both)
Cryptococcosis	Amphotericin + flucytosine
PCP (see page 222)	Septrin +/- steroids Pentamidine Primaquine + atovaquone + clindamycin (2nd line alternatives)

Further Reading

Beed M, Sherman R, Holden S. Fungal infections in critically ill adults. *Contin Educ Anaesth Crit Care Pain* 2014; **14**(6): 262–267

Chapter 35

Guillian-Barré Syndrome

What is Guillain-Barré syndrome?

Guillain-Barré syndrome (GBS) is an acute inflammatory demyelinating poly-neuropathy thought to be an autoimmune response to a preceding illness (*Campylobacter*, CMV, EBV, HSV, upper respiratory tract infection (URTI), *Mycoplasma*).

What types are there?

The types are summarised in Table 35.1.

How does GBS present?

It is characterised by an ascending, symmetrical, flaccid weakness with hypore-flexia, disordered sensation and autonomic disturbance. The onset may be heralded by severe intrascapular or lumbar back pain.

What is the differential diagnosis?

1 Infective
   – Botulism
   – Diphtheria
   – Poliomyelitis
   – Lyme disease
2 Autoimmune disease
   – Myasthenia gravis
3 Organophosphate poisoning
4 Inherited disease
   – Acute intermittent porphyria
   – Periodic paralysis
5 Vitamin B12 deficiency
6 Inflammatory
   – Transverse myelitis/other cord lesion
7 Brainstem pathology
8 Critical illness neuromyopathy

Table 35.1 Features of different variants of GBS

Type	Autoantibodies	Features	Pathology
Acute inflammatory demyelinating polyneuropathy (AIDP)	Anti-GM2 ganglioside	Most common variant (~85%)	Inflammatory demyelinating polyradiculopathy triggered by humoral and cell-mediated autoimmune response to sensitising event, e.g. URTI There is myelin disruption in the peripheral nervous system
Miller-Fischer syndrome	Anti-GQ1b ganglioside	Ophthalmoplegia Ataxia Areflexia	As above
Acute motor axonal neuropathy (AMAN)	Directed against motor nerves and nodes of Ranvier	Typically follows *C. jejuni* infection Recently associated with Zika virus Progressive flaccid symmetric paralysis with areflexia Sensation unaffected	Non-inflammatory axonopathy without demyelination
Acute motor and sensory axonal neuropathy (AMSAN)	Directed against sensory nerves	Clinically similar to classical GBS	Pathologically related to AMAN

What investigations would you perform?

1 Neuroimaging – CT/MRI to exclude raised ICP and organic pathology
2 Lumbar puncture – typically isolated raised CSF protein level
3 Spirometry – particularly vital capacity (VC)
   - Transfer to ITU when VC <20 ml/kg
   - Consider intubation when VC <15 ml/kg
4 Search for underlying cause
   - Serum antibodies for *C. jejuni*, CMV, EBV, HSV, HIV, *M. pneumonia* and atypical pneumonia
   - Serology for viral hepatitis and atypical pneumonia
   - Stool for *C. jejuni*
   - Autoantibodies to differentiate subtypes

5 Other tests:
  - B12 and folate
  - TFTs
  - Urinary porphyrins
  - Drug and toxin screen
6 Neurophysiology – nerve conduction studies differentiate between demyelination (slow conduction velocity) and axonal degeneration (decreased amplitude); however, this is not often practical or available

What criteria would you use for ICU admission and for intubation of these patients?

Indications for admission:

1 Respiratory failure – VC <20 ml/kg
2 Bulbar weakness
3 Autonomic instability

Tell me about dysautonomia and its implications

Autonomic dysfunction presents as significant lability in BP and dysrhythmias that may progress to sinus arrest. Gastric emptying may also be affected. Dysautonomia results from an imbalance between the sympathetic and parasympathetic nervous systems and is more common in the demyelinating (rather than the axonal) form of GBS. It is usually present if the condition is advanced enough to necessitated mechanical ventilation. Intensive care admission is warranted for invasive monitoring and infusions of short-acting vasoactive medications, e.g. esmolol/labetalol, GTN, noradrenaline.

What is the management of patients with GBS?

The patient with GBS should be managed with an ABCDE approach, treating abnormalities as they are found. Specific focus points include:

1 **Treatment of GBS**
  - IVIg 0.4 g/kg/day for 5 days
    - Expensive
    - Usually favoured as first line due to ease of administration and fewer side effects
  - Plasma exchange with 3–5 treatments over 5–7 days
    - Benefit greatest when started within 7 days of onset of symptomatology
    - Reduces the need for respiratory support and shortens the recovery period
  - There is no evidence that one treatment is superior to the other
  - Steroids are not helpful

2 **Intubation and ventilation**
   - Intubate if VC <15 ml/kg or if evidence of aspiration/bulbar palsy
   - Avoid suxamethonium (increased risk of hyperkalaemic cardiac arrest)
   - NIV is of limited use and is contraindicated in presence of bulbar palsy
   - Early tracheostomy should be considered due to likelihood of protracted wean
   - Be aware that autonomic dysfunction predisposes to increased risk of aspiration (delayed gastric emptying, oesophageal dysmotility, loss of airway reflexes)

3 **Cardiovascular support**
   - Cardiac arrhythmias and labile BP should be treated promptly
   - Resistant bradyarrhythmias may require pacing
   - Beware of profound bradyarrhythmias/asystole on suctioning or turning

4 **General supportive care**
   - Thromboprophylaxis
   - VAP bundles (head up, ETT with supraglottic suction, daily sedation holds, proton pump inhibitor (PPI) therapy and thromboprophylaxis, oral chlorhexidine)
   - Gut care: PPI, enteral feeding, laxatives (GBS patients are prone to ileus so may require parenteral nutrition (PN))
   - Physiotherapy
   - Meticulous care of pressure areas and eye care to prevent exposure keratitis in patients with facial palsy
   - Analgesia including atypical agents, e.g. TCAs, gabapentin/pregabalin
   - Psychiatric support including anxiolysis

What is the prognosis?

   - 80% of patients have a good outcome at 1 year
   - 5% mortality
   - 5–10% have an incomplete recovery with prolonged ICU stay
   - 10% relapse

Predictors of poor prognosis:

1 Need for mechanical ventilation
2 Axonal variant
3 Elderly patients
4 Significant neurology at presentation

Further Reading
Hughes R A C, Wijdicks E F, Benson E, et al. Supportive care for patients with Guillain-Barré Syndrome. *Arch Neurol* 2005; **62**: 1194–1198

Yuki N, Hartung H P. Guillain-Barré Syndrome. *New Engl J Med* 2012; **366**: 2294–2304

Chapter 36

Haematological Malignancy on the ICU

Why may patients with haematological malignancy require Critical Care admission?

Patients with haematological malignancy may develop critical illness as part of their first presentation with the illness, or following treatment such as chemotherapy or bone marrow transplant.

Causes of critical illness complicating haematological malignancy can be broadly categorised into the following:

1 Neutropenia and sepsis
2 Respiratory failure
   – Infection
   – Pulmonary oedema/haemorrhage
   – Infiltration by underlying disease
3 Tumour lysis syndrome
4 Graft vs host disease (GvHD)
5 Complications of chemotherapy and stem cell transplant
6 CNS dysfunction and seizures
   – Hyperviscosity syndrome
   – Intracerebral bleed/venous thrombosis
   – Underlying malignancy
   – Electrolyte imbalance
7 GI dysfunction including neutropenic enterocolitis (typhlitis)
8 Acute renal failure
   – Nephrotoxic drugs
   – Sepsis and hypoperfusion
   – Underlying disease

How are neutropenia and neutropenic sepsis defined?

As defined by NICE (CG151):

Neutropenia	Neutrophil count <0.5 x 10^9/l
Neutropenic sepsis	Neutrophil count <0.5 x 10^9/l + clinical signs of infection *or* a temperature ≥38°C

What precautions should be taken when caring for a neutropenic patient to reduce the risk of sepsis?

Precautions that should be taken when caring for a neutropenic patient include:

1 Reverse barrier nursing
2 Positive pressure side room isolation
3 Avoid invasive procedures such as bladder catheterisation, central venous access etc. where possible
4 Avoid rectal examination/rectal temperature probe insertion (risk of haematogenous spread of the patient's endogenous bowel flora)
5 Meticulous oral hygiene

What are the principles of management for a patient with neutropenic sepsis?

The patient with neutropenic sepsis should be managed with an ABCDE approach, treating abnormalities as they are found. Specific management pertaining to neutropenic sepsis involves:

1 History and examination
   - Detailed history including pets and animal exposure, hobbies, recent renovations, history of TB exposure, presence of indwelling lines etc.
   - Ensure the oropharynx, skin and perirectal areas are visualised and look specifically for abscesses
2 Follow *Surviving Sepsis* guidelines:
   - Immediate administration of appropriate antibiotics according to local protocols
   - Serum lactate
   - FBC, U+Es, LFTs
   - Blood cultures, including cultures from any indwelling lines and other sites of potential infection
   - Crystalloid administration as necessary +/- vasopressor support
3 Imaging
   - CXR and any necessary abdominal imaging

Broadly speaking, what should an empirical antibiotic regimen include for a patient with febrile neutropenia?

- An IV anti-pseudomonal β-lactam agent, such a piperacillin-tazobactam or meropenem should be administered
- Additional antibiotics (aminoglycosides, quinolones) may be added if Gram-negative or resistant organisms are suspected, or in the presence of hypotension or potential pulmonary infection

- In patients with IgE-mediated hypersensitivity reactions to penicillin, alternative therapeutic options include ciprofloxacin and clindamycin, or vancymycin and aztreonam
- Local policies reflect variations in organism resistance/susceptibility

What is tumour lysis syndrome?

Tumour lysis syndrome (TLS) is the result of metabolic abnormalities occurring when a large volume of tumour cells are lysed (usually following treatment with chemotherapy, but can occur spontaneously). It is most frequently associated with acute leukaemias and high-grade lymphomas particularly Burkitt's lymphoma.

The features of TLS are potentially life-threatening hyperkalaemia, metabolic acidosis and renal failure. Severe hypocalcaemia and hyperphosphataemia can occur, and increased serum and urinary urate levels are seen.

What is the treatment of tumour lysis syndrome?

Tumour lysis syndrome should be managed using an ABCDE approach, treating abnormalities as they are found. Specific treatment for TLS are as follows:

1 Aggressive fluid resuscitation
2 Treatment of hyperkalaemia (which may include RRT)
3 Rasburicase (a recombinant urate oxidase enzyme which reduces plasma uric acid concentrations)

The use of forced alkaline diuresis is declining due to questionable efficacy and risk of fluid overload.

What chemotherapeutic agents do you know of? How do they work and what complications are associated with their use?

Table 36.1 summarises some commonly used chemotherapy drugs.

What complications of allogenic haematopoietic cell transplantation may result in critical care admission?

Complications of allogenic haematopoietic cell transplantation (HCT) can be categorised into early and late (Table 36.2).

Table 36.1 Complications associated with chemotherapeutic agents

Drug group	Mechanism of Action	Examples	Serious complications
Alkylating agents	Cause DNA cross-links and prevent cell replication	Cyclophosphamide	Idiopathic interstitial pneumonitis Haemorrhagic cystitis
Anti-metabolites	Diverse mechanism of action: May interfere with nucleotide metabolism (and hence DNA synthesis and repair)	Methotrexate 5-FU	Pulmonary fibrosis, nephrotoxicity Cardiotoxicity, acute cerebellar syndrome
Antibiotics/ Topoisomerase interactive agents	Interact with topoisomerase enzymes causing DNA damage	Doxorubicin Bleomycin	Cardiotoxicity Pulmonary fibrosis – importantly, exposure to high FiO_2 causes rapid progression of fibrosis (target SpO_2 88–92% in these patients)
Anti-microtubule agents	Interfere with mitotic and non-mitotic processes	Paclitaxel Vincristine	Pulmonary and cardiotoxicity Peripheral neuropathy

Table 36.2 Complications of stem cell transplant

Early complications (<100 days)	Late complications (>100 days)
Infection	Chronic GvHD
Haemorrhage	Chronic pulmonary disease
Acute GvHD	Infections
Interstitial pneumonitis	Autoimmune disorders
Aplastic anaemia secondary to graft failure	

What is graft vs host disease?

Graft vs host disease is an immune-mediated disease following allogenic HCT (and transplantation of solid organs containing lymphoid tissue) that results from a complex interaction between donor and recipient adaptive immunity (antigen presenting cells of the recipient interact with the mature T-cells of the donor). It can occur even when the donor is perfectly matched (human leucocyte antigen (HLA)-identical).

Acute GvHD (<100 days post-HCT) typically presents with enteritis, hepatitis and dermatitis. Diagnosis can be histological (skin, rectal or liver biopsy) or by using a clinical diagnosis and staging system such as the Seattle Glucksberg criteria (Table 36.3).

Table 36.3 The Seattle Glucksberg staging system for acute GvHD

	Skin changes	Bilirubin (μmol/l)	GI fluid loss (ml/day)
Stage I	Skin rash over <25% of body	26–60	500–1000
Stage II	25–50% of skin surface involved	61–137	1000–1500
Stage III	>50% of skin surface involved Erythroderma	138–257	>1500
Stage IV	Bullous desquamation of the skin	>257	>2500 Ileus

The identification of GvHD as the cause of critical illness is not always straightforward, as the features can be the result of a number of other pathologies.

Chronic GvHD (>100 days post-HCT) is a diverse syndrome with varying clinical features resembling autoimmune disorders such as scleroderma, primary biliary cirrhosis, bronchiolitis obliterans and chronic immunodeficiency. Chronic GvHD may be an extension of acute GvHD or occur de novo.

What are the treatment options for GvHD?

Treatment options include:

1 High dose steroids
2 Immunosuppressants, e.g. ciclosporin
3 Parenteral nutrition may be required to facilitate gut rest where GI involvement is present (octreotide may be useful for severe diarrhoea)

What is typhlitis?

Typhlitis or neutropenic enterocolitis is a life-threatening gastrointestinal complication of chemotherapy. Symptoms include nausea, abdominal distension, pain and tenderness, fever and chills. Typhlitis has a poor prognosis and successful treatment depends on an early diagnosis achieved with a high index of suspicion and the use of CT imaging. Elective right hemicolectomy may be required to prevent recurrence.

Further Reading

Allan N, Siller C, Breen A. Anaesthetic implications of chemotherapy. *Contin Educ Anaesth Crit Care Pain* 2012; **12**(2): 52–56

Beed M, Levitt M, Bokhari S W. Intensive care management of patients with haematological malignancy. *Contin Educ Anaesth Crit Care Pain* 2010; **10**(6): 167–171

Dignan FL, Clark A, Amrolia P, et al. British Committee for Standards in Haematology and the British Society for Blood and Marrow Transplantation. Diagnosis and management of acute graft-versus-host disease. *Br J Haematol* 2012; **158**(1): 30–45

National Institute for Health and Care Excellence (NICE), 2011. Neutropenic sepsis. Clinical guideline 151 [online]. London: NICE. Available at: www.nice.org.uk/guidance/cg151 (Accessed: 4 December 2016)

Chapter 37

Haemoglobinopathies, Coagulopathies and Thrombophilia in the ICU

What is the pathophysiology of sickle cell disease?

Sickle cell disease (SCD) is due to a point mutation at position 6 on the β-haemoglobin gene on chromosome 11 (valine is substituted in place of glutamate), resulting in production of haemoglobin-S (HbS). It is an autosomal recessive condition and patients who are homozygous for the recessive allele (HbSS) have severe disease phenotype. Both the homozygous and the heterozygous genotype (sickle cell trait (HbAS)), confer resistance to malaria.

Haemoglobin-S is less soluble and more viscous compared to HbA, with a tendency to polymerise. This polymerisation is worsened by hypoxia. The HbS polymers form within the red cell, distorting its contour into the classical 'sickle' shape. Initially the sickling process is reversible, but once potassium and water are lost from the cell it becomes irreversible. These abnormal red cells break down more rapidly (causing haemolytic anaemia) and also cause microvascular occlusion, thrombosis and distal infarction (causing sickle crises). Homozygous cells sickle at SO_2 ≤85% (i.e. PO_2 5.2–6.5 kPa) and heterozygous cells will sickle at SO_2 ≤40% (i.e. PO_2 3.2–4.0 kPa: lower than that of venous blood).

The disease becomes clinically apparent between 3 and 6 months of age, when there is a change from fetal to adult haemoglobin.

What types of sickle crises are there?

The types of sickle crisis are outlined in Table 37.1. The types of crises most likely to necessitate critical care admission are acute chest syndrome, stroke and AKI.

What investigations should be performed in sickle cell disease?

1 FBC
   - Typically, a Hb of between 60–90 g/l with reticulocytosis is seen in HbSS (there may also be a reactive thrombocytosis and leucocytosis)
   - HbAS patients may have a normal haemoglobin level

Table 37.1 Types of sickle cell crises

	Presentation	Management

Vaso-occlusive	i Acute chest syndrome (due to pulmonary infarction)
	   – Acute illness with fever and/or respiratory symptoms in the presence of a new pulmonary infiltrate
	   – Presentation similar to pneumonia (cough, dyspnoea, haemoptysis)
	   – High risk of respiratory failure and progression to ARDS
	   – Leading cause of mortality in adults
	 ii Stroke
	   – Occurs in 10% of children with SCD
	   – Leading cause of paediatric mortality in SCD
	   – May be prevented by regular transfusions
	 iii Long bone ischaemia and avascular necrosis
	 iv Abdominal pain (due to visceral ischaemia)
	 v AKI
		Rest, oxygen, IV hydration, analgesia (patients are often opioid-tolerant so may need adjuncts)
		 +/– Broad spectrum antibiotics
		 Exchange transfusion

Sequestration	Occur mainly in the paediatric population Caused by sudden splenic sequestration Presents with worsening anaemia, hypotension and a rapidly enlarging spleen By adulthood, most patients have infarcted their spleen (auto-splenectomy) and require immunisation and antibiotic prophylaxis	Fluid resuscitation and cautious transfusion Aim to increase the Hb by 20–30 g/l
Aplastic	Red cell aplasia caused by parvovirus B19 infection or folate deficiency	Transfusion (increase Hb by 20–30 g/l)

2 Blood film
   – Sickling, target cells, Howell-Jolly bodies (small round inclusions seen within red cells – these cells are normally filtered out by a functioning spleen)
3 *Sickledex* test
   – Confirms the presence of HbS (but does not differentiate between disease and trait)
4 Haemoglobin electrophoresis
   – Gold standard
   – Detects different types of haemoglobin and provides relative proportions of each

Other investigations should be directed at the affected organ system, looking carefully for any complications. Sepsis is a common precipitant for crises and should be actively sought.

How would you manage a patient with acute chest syndrome?

The patient with acute chest syndrome should be managed with an ABCDE approach, treating abnormalities as they are found. General principles of management of acute crises are directed at preventing ongoing sickling (avoiding hypoxia, dehydration and acidosis) and providing adequate analgesia. Haematology involvement is mandatory.

Specific management of acute chest syndrome involves:

1. Oxygen and ventilatory support
   - NIV has been used successfully to reduce the need for intubation
   - Indications for intubation and ventilation are:
     i. Worsening hypoxia
     ii. Severe dyspnoea
     iii. Increasing hypercapnia with respiratory acidosis
2. Fluid resuscitation/rehydration
3. Broad-spectrum antibiotics
4. Bronchodilators and steroids in patients with wheeze or a history of asthma
5. Blood transfusion
   - Early 'top-up' transfusion is effective in milder cases if Hb <70 g/l
   - Exchange transfusion indicated in patients with:
     i. Deterioration despite treatment
     ii. High Hb levels
     iii. Marked hypoxia
   - Exchanges should be managed by the haematologists
   - Target Hb 90–100 g/l with <30% HbS

Indications for exchange transfusion include:

1. Acute chest syndrome
2. Stroke
3. Acute hepatic sequestration
4. Multi-organ failure

What is thalassaemia?

Thalassaemia is caused by abnormalities in the transcription of either α- or β-globin genes, leading to the excessive production of the other. These chains may precipitate within the red cell, causing haemolysis and anaemia.

In health, four α-globin genes and two β-globin exist. The diseases become clinically apparent between 3 and 6 months of age, when there is a change from fetal to adult haemoglobin.

α-thalassaemia results from the deletion of between one and all four of these genes, and clinical severity varies accordingly. Deletion of all four genes is incompatible with life.

β-thalassaemia is usually due to a single-gene mutation resulting in reduced production of β-globin chains. The excess α-globin chains combine with the available β-globin, δ-globin or γ-globin chains. As a result, abnormal amounts of HbA2 (δ chains) and HbF (γ chains) are formed. The heterozygous state is known as *minor* (mild hypochromic, microcytic anaemia with Hb 20–30 g/l below normal) and the homozygous state as *major* (profound anaemia that is transfusion-dependent).

What special considerations should be given to the critically ill patient with β-thalassaemia major?

1 Transfusion support
   – Usual transfusion threshold is Hb <95–100 g/l (this level suppresses innate ineffective erythropoiesis)
2 Infection prevention/control
   – Patients may have had a splenectomy to reduce transfusion requirements
   – Continue prophylaxis
   – Increased risk of overwhelming sepsis
3 *Yersinia* infection
   – May occur in the presence of iron overload
   – Have high index of suspicion in patients with diarrhoea
4 Iron-overload
   – May be associated with underlying hepatic impairment and cardiomyopathy
   – Treat with desferrioxamine to chelate the iron

What is factor V Leiden?

Factor V is an essential protein in the coagulation cascade and is required to produce thrombin. It is usually inactivated by activated protein C (APC), thus preventing excessive clot production. Factor V Leiden is an autosomal dominant condition with incomplete penetrance in which the sufferer produces a mutated form of factor V. Activated protein C is unable to degrade this abnormal form and this results in ongoing clot formation, i.e. thrombophilia. Patients typically present with venous thromboembolism; arterial thrombosis is rare.

What is antiphospholipid syndrome?

Antiphospholipid syndrome (APS) is an autoimmune hypercoagulable state caused by the presence of antiphospholipid antibodies. It typically presents with arterial or venous thromboses, or pregnancy-related complications (e.g. recurrent miscarriage, still birth, intra-uterine growth retardation, pre-term labour, pre-eclampsia). In rare cases of catastrophic APS severe generalised thrombosis occurs, resulting in multi-organ failure and a high mortality.

Antiphospholipid syndrome may be primary or secondary to other autoimmune disease, particularly systemic lupus erythematosus (SLE). The diagnostic criteria are:

1 One clinical event (thrombotic or pregnancy-related)
2 Two antibody tests at least 3 months apart that confirm the presence of either:
  i Lupus anticoagulant
  ii Anti-β_2-glycoprotein-1 antibodies (subset of anticardiolipin antibodies)

It is managed with aspirin or anticoagulation, and plasma exchange in catastrophic APS.

What is the pathophysiology of haemophilia?

The haemophilias are associated with deficiency of specific coagulation factors and are inherited in an X-linked recessive fashion, hence only affect males. There are two types: A (deficiency of factor VIII (fVIII)) and B (deficiency of factor IX). Disease severity is based on quantification of clotting factor levels (mild 5–50%, moderate 1–5%, severe <1%).

How do patients with haemophilia present to the ICU?

In addition to the conditions that affect the general population, patients with haemophilia may present with severe bleeding (e.g. post-operatively, following trauma) and the complications of haemorrhage, or massive transfusion. The most common presentations are haemarthroses and muscle haematomas.

How are haemophiliacs managed on ICU?

Even in the absence of bleeding, patients with haemophilia should continue to receive their usual clotting factor concentrate prophylaxis to maintain clotting factor levels >50%. This is usually given as bolus doses but may be administered by infusion. If interventions are planned, the dose should be increased to target levels >100%. Additionally, tranexamic acid (TXA) has been used with good effect, and DDAVP (desmopressin) may be used to increase fVIII levels in patients with mild haemophilia A (DDAVP has no effect in haemophilia B).

What is Von Willebrand's disease?

Von Willebrand's disease (vWD) is the most frequently occurring hereditary coagulopathy. It is present in 1% of the population, although only a minority are symptomatic. It typically exhibits autosomal dominant inheritance and is characterised by a quantitative or, more rarely, qualitative deficiency of vWF. Under normal circumstances, vWF is produced by platelets and vascular endothelium. It is required for platelet adhesion to the subendothelium and also binds to fVIII and prevents its breakdown.

There are three types (see Table 37.2).

Table 37.2 Types of von Willebrand's disease

	Type 1	Type 2	Type 3
Inheritance	Autosomal dominant	Autosomal dominant	Autosomal recessive
Incidence	85%	~15%	Rare
Defect	Mild-moderate deficiency of vWF	Functional defect of vWF Subclassified into type 2A (10%), 2B (5%), 2 M (rare) and 2 N (rare)	Severe deficiency of vWF (<1%)

Von Willebrand's disease usually presents with mucosal bleeding, e.g. dental extractions, epistaxis, menorrhagia, post-partum haemorrhage. It is managed with prophylactic DDAVP (0.3 mcg/kg) and fVIII concentrate.

What is disseminated intravascular coagulation?

Disseminated intravascular coagulation is a dysregulated host response to various triggers. It may be defined as:

> An acquired syndrome characterised by the intravascular activation of coagulation with loss of localisation arising from different causes. It can originate from and cause damage to the microvasculature, which if sufficiently severe, can produce organ dysfunction.

What are the conditions that trigger DIC most commonly?

1 Sepsis
2 Trauma (including burns and rhabdomyolysis)
3 Obstetric causes (AFE, placental abruption, pre-eclampsia, septic abortion, post-partum haemorrhage)

Describe the pathophysiology of DIC

The pathophysiological hallmark of DIC is excessive thrombin generation. Accelerated thrombogenesis occurs alongside excessive fibrinolysis, resulting in a heterogeneous clinical presentation involving simultaneous thrombosis and bleeding.

In health, thrombin regulates pro- and anticoagulant activity as well as the fibrinolytic and antifibrinolytic pathways. In the presence of a severe and persisting trigger, thrombin generation becomes excessive and normal regulatory mechanisms are overwhelmed. The localisation of thrombogenesis is lost and clot is disseminated systemically. Additionally, the underlying trigger often causes endothelial dysfunction with nitric oxide depletion, which results in uninhibited platelet activation. The fibrinolytic pathway works desperately to counteract this clot formation, and plasmin activation results in the generation of large numbers of fibrin-degradation products (FDPs).

What are the clinical features of DIC?

The features of the primary insult frequently confuse the clinical presentation. There is usually bleeding, which can range from mild episodic bleeding to severe haemorrhage, as the result of consumption of clotting factors and platelets. Thrombotic phenomena are often seen in combination with bleeding, and organ dysfunction may result.

Bleeding-related
1 The *skin* is the first organ that manifests changes of DIC
   - Ecchymoses and petechiae may become widespread
   - Bleeding from venepuncture sites or wounds
2 Mucosal bleeding may occur due to hyperfibrinolysis and can result in GI or urinary tract haemorrhage

Thrombosis-related
1 AKI (28%)
2 Hepatic dysfunction (18%)
3 Respiratory failure (16%)
   - Alveolar haemorrhage
   - Pulmonary emboli
   - ARDS (may be caused by underlying triggering disease)
4 CNS dysfunction (1.4%)
   - Large vessel occlusion
   - Neurological obtundation/coma
   - Subarachnoid haemorrhage
   - Multiple cortical and brainstem haemorrhages and infarcts

How is DIC diagnosed?

The International Society on Thrombosis and Haemostasis (ISTH) has described criteria for the diagnosis of DIC (Table 37.3). It is diagnosed if the score is ≥5.

In addition, near-patient viscoelastic haemostatic assays (VHAs), e.g. Thromboelastography (TEG®), may be useful. In early DIC, the trace will reveal

Table 37.3 The ISTH diagnostic criteria for DIC

Underlying predisposing clinical condition	Essential	
Platelet count (x 10^9/l)	50–100	1 point
	<50	2 points
FDP / D-dimer	Moderate increase	2 points
	Marked increase	3 points
Fibrinogen	<1	1 point
Prothrombin time prolongation	3–6 s	1 point
	>6s	2 points

hypercoagulability (short R time, increased α angle, increased maximum amplitude (MA) with secondary fibrinolysis (high Ly30/Ly60). Later, the patient will be hypocoagulable (prolonged R time, reduced α angle, low MA). Please see the 'Trauma' topic (page 471) for a full explanation of VHAs.

How is DIC managed?

The patient with DIC should be managed with an ABCDE approach, treating abnormalities as they are found. Treatment is centred around that of the underlying condition and the provision of blood product support *only* if the patient is bleeding.

1 **Blood products**
   - Packed RBCs (aim Hb ≥90 g/l in the acutely bleeding patient)
   - Fresh frozen plasma (FFP, 15–20 ml/kg) should be administered in the bleeding patient with an INR or APTT ratio > 1.5
   - Platelets should be considered if platelet count <50 x 10^9/l
   - Cryoprecipitate (two pools) or fibrinogen concentrate (3 g) if fibrinogen <1.5 g/l (some sources say <1.0 g/l)
2 **Thromboprophylaxis** should be seriously considered in critically ill patients who are high risk of venous thromboembolism
   - If the risk of bleeding is high, unfractionated heparin can be used
3 **Tranexamic acid should be avoided**
   - Hyperfibrinolysis is secondary to excess thrombin generation and is a physiological response to mitigate the uncontrolled thrombin generation
   - Inhibiting excessive fibrinolysis with antifibrinolytic agents may be harmful in DIC

Further Reading

Martlew V. Critical care of patients with a congenital bleeding disorder. In: Thachil J, Hill Q A, eds. *Haematology in Critical Care: A Practical Handbook*. John Wiley & Sons Ltd, 2014; 69–73

Retter A, Howard J. Sickle cell disease and thalassaemia in the critical care setting. In: Thachil J, Hill Q A, eds. *Haematology in Critical Care: A Practical Handbook*. John Wiley & Sons Ltd, 2014; 112–117

Thachil J. Disseminated intravascular coagulation. In: Thachil J, Hill Q A, eds. *Haematology in Critical Care: A Practical Handbook.* John Wiley & Sons Ltd, 2014; 52–57

Thomas C, Lumb A B. Physiology of haemoglobin. *Contin Educ Anaesth Crit Care Pain* 2012; **12**(5): 251–256

Wada H, et al for the Scientific and Standardization Committee on DIC of the ISTH. Guidance for diagnosis and treatment of disseminated intravascular coagulation from harmonization of the recommendations from three guidelines. *J Thromb Haemost* 2013; **11**: 761–767

Wilson M, Forsyth P, Whiteside J. Haemoglobinopathy and sickle cell disease. *Contin Educ Anaesth Crit Care Pain* 2010; **10**(1): 24–28

Chapter 38

Haemolytic Uraemic Syndrome and Thrombotic Thrombocytopenic Purpura

What is haemolytic uraemic syndrome?

Haemolytic uraemic syndrome (HUS) is a triad of:

1 Microangiopathic haemolytic anaemia (MAHA)
2 Thrombocytopenia
3 Renal failure

What are the causes?

There are two causes for HUS: epidemic and atypical. The epidemic form is associated with a prodromal illness and bloody diarrhoea following infection with verotoxin-producing enterococci (*E. coli* 0157) or *Shigella*.

Atypical HUS is much rarer and has a poorer prognosis. It may occur following:

1 *Strep. pneumoniae*, CMV or HIV infection
2 Bone marrow transplant/solid organ transplantation
3 Drug exposure, e.g. quinine, heroin and ciclosporin
4 Malignancy
5 Pregnancy

What is the pathophysiology?

Following ingestion of the toxin, bloody diarrhoea occurs as a result of haemorrhagic colitis. Over the subsequent days to one week, an AKI develops which is a result of direct injury of the renal vascular endothelium secondary to toxin production. This leads to excessive platelet aggregation, platelet microvascular thrombi and ultimately AKI. Subsequent hypertension and fluid overload are common.

In atypical HUS, there is often dysregulation of the complement system, e.g. factor H and I deficiency.

What investigations would you perform?

1 Blood tests
   - FBC and film (looking for reticulocytes, evidence of haemolysis and thrombocytopenia)
   - Direct Coombs test (differentiate between immune and non-immune mediated)
   - Lactate dehydrogenase (LDH, raised in haemolysis)
   - U+Es (AKI)
   - LFTs including split bilirubin
   - Clotting including fibrinogen and D-dimers
   - HIV and hepatitis serology
   - Full renal screen (autoimmune and vasculitis screen)
2 Stool MC+S is mandatory
3 Urinalysis
4 Consider renal imaging to rule out other causes of AKI

How would you manage a patient with HUS?

The patient with HUS should be managed with an ABCDE approach, treating abnormalities as they are found. Specific management involves:

1 Administer 100% oxygen
2 Careful fluid therapy and electrolyte balance (GI losses, renal impairment)
3 Cardiovascular support/BP control
4 Renal and haematology input early
5 Treat the cause
   - Ciprofloxacin for *E. coli* and *Shigella*
6 Plasma exchange (PEx)
   - PEx is often used as HUS can be difficult to distinguish from thrombotic thrombocytopenic purpura (TTP) initially
   - Recommended in atypical HUS
   - In epidemic HUS, PEx, IVIg, steroids, antiplatelets have *not* proved beneficial.

What is the prognosis?

The mortality rate for HUS is 3–5%. Approximately 70–85% of patients with epidemic HUS recover normal renal function. Atypical HUS has a poorer prognosis with an initial mortality of ~25% and up to 50% of patients progressing to ESRD.

How does HUS differ clinically from TTP?

They are considered to be a spectrum of the same disease process. TTP is a malignant condition with a mortality of >90% if untreated.

Thrombotic thrombocytopenic purpura is a clinical diagnosis characterised by a pentad of:

1 Thrombocytopenia
2 MAHA
3 Fluctuating neurological signs (due to endothelial injury in the cerebral circulation)
4 Renal impairment
5 Fever

Clotting is usually normal – DIC is a late, ominous sign.

What is the underlying pathology in TTP?

The pathological hallmark in TTP is deficiency of von Willebrand factor-cleaving protease (vWF-CP), or ADAMTS13. This may be genetic (absence of enzyme) or acquired (presence of autoantibody).

vWF is a large glycoprotein present in the plasma whose functions include binding factor VIII, and activating and binding platelets in response to endothelial injury. It is produced in the endothelium as ultra-large multimers that are inactivated when cleaved by vWF-CP. In TTP, these multimers are not cleaved and there is uncontrolled platelet activation. Fibrin is deposited and thrombus propogated creating ischaemia distally, and red cells are shredded as they pass the fibrin/platelet mesh (i.e. MAHA).

How is TTP managed?

The treatment of TTP is more clearly defined than that of HUS. Specific interventions recommended by the British Committee for Standards in Haematology include:

1 **PEx** using Octaplas (solvent-detergent prepared FFP deficient in ultra-large multimeric vWF)
   - Daily PEx should continue for at least 2 days after platelet recovery (i.e. plts >150 x 10^9/l)
   - This removes the autoantibodies from the patient's circulation, and replaces their plasma with plasma containing normal levels of vWF-CP
2 Adjuvant high-dose pulsed **methylprednisolone** can be considered
   - Has been shown to be associated with an improved patient outcome and usually has minimal side effects
   - No RCT addressing whether a combination of PEx and corticosteroids is superior to PEx alone
3 **Rituximab** (monoclonal antibody against CD20, found on the surface of B cells)
   - Used in acute, life-threatening TTP and in patients with refractory or relapsing disease

4 Low dose **aspirin** should be commenced once plts >50 x 10^9/l
5 Supportive measures:
   – Red cell transfusion and folate supplementation during active haemolysis (higher transfusion trigger may be needed in patients with evidence of cardiac involvement)
   – Platelet transfusions are contraindicated unless there is life-threatening haemorrhage, as this will worsen thrombosis
   – Routine thromboprophylaxis should be given once plts >50 x 10^9/l

Further Reading

Scully M, et al. On behalf of the British Committee for Standards in Haematology. Guidelines on the diagnosis and management of thrombotic thrombocytopenic purpura and other thrombotic microangiopathies. *Brit J Haematol* 2012; **158**: 323–335

Chapter 39

The High-Risk Surgical Patient

What is a high-risk general surgical patient?

The term *high-risk surgical patient* is poorly defined. There are many differing descriptions, scoring systems and tests proposed in the literature that attempt to predict patients at high risk of postoperative morbidity and mortality.

A high-risk surgical patient has an expected mortality risk of >5% or twice the average risk of the population undergoing that procedure. A high-risk procedure is one with mortality >5%.

What factors are associated with increased perioperative risk?

Risk factors can be categorised into patient, institutional and surgery-specific factors (Table 39.1).

Table 39.1 Factors associated with increased perioperative risk

Patient factors	Institutional factors	Surgical factors
Age > 65 years	Poor preoperative evaluation	Emergency body cavity surgery
Male gender (men are 1.7x more likely to die than women of the same age)	Limited access to critical care	Complex surgery (i.e. open aortic, major vascular)
Frailty	Delayed surgery	Intra-operative events
Poor nutritional status	Inadequate senior supervision	
Comorbidity (CCF and cirrhosis pose particular threats)		

What perioperative methods (scoring systems) are you aware of for the prediction of post-operative outcomes?

Several classification systems have been described to stratify the risk of surgery:

1 *American Society of Anaesthesiologists (ASA) Classification* (Table 39.2)
   Devised in the 1960's, this quick and simple scoring system was used to assess the preoperative fitness of patients and predict risk.

   The ASA score is widely used, but is subject to high interobserver variability and lacks discriminatory power.

Table 39.2 ASA classification

I	A normal healthy patient
II	A patient with mild systemic disease
III	A patient with severe systemic disease
IV	A patient with severe systemic disease that is a constant threat to life
V	A moribund patient who is not expected to survive without the operation
VI	A declared brain-dead person whose organs are being removed for donor purposes

2 *Lee's revised cardiac risk index* (RCRI, Table 39.3)
   Lee's RCRI is a tool to stratify patients into risk categories for cardiac complications after non-cardiac surgery. It incorporates six factors (easily remembered by the mnemonic 'HICUPS'), the presence of each scores one point.
   H – High-risk surgery, i.e. intraperitoneal, intrathoracic, major vascular surgery
   I – IHD
   C – History of CCF
   U – (U+Es) Preoperative creatinine level >176 μmol/l
   P – Previous insulin therapy for DM
   S – History of stroke

Table 39.3 Lee's Revised Cardiac Risk Index

Score	Incidence of Major Cardiac Complications / Death
0	0.4%
1	0.9%
2	6.6%
≥3	11%

3 *Duke activity status index* (DASI)

The DASI is a functional status assessment and consists of a 12-item questionnaire that utilises self-reported physical work capacity to estimate peak metabolic equivalents (METs). One MET = 3.5 ml/kg/min VO_2, which is equivalent to the oxygen requirement when sitting quietly.

Activity tolerance of <4 METs is considered poor exercise tolerance and is associated with an increased risk of cardiac complications in non-cardiac surgery. Walking on level ground at around 4 miles per hour or walking up a flight of stairs expends approximately 4 METs of activity.

4 *Cardiopulmonary exercise testing* (CPET)

CPET is a test of dynamic cardiac function and gives an objective assessment of functional capacity.

  i *Anaerobic threshold* (AT)

  The AT is the oxygen consumption above which aerobic energy production is supplemented by anaerobic mechanisms, causing a sustained increase in lactate and a metabolic acidosis (Wasserman K, 1986). The oxygen consumption at the AT depends on factors that affect oxygen delivery to the tissues and hence it is an important functional demarcation.

  An AT <11 ml/kg/min predicts increased mortality secondary to cardio-respiratory events and is an indication for post-operative care in a level 2/3 environment.

  ii *Ventilatory efficiency* (VE/VCO_2)

  Measurements of ventilatory efficiency are useful in assessing the presence and severity of both heart and lung diseases. With mismatching, efficiency of pulmonary gas exchange is reduced, necessitating an increase in minute ventilation (VE) for a given CO_2 output (VCO_2).

  VE/VCO_2 slope >34 predicts a higher risk.

  iii *Peak oxygen consumption* (VO_2 peak)

  <15 ml/kg/min (which corresponds to ~4 METs) predicts the risk of functional heart failure after surgery.

What other specific risk scoring systems are you aware of?

P-POSSUM (Physiological and Operative Severity Score for the enUmeration of Mortality and morbidity) is a score that is calculated perioperatively, utilising 12 physiological and 6 operative variables. It has been validated for use in general and vascular surgery patients. Its main limitation is the fact that it requires detail from the operation itself, meaning it is not suitable for pre-operative risk prediction.

Are there any other tests that can be requested preoperatively to better enable us to assess risk?

1 ECG
2 Echocardiography to assess global function
3 Dynamic stress testing to detect inducible myocardial ischaemia
   i Dobutamine stress echo
   ii Myocardial perfusion scanning
   iii Exercise tolerance test
4 CPET (see above)
5 Biomarkers, e.g. BNP levels

Further Reading

Boyd O, Jackson N. How is risk defined in high-risk surgical patient management? *Crit Care* 2005; 9(4): 390–396

Minti G, Biccard B. Assessment of the high-risk perioperative patient. *Contin Educ Anaesth Crit Care Pain.* (2014) **14** (1): 12–17

Pearse R M, Holt P J, Grocott M P. Managing perioperative risk in patients undergoing elective non-cardiac surgery. *Br Med J* 2011; **343**: d5759

Prytherch D, Whiteley M S, Higgins B et al. POSSUM and Portsmouth POSSUM for predicting mortality. *Br J Surg* 1998; **85**: 1217–1220

Chapter 40

HIV in Critical Care

What is HIV?

Human immunodeficiency virus (HIV) is a cytopathic retrovirus that preferentially infects CD4-receptor positive (CD4+) T-helper cells, resulting in reduced immune surveillance and increased susceptibility to opportunistic infection and malignancy. HIV is transmitted by sexual contact, contact with infected blood or blood products, and vertically from mother to child. Heterosexual transmission currently accounts for the majority of new HIV infection worldwide.

Acquired immunodeficiency syndrome (AIDS, now called HIV-related disease) is defined as a CD4 count <200 cells/mm^3 (or CD4 percentage <14%) in a person infected with HIV, or the presence of an AIDS-defining illness.

How is HIV classified?

The Centers for Disease Control and Prevention (CDC) classification system is most commonly used, and identifies four groups of patients, which are described in Table 40.1.

Table 40.1 CDC classification of HIV

Group I	*Acute seroconversion illness*
	This occurs soon after infection, although most patients are asymptomatic
	There is a high viral load, but there is a three-month period during which anti-HIV IgG antibodies are not detectable in the blood
Group II	*Asymptomatic infection*
	Most people with HIV remain asymptomatic, the virus reproduces at a slow rate
	Approximately 10% will go on to develop AIDS within the first three years
	The remainder progress to AIDS in a median of 10 years
Group III	*Persistent generalised lymphadenopathy*
Group IV	*Symptomatic HIV infection*
	Diagnosed when CD4 count <200 cells/mm^3 or in the presence of certain opportunistic infections
	Untreated patients with AIDS typically survive 3 years

How do patients with HIV present to critical care?

Following the introduction of highly active antiretroviral therapy (HAART), there has been a dramatic increase in people living with HIV and a fall in mortality from AIDS. The lifespan of a person with HIV is now only slightly less than that of a person without it, and as such it is deemed a manageable chronic condition. The spectrum of presentation to the ICU and prognosis of those conditions has changed. Non-AIDS-associated diagnoses are increasing and are associated with outcomes approaching those of patients without HIV.

1 *Respiratory failure* is the most common presentation to ICU
   - Pneumocystis jirovecii pneumonia (PCP) makes up 25–50% of these presentations
   - Acute exacerbations of chronic lung disease including asthma and COPD are also common
   - Bacterial pneumonia with organisms including *Pseudomonas* and *S. aureus*
2 *Tuberculosis*
   - This may present in an unusual manner, and is associated with a poorer prognosis than in patients without HIV
3 *Cardiovascular disease*
   - Ischaemic heart disease is common in HIV patients, and may be attributable to the atherogenic side effects of some of the HAART therapies
   - Endocarditis and myocarditis (especially in intravenous drug users (IVDUs))
4 *Liver failure*
   - Often due to co-infection with hepatitis B and C
   - Treatment with nucleoside reverse transcriptase inhibitors (NRTIs) and non-nucleoside reverse transcriptase inhibitors (NNRTIs) may cause hepatotoxicity
5 *Gastroenterological*
   - CMV colitis and cryptosporidial diarrhoea may cause dehydration and electrolyte imbalance
   - GI bleeding secondary to peptic ulceration, Kaposi's sarcoma or lymphoma
   - Perforation due to CMV colitis, TB or malignancy, or non-HIV-related causes
   - AIDS cholangiopathy
   - Acute pancreatitis
6 *Renal failure*
   - HIV-associated nephropathy (HIVAN) is a disease of progressive renal impairment with both microcystic tubulointerstitial disease and focal segmental glomerulosclerosis
   - Diabetic and hypertensive nephropathy are common in this population
   - Appropriate patients should be considered for RRT and/or transplantation
7 *Neurological complications* including status epilepticus and coma as a result of many disease processes:
   - Bacterial, viral, tuberculous or fungal meningoencephalitis
   - Space occupying lesions such as toxoplasmosis (ring enhancing lesions), aspergillomas, abscesses or lymphoma
   - Progressive multifocal leucoencephalopathy

What is the prognosis of patients with HIV admitted to ICU?

A poor prognosis is associated with:

1 High APACHE II score
2 Organ failure, especially requiring mechanical ventilation
3 AIDS-defining illness
4 Sepsis, especially associated with PCP

What is PCP?

Pneumocystis pneumonia (PCP) is caused by the yeast-like fungus *Pneumocystis jirovecii*. It has a slow and indolent course, presenting with progressive shortness of breath, fever and a dry cough. Examination findings are often unremarkable, although ABG may show moderate hypoxaemia and CXR may reveal diffuse granular opacities resembling ARDS, pneumatocoeles or pneumothoraces (especially in patients taking nebulised pentamidine). Definitive diagnosis is based on the presence of the organism in samples of induced sputum or from BAL or lung biopsy. The treatment options are detailed in Table 40.2.

Table 40.2 Treatment of PCP

First line	IV co-trimoxazole 120 mg/kg per day in divided doses for 2–3 weeks +/– IV pentamidine 4 mg/kg per day
Second line	Primaquine + clindamycin Atovaquone Trimethoprim + dapsone

Steroids given within 48–72 hours of diagnosis reduce the risk of respiratory failure, mechanical ventilation and death and are indicated if:

1 PaO_2 <9 kPa
2 A:a gradient >5 kPa

Intensive, early NIV has been used successfully in patients with PCP-induced respiratory failure, and invasive ventilation is reserved for those who fail a trial of NIV. The prognosis of patients with PCP complicated by pneumothorax is poor.

How is HIV treated? Can you name the different types of drugs used? Tell me some of the more common side effects

A typical HAART regimen usually involves a combination of three antiretroviral (ARV) drugs, most commonly two NRTIs plus a protease inhibitor (PI) or an NNRTI. Table 40.3 outlines each of the main classes of drug used.

Table 40.3 Types of antiretroviral therapy

Drug	Example	Mechanism of Action	Side Effects
Nucleoside reverse transcriptase inhibitors	Lamivudine, zidovudine	Acts as a false nucleotide and functions as a competitive inhibitor	Lactic acidosis Hepatic steatosis Zidovudine causes rhabdomyolysis
Non-nucleoside reverse transcriptase inhibitors	Nevirapine	Binds to reverse transcriptase and inhibits enzyme activity	Hepatotoxicity
Protease inhibitors	Saquinavir	Prevents processing of viral proteins	Stevens-Johnson syndrome (SJS) Dyslipidaemias
Fusion inhibitors	Enfurviratide	Blocks fusion of HIV virus with host cell membranes	GI side effects

What are the challenges of HIV treatment on the ICU?

Generally, HAART in HIV patients should be managed on a case-by-case basis with input from the infectious diseases team and the HIV pharmacist. The viral load should be monitored if possible. If the patient is taking HAART pre-ICU then it should be continued, although treatment could be deferred if the CD4 count is >200 cells/mm^3 and the patient has a non-HIV related illness. It is important that *all* elements of the HAART regime are continued so as not to encourage resistance.

There are numerous challenges associated with treatment of HIV on the ICU.

1 Drug delivery
   - Only zidovudine has an IV preparation
   - Others are mostly capsules or tablets, which can be opened and/or crushed and administered enterally if they are not enteric-coated / modified-release preparations
2 Absorption may be affected by various pathological states or procedural techniques performed on the ICU
   - Decreased gastric motility
   - Continuous enteral feeding (has to be interrupted to administer certain ARVs)
   - Gastric alkalinisation with PPIs or H$_2$-receptor antagonists (H$_2$RAs) is contra-indicated with some ARVs
   - Nasogastric suctioning
3 Dosing
   - Hepatic insufficiency will reduce metabolism of NNRTIs

    – Renal impairment will reduce clearance of nearly all NRTIs (except abacavir)

4 Interactions

    – Benzodiazepines should be used with caution with NNRTIs

    – NRTIs interact with numerous agents including benzodiazepines, amiodarone, PPIs and H_2RAs

5 Toxicity

    – ARV therapy can result in severe and life threatening side effects which may lead to, or complicate, ICU admission, including Stevens-Johnson syndrome, hepatic necrosis, pancreatitis and lactic acidosis

6 Immune reconstitution inflammatory syndrome (IRIS)

HAART should be initiated if:

1 The patient has an AIDS-defining illness

2 CD4 count <200 cells/mm^3

3 Anticipated prolonged ICU stay

4 Deterioration despite optimal ICU management

Which patients can we test for HIV on the ICU?

In critically ill patients there is a balance to be reached between informed consent (which is often not possible in this patient group) and the best interests of the patient. It can be argued that knowledge of HIV status is useful in all patients and helps to guide investigation and treatment. Indeed, some units in areas where HIV is prevalent perform the test as part of their routine admission bloods. If knowledge of HIV status would make a difference to the treatment of a patient without capacity, then a test should be performed.

Diagnosis is based on detection of anti-HIV IgG antibodies, which may not become positive for up to 12 weeks after infection. Viral load and p24 antigen levels can also be measured.

What is immune reconstitution syndrome and how do we manage it?

There is a risk of precipitating IRIS following the initiation of HAART. The immune function begins to recover and then responds to the previously acquired opportunistic infection with an overwhelming inflammatory response, which may be associated with a paradoxical worsening of the clinical picture.

If IRIS unmasks a previously occult opportunistic infection, then treatment should be initiated against the offending organism. If there is paradoxical worsening in a patient with previously treated infection, then supportive management is advocated. Steroids are given in severe cases.

Further Reading

Dhasmana DJ, Dheda K, Ravn P. Immune reconstitution. Inflammatory syndrome in HIV-infected patients receiving antiretroviral therapy. *Drugs* 2008; **68**: 191–208

Huang L, Quartin A, Jones D, Havlir D V. Intensive care of patients with HIV infection. *N Engl J Med* 2006; **355**: 173–181

Prout J, Agarwal B. Anaesthesia and critical care for patients with HIV infection. *Contin Educ Anaesth Crit Care Pain* 2005; **5**: 153–156

Chapter 41

Hypertension

Define hypertension

Hypertension is defined as a systolic BP >140 mmHg or a diastolic BP >90 mmHg. The British Hypertension Society grades hypertension based on severity:

Grade 1   140/90 – 159/99 mmHg
Grade 2   160/100 – 179/109 mmHg
Grade 3   ≥180/110 mmHg

What are the causes of hypertension?

Hypertension is classified as either primary (also known as essential or idiopathic), or secondary. Essential hypertension constitutes approximately 90% of cases. Secondary causes are outlined in Table 41.1.

What is malignant hypertension?

Malignant hypertension is a hypertensive emergency most commonly seen in untreated essential hypertension, but also occurs in RAS or phaeochromocytoma. It is severe hypertension associated with retinopathy, papilloedema, encephalopathy, microangiopathic haemolytic anaemia and nephropathy. The pathological hallmark is arteriolar fibrinoid necrosis. There is arterial myointimal proliferation, platelet and fibrin deposition, MAHA and abnormal vascular autoregulation producing widespread endothelial injury and vasoconstriction. End-organ ischaemia results and there is a compensatory activation of the RAA system, which worsens the hypertension and a vicious cycle ensues. The profound hypertension triggers natriuresis, and the resulting intravascular depletion may be unmasked as the blood pressure is brought under control.

How is hypertension investigated?

A full work-up is needed to ensure that a secondary treatable cause is excluded, before the diagnosis of essential hypertension can be made. A full history and examination should be performed, including fundoscopy. It is also

Table 41.1 Secondary causes of hypertension

Renal ~80% of secondary causes	Diabetic nephropathy Renovascular disease Glomerulonephritides Polycystic kidney disease
Congenital	Coarctation of the aorta
Endocrine	Phaeochromocytoma Acromegaly Cushing's syndrome/disease Conn's syndrome Hyperthyroidism
Drugs	Steroids NSAIDs Ciclosporin MAOIs
Toxins	MDMA Cocaine Serotonin syndrome
Pregnancy-related	Pregnancy-induced hypertension Pre-eclampsia
Causes on the ICU	Inadequate sedation, anxiety, pain Hypoxia, hypercapnia, hypothermia Vasoactive medications Fluid overload Increased ICP

important to look for objective evidence of end-organ dysfunction. Investigations include:

1 Blood tests
   - FBC, U+Es, glucose, cholesterol and triglycerides
   - TFTs
   - Aldosterone and renin levels
   - Cortisol level
2 Urinalysis
   - Dipstick for blood and protein
   - Microscopy to look for casts (glomerulonephritis)
   - 24-hour urinary collection for metanephrines and catecholamines (phaeochromocytoma)
3 Radiology
   - CXR
     - Evidence of cardiac failure
     - Rib notching may be seen in aortic coarctation

- CT brain may be indicated, especially in malignant hypertension to differentiate causes of encephalopathy, visual disturbance and headache, and to look for intracranial haemorrhage
- Renal imaging
  - Renal ultrasound in the first instance
  - MRI/MRA may be required in renovascular disease
4 ECG: Performed to look for evidence of left ventricular hypertrophy (LVH) or strain
5 Echocardiography: To assess LV systolic and diastolic function

What is the management of malignant hypertension?

Patients with malignant hypertension should be managed in a high-dependency environment. An ABCDE approach should be used and abnormalities treated as they are found. Short-acting drugs are preferred: intravenous beta-blockers (e.g. labetalol, esmolol), GTN and SNP are the agents of choice. Specific management goals are:

1 Diastolic BP should be lowered to 100–105 mmHg over a period of 2–6 hours
   - There should not be more than a 25% reduction in MAP (compensatory autoregulatory changes mean that organ dysfunction is a potential risk if BP is lowered more quickly than this)
2 Further gradual reductions should be made over the ensuing 24 hours

How do you treat essential hypertension?

In the non-emergent situation, the treatment is focussed on lifestyle changes including smoking cessation, improving diet, exercise and weight loss, and reducing salt and alcohol intake. Pharmacological therapy is dependent on patient population (Figure 41.1).

What is posterior reversible encephalopathy syndrome (PRES)?

PRES is associated with an abrupt increase in blood pressure, and is most commonly seen in association with renal disease, pre-eclampsia and some drugs, e.g. ciclosporin. It is a syndrome of headache, confusion, seizures and visual disturbance. It is characterised radiologically by oedematous lesions within the parietal and occipital lobes, seen as diffuse hyperintense lesions in the white matter on T2-weighted MRI. Rapid control of the hypertension will reverse the changes.

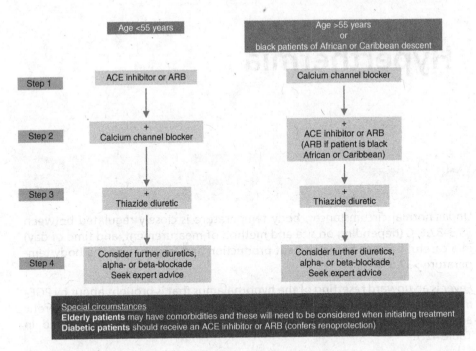

Figure 41.1 The British Hypertension Society/NICE guidelines for the treatment of hypertension

Further Reading

Mancia G, Fagard R, Narkiewicz K et al. ESH/ESC guidelines for the management of arterial hypertension: The task force for the management of arterial hypertension of the European Society of Hypertension (ESH) and the European Society of Cardiology (ESC). *Eur Heart J* 2013; **34**: 2159–2219

National Institute for Health and Care Excellence (NICE), 2011. Hypertension in adults: diagnosis and management. Clinical guideline 127 [online]. London: NICE. Available at: www.nice.org.uk/guidance/CG127 (Accessed: 4 December 2016)

Chapter 42

Hyperthermia

What is the difference between fever, hyperpyrexia and hyperthermia?

Under normal circumstances, body temperature is closely regulated between 35.5–37.5°C (depending on site and method of measurement, and time of day) in a careful balance between heat production and loss. *Pyrexia* is a body temperature >37.5°C.

Fever is an upward resetting of the hypothalamus that is brought about by PGE_2 in response to infectious or non-infectious causes. It may respond to antipyretic agents, e.g. paracetamol, NSAIDs. The causes of fever are summarised in Table 42.1.

Table 42.1 Causes of fever

Infectious	Non-Infectious
Bacterial	Burns
Viral	Acute pancreatitis
Fungal	Transfusion reactions
	Malignancy
	Rheumatological disease, e.g. vasculitis, RA, gout
	Intracranial pathology, e.g. TBI, stroke, haemorrhage, infection, tumour

Hyperpyrexia describes a situation in which body temperature is extremely high (>41°C), and is associated with severe infections or following head injury.

Hyperthermia is a core body temperature >37.5°C with a normal hypothalamic set point, and indicates an imbalance between heat production and loss. There is no response to antipyretic therapy.

What are the causes of hyperthermia?

The causes of hyperthermia can be divided into those related to increased heat production and those related to reduced heat loss (Table 42.2).

Table 42.2 Causes of hyperthermia

Increased heat production	Drugs (either in overdose or as an abnormal reaction to normal / therapeutic dose)	Amphetamine MDMA Cocaine MAOIs TCAs
	Malignant hyperthermia	Suxamethonium, volatile anaesthetic agents
	Serotonin syndrome	
	Neuroleptic malignant syndrome	
	Endocrinological disease	Phaemochromocytoma, hyperthyroidism
Reduced heat loss	Increased heat conservation	Neonates, infants
	Non-exertional (environmental) heat stroke	
	Exertional heat stroke	
	Drugs	Anticholinergic agents

How can we cool hyperthermic patients?

Patients may be cooled passively or actively (Table 42.3).

Table 42.3 Methods of cooling in hyperthermia

Passive	Active
Reduce ambient temperature	Cool IV fluids
Remove clothing	Cold peritoneal lavage
Moisten skin	Intravascular cooling devices
Cool air/fans	Extracorporeal circuits, e.g. CVVHF, bypass, ECMO
Cooling blankets	
Ice packs	

What is malignant hyperthermia? Describe the genetics, pathogenesis and presentation

Malignant hyperthermia (MH) is a rare inherited syndrome with an incidence of 1:10 000 to 1:200 000. It exhibits autosomal dominant inheritance with variable penetrance. The primary defect is in the ryanodine receptor on the sarcoplasmic reticulum, the gene for which is on the long arm of chromosome 19. The RYR1 channel in skeletal muscle allows calcium stored in the sarcoplasm to pass into the cytoplasm. In MH, an abnormal RYR1 allows excessive calcium release following exposure to trigger agents (halogenated volatile anaesthetics and suxamethonium). This causes sustained skeletal muscle contraction resulting from ATP depletion (ATP is needed for muscle relaxation) leading to muscle rigidity, a combined metabolic and respiratory acidosis and ultimately hyperthermia. There is increased metabolic rate, with increased oxygen consumption, and CO_2 and heat production.

How is MH managed?

Malignant hyperthermia usually presents soon after induction of anaesthesia. The patient with suspected MH should be managed with an ABCDE approach, and abnormalities treated as they are found. Specific management involves:

1 Stop all potential trigger agents
   - Maintain anaesthesia with an intravenous infusion such as propofol
   - Maintain oxygenation using a Water's circuit or bag-valve-mask connected to wall oxygen whilst sourcing a *gas-free* anaesthetic machine
2 Finish or abandon surgery as soon as possible
3 Start preparing **dantrolene** immediately (this will usually need at least one extra member of staff as it is laborious and takes time to dissolve)
   - Dantrolene uncouples excitation and contraction
   - Give dantrolene in boluses of 1 mg/kg, repeated every 10 minutes, to a maximum of 10 mg/kg
4 **Hyperventilate** with 100% oxygen
5 Instigate **cooling**
   - Cold IV fluids, external and intravascular cooling devices
   - Ask the surgeons to pour cool fluid into the abdominal cavity if it is open
   - Extracorporeal cooling may be required, e.g. with CVVHF
6 Monitor electrolytes and treat hyperkalaemia aggressively
7 Monitor serum creatine kinase (CK), urine output and myoglobin levels
   - Have a low threshold to start high volume fluid therapy for rhabdomyolysis
8 Transfer to ICU and explain events to next of kin
9 Following recovery, refer the patient and their relatives for genetic testing

The AAGBI have produced guidelines on the management of an MH crisis (Figure 42.1).

How does MDMA toxicity present?

The effects of MDMA are idiosyncratic. Pathologically, there is increased neuronal serotonin release causing sympathetic overactivity, which produces tachycardia and hypertension. Intracranial haemorrhage and sudden cardiac death may result. There is psychomotor agitation with increased muscle activity.

Malignant Hyperthermia Crisis

AAGBI Safety Guideline

Successful management of malignant hyperthermia depends upon early diagnosis and treatment; onset can be within minutes of induction or may be insidious. The standard operating procedure below is intended to ease the burden of managing this rare but life threatening emergency.

1 Recognition

- Unexplained increase in ETCO$_2$ **AND**
- Unexplained tachycardia **AND**
- Unexplained increase in oxygen requirement
  (Previous uneventful anaesthesia does **not** rule out MH)
- Temperature changes are a late sign

2 Immediate management

- **STOP** all trigger agents
- **CALL FOR HELP.** Allocate specific tasks (action plan in MH kit)
- Install clean breathing system and **HYPERVENTILATE** with **100% O$_2$ high flow**
- Maintain anaesthesia with intravenous agent
- **ABANDON/FINISH** surgery as soon as possible
- Muscle relaxation with non-depolarising neuromuscular blocking drug

3 Monitoring & treatment

- Give **dantrolene**
- Initiate active **cooling** avoiding vasoconstriction
- **TREAT:**
  - **Hyperkalaemia:** calcium chloride, glucose/insulin, NaHCO$_3^-$
  - **Arrhythmias:** magnesium/amiodarone/metoprolol **AVOID** calcium channel blockers - interaction with dantrolene
  - **Metabolic acidosis:** hyperventilate, NaHCO$_3^-$
  - **Myoglobinaemia:** forced alkaline diuresis (mannitol/furosemide + NaHCO$_3^-$); may require renal replacement therapy later
  - **DIC:** FFP, cryoprecipitiate, platelets
- Check plasma CK as soon as able

DANTROLENE
2.5mg/kg immediate iv bolus.
Repeat 1mg/kg boluses as required to max 10mg/kg

For a 70kg adult

- **Initial bolus: 9 vials dantrolene** 20mg (each vial mixed with 60ml sterile water)
- Further boluses of 4 vials dantrolene 20mg repeated up to 7 times.

Continuous monitoring
Core & peripheral temperature
ETCO$_2$
SpO$_2$
ECG
Invasive blood pressure
CVP

Repeated bloods
ABG
U&Es (potassium)
FBC (haematocrit/platelets)
Coagulation

4 Follow-up

- Continue monitoring on ICU, repeat dantrolene as necessary
- Monitor for acute kidney injury and compartment syndrome
- Repeat CK
- Consider alternative diagnoses (sepsis, phaeochromocytoma, thyroid storm, myopathy)
- Counsel patient & family members
- Refer to MH unit (see contact details below)

The UK MH Investigation Unit, Academic Unit of Anaesthesia, Clinical Sciences Building, Leeds Teaching Hospitals NHS Trust, Leeds LS9 7TF. Direct line: 0113 206 5270. Fax: 0113 206 4140. Emergency Hotline: 07947 609601 (usually available outside office hours). Alternatively, contact Prof P Hopkins, Dr E Watkins or Dr P Gupta through hospital switchboard: 0113 243 3144.

Your nearest MH kit is stored ....

This guideline is not a standard of medical care. The ultimate judgement with regard to a particular clinical procedure or treatment plan must be made by the clinician in the light of the clinical data presented and the diagnostic and treatment options available.
© The Association of Anaesthetists of Great Britain & Ireland 2011

Figure 42.1 Guideline for management of malignant hyperthermia crisis
Reproduced with kind permission from the AAGBI

Generalised seizures are common. Hyperpyrexia results from increased sympathetic activity and disturbance in central thermoregulation, and should be treated aggressively. Rhabdomyolysis, AKI, DIC and death may occur.

In addition to supportive care, the management involves active cooling and dantrolene administration. Serotonin antagonists, e.g. cyproheptadine, can be used.

What is neuroleptic malignant syndrome?

Neuroleptic malignant syndrome (NMS) is a potentially fatal idiosyncratic reaction to antipsychotic agents such as butyrophenones (e.g. haloperidol) and phenothiazines (e.g. chlorpromazine, prochlorperazine). It results from dopamine antagonism in the striatum and the hypothalamus.

The patient typically presents within the first week of instigation of antipsychotic therapy with altered mental status, features of autonomic disturbance (including hyperthermia) and extrapyramidal signs (profound bradykinesia and muscular rigidity, which may be so severe as to cause rhabdomyolysis).

In addition to supportive therapy and cooling, the offending agent should be withdrawn. Bromocriptine (a dopamine agonist) and dantrolene can be used as treatment. A period of two weeks should be allowed before restarting any antipsychotic medications. The likelihood of recurrence is approximately 30%.

What is serotonin syndrome?

Serotonin syndrome can result from the interaction of two serotonin-enhancing medications. It may also occur following overdose of a serotonergic drug, or in patients taking MAOIs who eat tyramine-containing foods. Serotonergic drugs fall into five classes:

1 Serotonin precursors, e.g. tryptophan, L-3,4-dihydroxyphenylalanine (L-DOPA)
2 Serotonin agonists, e.g. LSD, norpethidine (breakdown product of pethidine)
3 Enhance serotonin activity, e.g. MDMA
4 Prevent serotonin reuptake, e.g. SSRIs, tramadol
5 Prevent serotonin breakdown, e.g. MAOIs

The syndrome is classically of rapid onset and presents as a triad of altered mental status, autonomic disturbance (including hyperthermia) and neuromuscular excitability (e.g. tremor, myoclonus, hyperreflexia). Management is both supportive and specific, involving withdrawal of the offending agents, cooling, symptomatic treatment with benzodiazepines and propranolol, and consideration of dantrolene and serotonin antagonists such as cyproheptadine.

Table 42.4 compares NMS and serotonin syndrome.

Table 42.4 Comparison of features of neuroleptic malignant syndrome and serotonin syndrome

	Neuroleptic Malignant Syndrome	Serotonin Syndrome
Pathophysiology	Dopamine-receptor antagonism	Excessive serotonergic activity
Causes	Butyrophenones, e.g. haloperidol Phenothiazines, e.g. chlorpromazine, prochlorperazine	The addition of a serotonergic drug to a regimen that already includes serotonin-enhancing drugs Following overdose of serotonergic drugs The 'cheese effect' – ingestion of tyramine-containing foods by patients taking MAOIs
Onset	More indolent onset, typically within the first week of starting or increasing medication	Rapid (hours)
Features	Altered mental status Autonomic disturbance including hyperthermia Extrapyramidal effects May be associated with multi-organ failure	Altered mental status Autonomic disturbance including hyperthermia Neuromuscular excitability
Management	Withdrawal of antipsychotic Bromocriptine Dantrolene	Withdrawal of precipitating agents Benzodiazepines Propranolol Serotonin antagonists Dantrolene

What is heat stroke? What different types are there?

Heat stroke occurs when normal physiological methods for heat loss are overwhelmed. It is defined as altered mental status, anhydrosis and a core temperature >40.6°C.

Classical (non-exertional) heat stroke usually occurs over a period of days is typically seen in patients with reduced capacity for thermoregulation, such as those at extremes of age.

Exertional heat stroke occurs in fit and healthy individuals as a result of strenuous exercise or overexertion.

Further Reading

The Association of Anaesthetists of Great Britain and Ireland (AAGBI), 2011. Malignant hyperthermia crisis: AAGBI safety guideline [online]. London: AAGBI. Available at: www.aagbi.org/publications/publications-guidelines/malignant-hyperthermia-crisis (Accessed on 2 January 2017)

Chinniah S, French J L H, Levy D M. Serotonin and anaesthesia. *Contin Educ Anaesth Crit Care Pain* 2008; **8**(2): 43–45

Faulds N, Meekings T. Temperature management in critically ill patients. *Contin Educ Anaesth Crit Care Pain* 2013; **13**(3): 75–79

Chapter 43

Hyponatraemia

Sodium is the principal extracellular cation.

Table 43.1 Sodium homeostasis

Normal serum Na$^+$	135–145 mmol/l
Total body sodium	60 mmol/kg
Average daily requirement	1–2 mmol/kg/day
Absorption	Small intestine

Homeostasis	70% is exchangeable (90% for potassium)
	 Sodium reabsorption is influenced by:
	   i Renin-angiotensin-aldosterone system
	   ii ADH
	   iii Thirst
	   iv β-adrenoceptor stimulation at the proximal convoluted tubule (PCT)

Excretion	>99% of sodium is reabsorbed by the kidney: – 70% in the PCT – 20% in the thick ascending loop of Henle – 5% in the DCT – 3% in the collecting duct
Roles	Regulation of extracellular volume Preservation of osmolality, i.e. guarantees cellular integrity Tubuloglomerular function (maintenance of the hypertonic medullary interstitium)

What is the normal range of sodium?

135–145 mmol/l.

How can you classify hyponatraemia?

Hyponatraemia is typically classified according to the tonicity of the extracellular fluid/plasma osmolality and the patient's volume status; specifically, hypervolaemic, euvolaemic and hypovolaemic causes.

True hyponatraemia is regarded as a low sodium level in the presence of hypo-osmolality. Further classification is according to volume status (see below); however, assessment can be difficult. Hyponatraemia occurring without hypo-osmolality is referred to as pseudohyponatraemia (occurs secondary to elevated levels of lipids or proteins).

1 *Hypovolaemic hyponatraemia*

   Total body water and total body sodium are both low, but there is disproportionate loss of sodium compared to water, e.g. increased ADH secretion in hypovolaemic states (vomiting, diarrhoea, excessive sweating etc.)

   – Urinary sodium differentiates renal vs extra-renal losses: urinary sodium <20 mEq/l suggests an extra renal cause

2 *Euvolaemic hyponatraemia*

   This is the most common category of hyponatraemia seen in hospital inpatients

   Causes include:

   i Syndrome of inappropriate ADH (SIADH)
   ii Glucocorticoid deficiency
   iii Hypothyroidism
   iv Low solute intake (e.g. beer potomania)
   v Psychogenic polydipsia

3 *Hypervolaemic hyponatraemia*

   Essentially dilutional hyponatraemia

   – Oedema is seen as a result of impairment of the kidneys' ability to excrete water maximally
   – There is a paradoxical increase in total body sodium, but a simultaneous and proportionally larger increase in total body water

   Causes include:

   i Nephrotic syndrome
   ii Congestive cardiac failure
   iii Cirrhotic liver disease

A diagnostic algorithm is illustrated in the Figure 43.1.

What is the pathophysiology of the neurological signs seen in severe hyponatraemia?

Neurological signs result from the change in osmotic gradient that develops between the intracellular and the extracellular fluid compartments producing tissue oedema. The effects of this tissue swelling are clinically most pronounced in the brain, where the non-compliant skull combined with lack of adaptive mechanisms means raised ICP can be rapidly devastating. This is particularly important in patients with severe hyponatraemia that has occurred over hours, when convulsions, coma and death secondary to cerebral herniation can result.

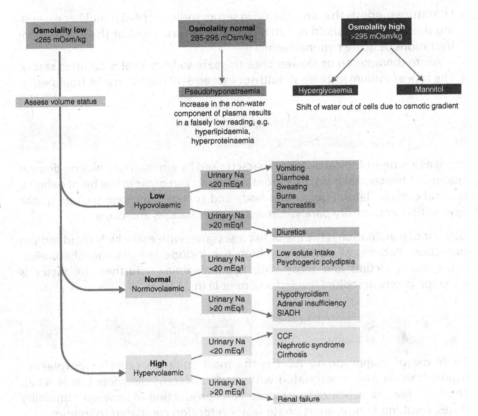

Figure 43.1 Hyponatraemia diagnostic algorithm

How would you manage a severely hyponatraemic patient presenting with seizures?

A difficult therapeutic dilemma is posed by patients with neurological symptoms and hyponatraemia of unknown duration. Overaggressive replacement may risk a serious demyelinating disorder, whereas the consequences of delaying treatment may allow the development of further oedema resulting in death.

Management of this emergency situation should follow an ABCDE approach, treating abnormalities as they are found. Specific management involves:

1 Administer hypertonic (3%) saline (and furosemide if necessary to promote free water excretion) until symptoms subside
   - The aim is to address cerebral oedema, but not to normalise sodium concentration
   - It is possible to calculate the expected change in serum sodium concentration on the basis of the volume of and rate at which the hypertonic saline is infused
2 Admit to critical care and monitor sodium level 1–2 hourly

3 Literature suggests that an increase in serum sodium of 4–6 mmol/l or exceeding the seizure threshold of 120 mmol/l can reverse most of the severe manifestations of acute hyponatraemia
  – Acute therapy can be slowed once this safe sodium level is attained stably
4 The rate of sodium increase should not exceed 8-10 mmol/l in a 24-hour period

What is central pontine myelinolysis?

This is a rare neurological disorder characterised by symmetrical midline demyelination of the central pons. Extrapontine lesions can occur in the basal ganglia, internal capsule, lateral geniculate body and cortex. Symptoms include motor dysfunction, respiratory paralysis, mental state changes and coma.

Osmotic demyelination is the major risk associated with excessively rapid sodium correction. Patients at particularly high risk include the malnourished, alcoholics, burns victims and those with hypokalaemia. A further risk factor is a change in serum sodium level of >12 mmol/l in 24 hours.

What is SIADH and what are the causes?

Syndrome of inappropriate ADH is the most common cause of euvolaemic hyponatraemia and is associated with many different disorders (Table 43.2). The main feature is failure to suppress ADH production in lowered osmolality states, resulting in disproportionate water retention compared to sodium.

Table 43.2 Causes of SIADH

Drugs	Hypoglycaemic agents
	Psychotropics (i.e. antipsychotics, antidepressants)
	Chemotherapeutic agents (especially vincristine and cyclophosphamide)
Malignancy	Lung (especially small cell lung cancer)
	Brain
	Neck
	Duodenum
	Pancreas
CNS disorders	Infection
	Trauma
	Ischaemia
	Haemorrhage
Pulmonary disorders	Pneumonia
	Acute respiratory failure
Pain	Can mediate an increase in ADH secretion post-op

How do you treat SIADH?

1 Fluid restriction, aiming for a slow rise in serum sodium of 1–1.5 mmol/l/day
2 In symptomatic patients, hypertonic saline (1.8%) can be administered via a central line
3 Demeclocycline 600–1200 mg/day to inhibit the renal response to ADH (i.e. it induces nephrogenic DI)
4 ADH receptor antagonists are available (e.g. conivaptan)

Further Reading

Bradshaw K, Smith M. Disorders of sodium balance after brain injury. *Contin Educ Anaesth Crit Care Pain* 2008; 8: 129–33

Ellison D H, Berl T. The syndrome of inappropriate antidiuresis. *N Engl J Med* 2007; 356: 2064–2072

Verbalis J G, Goldsmith S R, Greenberg A, et al. Diagnosis, evaluation and treatment of hyponatraemia: expert panel recommendations. *Am J Med* 2013; 126(10): S1–S42

Chapter 44

Hypothermia

What is normal core body temperature?

Normal core temperature fluctuates between 35.5–37.5°C.

Define hypothermia

Hypothermia is defined as a core body temperature <35°C. It may be subclassified into mild (32-35°C), moderate (28-32°C) and severe (<28°C).

Note that NICE define *perioperative hypothermia* differently: mild (35–35.9°C), moderate (34–34.9°C) and severe (<34°C).

How is heat lost from the body?

Heat loss occurs via five routes:

1 Radiation (40%)
2 Convection (30%)
3 Evaporation (15%)
4 Conduction (5%)
5 Respiration (10%)

What are the mechanisms by which a person may become hypothermic?

The mechanisms by which hypothermia occurs are shown in Table 44.1.

What are the risk factors for hypothermia?

The most common risk factors for developing hypothermia are:

1 Extremes of age
   - Lack the ability to increase their basal metabolic rate to compensate for changes in ambient temperature, e.g. by shivering

Table 44.1 The causes of hypothermia

Increased heat loss	Trauma (prolonged exposure on scene and in hospital during primary and secondary surveys, open body cavities, may be wet or have neurogenic shock following spinal cord injury)
	Surgery (open body cavities with increased evaporative losses)
	General or regional anaesthesia (predominantly via vasodilatation and loss of behavioural and physiological compensatory mechanisms)
	Immersion in cool/cold water
	Burns (large surface area for evaporative loss, vasodilatation)
Decreased thermogenesis	Hypothyroidism, hypoadrenalism
	Elderly patients
	Malnutrition
Impaired thermoregulation	Drugs that directly impair the body's thermoregulatory mechanisms, e.g. anaesthetic agents, vasodilators
	Drugs that impair behaviour (covering bare skin) and physiological compensatory mechanisms (shivering) e.g. sedative agents and alcohol
	Hypothalamic impairment that may occur as a result of any CNS pathology, e.g. stroke, trauma, tumours, encephalopathy
Altered hypothalamic set point	The patient is effectively hypothermic at normal core body temperature, e.g. sepsis, burns

2 Low socio-economic status
3 Trauma
  – Approximately 13% of patients with major trauma are hypothermic (this is associated with a threefold increased risk of mortality in this group)
  – The mortality of trauma patients with a core temperature <32°C is 100%
4 Surgery
  – Inadvertent perioperative hypothermia is associated with an increased morbidity, mortality and LOS in recovery and in hospital

What are the complications of hypothermia?

Cardiovascular

- The initial catecholamine surge causes hypertension and tachycardia, with increased CO
- There is widespread peripheral vasoconstriction
- Decreasing temperature is subsequently accompanied by bradycardia
- Below 33°C the ECG may show *J (Osborn) waves* – positive deflection at the J point (just after the QRS complex), roughly proportional in size to the degree of hypothermia and more prominent in the chest leads (Figure 44.1)

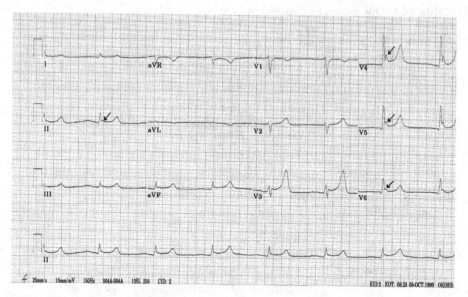

Figure 44.1 The ECG in hypothermia showing sinus bradycardia and J waves
Reproduced with permission from Alhaddad IA, et al. (*Circulation* 2000)

- Bradyarrhythmias, particularly AF, are common
- Below 28°C the heart becomes susceptible to developing ventricular tachyar-rhythmias, particularly resistant VF
- Asystole occurs at core temperatures <20°C

Respiratory

- There is depression of the normal ventilatory responses, with progressive bradypnoea
- The cough reflex is lost and the patient develops profound bronchorrhoea
- Apnoea occurs <24°C

Neurological

- Hypothermia has a CNS depressant effect, with reduced GCS, confusion and lethargy
- Tendon reflexes are diminished and lost once core temperature drops below 28°C
- Coma ensues and the pupils are fixed and dilated below 30°C
- The EEG is isoelectric at temperatures <20°C

Renal

- The initial profound vasoconstriction results in a *cold diuresis* in response to the apparent increase in central intravascular volume – the ensuing hypovo-laemia becomes clinically apparent as the patient is rewarmed

- Hypothermia impairs ADH secretion and increases resistance to its action, worsening the polyuria

Gastrointestinal

- Gastric motility is impaired (increased aspiration risk)
- Hepatic blood flow is reduced, slowing drug metabolism

Metabolic/endocrine

- The basal metabolic rate (BMR) decreases by 7% for every 1°C drop in core temperature
- There is reduced oxygen consumption, CO_2 production, and glucose and fat metabolism
- There is a metabolic acidosis with accompanying hyperkalaemia, hypermagnesaemia and hyperglycaemia
- Shivering occurs (temporarily increases the BMR by a factor of five) – it is maximal at 35°C and decreases as temperature drops further. It ceases completely once hepatic glycogen stores are exhausted, and muscles stiffen (<32°C)
- Hypothermia causes pancreatitis and increases insulin resistance

Haematological

- There is thrombocytopenia due to sequestration, bone marrow depression and consumption
- A progressive coagulopathy develops, eventually resulting in DIC (the coagulation cascade contains numerous temperature-sensitive enzyme systems)
- Blood viscosity increases as temperature drops – this may be compounded by the cold diuresis
- WCC drops and immunity is impaired – wound and respiratory tract infections are more common

How would you manage the hypothermic patient?

The patient with hypothermia should be managed with an ABCDE approach and abnormalities treated as they are found. The specific management should involve:

1 **Resuscitation**
   - Pulse check (may be very difficult and necessitate echo to confirm) – do not delay CPR
   - For hypothermia-associated cardiac arrest:
     - Defibrillation unlikely to be successful in VF – up to three defibrillation attempts permitted and if unsuccessful, delay further attempts until core temperature >30°C

- Avoid giving ALS drugs until core temperature >30°C. Double the dosing intervals at core temperatures of 30–35°C
- Patient movement and procedures (especially intubation) should be undertaken *cautiously* to avoid precipitating VF
- Remember: *you are not dead, until you are warm and dead* (i.e. core temperature >32°C)

2 **Manage the hypothermia** – for acute hypothermia, rewarming can occur fairly rapidly at 2–3°C per hour
  - i Passive rewarming (for mild hypothermia)
    - Remove wet clothing and dry the patient
    - Increase ambient temperature (particularly important in trauma theatre)
    - Blankets, aluminium foil, hat
    - Encourage mobilisation if the patient is conscious and cardiovascularly stable
  - ii Active external rewarming
    - Forced air warmers, radiant heaters
  - iii Active internal rewarming
    - Warm IV fluids
    - Warm, humidified inspired gases
    - Peritoneal or intravesical lavage with warm fluid
    - Central venous heat exchange catheters
    - Extracorporeal methods, e.g. RRT, ECMO, bypass
  - iv Monitoring – usual monitoring + core temperature (oesophageal probe) monitoring with a low-reading thermometer
  - v Serial ABGs (use temperature uncorrected values)
  - vi Patients with core temperature <32°C will require intubation and ventilation
    - Muscle rigidity may make laryngoscopy and mechanical ventilation difficult
    - Frequent endobronchial suctioning is necessary due to bronchorrhoea

3 Treat any **underlying cause**
4 Manage **complications of hypothermia**

What are the complications associated with rewarming?

1 *Afterdrop*
  - Vasodilatation and release of cold blood from the peripheries into the core may cause a second drop in temperature
  - Usually not clinically significant
2 Acidosis and hyperkalaemia
  - Consequence of reperfusion injury
3 Shock (multifactorial)
  - Hypovolaemia as a result of vasoconstriction and subsequent cold diuresis
  - Cardiogenic shock due to myocardial depression
  - Distributive shock due to vasodilatation on rewarming

In which situations on the ICU would you consider inducing therapeutic hypothermia? Outline any evidence for this practice

Controlled, induced therapeutic hypothermia (TH) has been advocated to prevent or mitigate neurological injury in a number of situations.

1 *Post-cardiac arrest*
   In 2002, two RCTs in the NEJM (**Bernard *et al*; HACA** trial) of TH after out-of-hospital cardiac arrest (OOHCA) demonstrated significantly improved neurological outcomes. As a result of this, the International Liaison Committee on Resuscitation (ILCOR) recommended that all unconscious patients who have suffered an OOHCA where the rhythm was shockable should receive 24 hours of TH to 32–34°C. The 2010 UK Resuscitation Council guidelines extrapolated this, recommending that TH be considered in all patients, in- and out-of-hospital, following cardiac arrest regardless of underlying rhythm.

   However, in 2013 the **TTM** trial (NEJM) compared targeted temperature management to either 33°C or 36°C in patients who had suffered an OOHCA. There was no difference in neurological outcome or all-cause mortality between the two groups. Interestingly, there was no significant difference in the incidence of adverse effects.

   Although the most recent trial has shown no additional benefit to cooling to 33°C, many argue that this does not necessarily imply that 36°C is equivalent to 33°C. As such, the use of TH is still commonplace with many units targeting 33°C unless side effects are problematic. There is agreement, however, that *hyperthermia* should be avoided.

2 *Following traumatic brain injury*
   The **Eurotherm3235** trial (NEJM, 2015) looked at the induction of TH to 32–35°C for 48 hours in trauma patients with raised ICP. The trial was stopped early due to a concern of harm: a favourable outcome was more common in the control group and the risk of death was higher in the intervention group. It is not clear whether the hypothermia itself is harmful, or whether the resulting delay in instigating other therapies, e.g. hyperosmolar therapy or barbiturate coma, is harmful.

3 *Following perinatal hypoxia*
   There have been ten RCTs that have shown that the institution of TH in neonates who have suffered hypoxic brain injury for 72 hours is associated with a reduction in poor outcome.

   NICE recommends the use of TH in these cases.

4 TH is also used in deep hypothermic arrest for aortic root surgery.

How would you institute therapeutic hypothermia?

Induction of TH should be achieved as quickly as possible and is usually instigated before arrival on the ICU.

1 Initial strategies include:
   - Covered ice packs to head, neck, axillae and groin
   - Evaporative cooling with fans
   - Administration of cold IV fluids (unless there are signs of significant volume overload)
2 Additional strategies (and maintenance of TH):
   - Surface cooling, e.g. circulating water blankets or suits, helmets or caps in cases of perinatal hypoxia
   - Core cooling, e.g. CoolGard™ intravascular cooling device

Shivering should be prevented during TH as it increases oxygen demand and heat production. This is achieved using sedation and NMBAs. Once the temperature is <33.5°C, the shivering reflex is obtunded.

In TH following cardiac arrest, the target temperature should be maintained for 12–24 hours (from the time target temperature was reached) and the patient should then be rewarmed in a controlled fashion at a rate of 0.5–1°C per hour.

Further Reading

Alhaddad I A, Khalil M, Brown E J. Osborn Waves of Hypothermia. *Circulation* 2000; **101**: e233–e244

Faulds M, Meekings T. Temperature management in critically ill patients. *Contin Educ Anaesth Crit Care Pain* 2013; **13**(3): 75–79

Polderman K H, Herold I. Therapeutic hypothermia and controlled normothermia in the intensive care unit: Practical considerations, side effects, and cooling methods. *Crit Care Med* 2009; **37**(3): 1101–1120

Chapter 45

ICU-Acquired Weakness

Define ICU-acquired weakness

The definition of ICUAW is clinically detected weakness in critically ill patients in whom there is no plausible aetiology other than critical illness. It describes a spectrum of disorders leading to muscle weakness. The underlying pathology may be myopathy (critical illness myopathy, CIM), neuropathy (critical illness polyneuropathy, CIPN) or a mixture of both (critical illness neuromyopathy, CINM). The clinical presentations of each are indistinguishable.

What are the risk factors for ICU-acquired weakness?

The aetiology of ICUAW is uncertain. The main postulated risk factors are:

1 Severe sepsis and multiple organ failure
2 Prolonged mechanical ventilation
3 Excessive sedation
4 Muscle immobilisation
5 Use of corticosteroids
6 Neuromuscular blockade
7 Hyperglycaemia

Other possible risk factors include: female gender, PN, neurological disease and the elderly.

How is muscle weakness assessed?

Symmetrical, flaccid tetraparesis with sparing of the facial muscles is typical of ICUAW.

Motor weakness can be assessed using the Medical Research Council (MRC) sum-score (Table 45.1). Three muscles in both upper and both lower limbs are assessed and each graded from 0 to 5. The score ranges from 0 (tetraplegia) to 60. A sum-score of <48 suggests polyneuromyopathy.

Table 45.1 MRC sum-score

Movement tested on each side	Score for each movement
Arm abduction	0 = no movement
Flexion at the elbow	1 = flicker of movement
Wrist extension	2 = movement with gravity eliminated
Hip flexion	3 = movement against gravity
Extension at the knee	4 = movement against resistance
Foot dorsiflexion	5 = normal power

What is the differential diagnosis of ICU-acquired weakness?

The differential diagnoses of ICU-acquired weakness include:

1 Guillain-Barre syndrome
2 Myasthenia gravis
3 Lambert-Eaton syndrome
4 Motor neurone disease
5 Spinal cord injury
6 Rhabdomyolysis
7 Drug-induced weakness
8 Myopathy/myositis
9 Infective causes, including botulism

How is ICU-acquired weakness investigated?

1 Laboratory tests
  i Blood tests
    – Inflammatory markers
    – Electrolytes
    – ESR
    – Creatine kinase (mildly elevated in CIM)
    – Auto-antibodies
    – B_{12} level
  ii Lumbar puncture
2 Imaging: MRI of the brainstem and spine
3 Neurophysiological investigation
  i Nerve conduction studies (NCS)
    – CIM: normal
    – CIPN: decreased compound muscle action potential (CMAP) and sensory action potentials with normal conduction velocity

ii Electromyography (EMG)
- Requires a fully cooperative patient; often not the case for ventilated and sedated patients
- Typical patterns of myopathic EMGs are motor unit potentials with small amplitudes and short durations

iii Muscle biopsy
- Only indicated where there is diagnostic uncertainty
- Excludes other diagnoses, e.g. demyelination
- Allows subclassification into three morphological subtypes of CIM:
  1 Unspecific and uncomplicated CIM (distinct calibre variations and angulations, internalised nuclei)
  2 Thick-filament myopathy (selective proteolysis and loss of myosin filaments)
  3 Acute necrotising myopathy

How is ICU-acquired weakness managed?

Management involves a multidisciplinary supportive approach, focussing on prevention and avoidance of risk factors. Early mobilisation coupled with an aggressive sedation weaning protocol, and daily physical and occupational therapy are important to shorten ventilator time. Optimising nutrition and ensuring electrolyte replacement alongside minimising the use of corticosteroids and neuromuscular blockade is also important. Strict glycaemic control using insulin is the only strategy that has been shown to reduce the incidence of critical illness polyneuromyopathy, although this is in conflict with the conclusions drawn from the **NICE-SUGAR** trial (see page 321).

Research indicates that daily electrical muscular stimulation can prevent the onset of ICUAW.

Further Reading
Appleton R. Intensive care unit-acquired weakness. *Contin Educ Anaesth Crit Care Pain* 2012; **12**(2): 62–66

de Jonghe B, Lacherade J C, Sharshar T, Outin H. Intensive care unit-acquired weakness: risk factors and prevention. *Crit Care Med* 2009; **37**: S309–315

Stevens R D, Marshall S A, Cornblath D R, et al. A framework for diagnosing and classifying intensive care unit-acquired weakness. *Crit Care Med* 2009; **37**(10): S299–S308

Chapter 46

Infective Endocarditis

What is infective endocarditis?

Infective endocarditis (IE) is a microbial infection of a native or prosthetic heart valve or the mural endocardium, leading to the formation of vegetations and subsequent tissue destruction. It is essentially a multi-system disorder given the propensity for haematogenous spread.

Historically, endocarditis has been divided into acute and subacute presentations. Acute bacterial endocarditis has a fulminant course over days to weeks. It is more likely to be secondary to *S. aureus* and to result in haematogenous spread. Subacute bacterial endocarditis progresses slowly over weeks to months and is less likely than the acute form to cause metastatic infection.

What are the risk factors for infective endocarditis?

Risk factors for endocarditis include:

1 Prosthetic heart valves
2 History of intravenous drug abuse
3 Congenital heart disease
4 History of endocarditis
5 Damaged heart valves (e.g. following rheumatic fever)

Describe the clinical manifestations of endocarditis

The clinical presentation of IE is highly variable: nonspecific symptoms including a history of anorexia and weight loss, night sweats, malaise, nausea, vomiting and weakness are frequently described. The other clinical signs and symptoms of endocarditis are the result of several processes (see below). The incidence of peripheral manifestations has decreased (and are usually not specific to IE, but they are listed below for completeness):

1 *Valvular involvement*
  – New heart murmur
  – Congestive heart failure due to valvular incompetence (the severity of valvular destruction varies with virulence of the infecting organism and duration of the infection)

2 *Bacteraemia*
   – Fever
   – Elevated CRP
3 *Embolisation*
   – Septic emboli may affect the spleen, kidneys, heart, brain and other major organs
   – Symptoms are determined by location:
      i Splenic emboli: left upper quadrant pain, left-sided pleural effusion or rub
      ii Renal emboli: renal infarction, haematuria and flank pain
      iii Coronary emboli: myocardial infarction and arrhythmias
      iv Cerebral emboli: focal neurological complaints and stroke syndromes
      v Pulmonary emboli: dyspnoea and cough (right heart involvement)
   – *Janeway lesions* (macular, painless plaques on the palms and soles)
   – Splinter haemorrhages (tiny linear lesions in the nail bed)
4 *Immune complex formation*
   – Interstitial nephritis or proliferative glomerulonephritis secondary to the deposition of circulating immune complexes in the kidney
   – Immunologically mediated synovitis: musculoskeletal symptoms
   – Immune-mediated myocarditis: palpitations
   – *Osler nodes*: immune complex deposition on hands and feet (painful, red raised lesions)
   – *Roth's spots*: retinal immune complex mediated vasculitis (retinal haemorrhages with white or pale centres)

What are the causative organisms?

The majority of cases of IE are caused by gram positive bacteria; the commonest organism overall being *S. aureus* (now more common than oral streptococci). The organisms causing endocarditis can be broadly divided into those affecting either native or prosthetic valves.

Causative organisms for native valve endocarditis include:

1 Streptococci
   – *Streptococcus bovis* is frequently associated with malignancy
2 Staphlococcus aureus
   – MSSA is more frequently isolated in community-acquired IE
   – MRSA IE is predominantly related to nosocomial infection, wound infection, intravenous lines, or surgical intervention in the previous 6 months
3 Enterococci
4 Gram-negative bacilli
5 HACEK organisms
   – *Haemophilus*
   – *Actinobacillus actinomycetemcomitans*
   – *Cardiobacterium hominis*
   – *Eikenella corrodens*
   – *Kingella kingae*

6 Rare organisms
  – *Rickettsia* (Q fever)
  – *Mycoplasma*
  – *Legionella*

In addition, *Pseudomonas aeruginosa* and fungal infections are seen in intravenous drug abusers.

Causative organisms for prosthetic valve endocarditis can be divided by timing of infection (Table 46.1):

– Early (within 60 days of valve insertion)
– Late (after 60 days of valve insertion)

Table 46.1 Organisms causing prosthetic valve IE

Early	Late
Staphylococcus aureus	*Staphylococcus aureus*
Coagulase-negative staphylococci	Coagulase-negative staphylococci
Enterococci	Streptococci
Fungi (Candida and Aspergillus mainly)	Enterococci
Gram-negative organisms	Gram-negative organisms

How is infective endocarditis diagnosed?

The modified Duke criteria (Table 46.2) are based on clinical, microbiological, and echocardiographic findings and have a sensitivity and specificity of around 80% when applied to patients with native valve IE with positive blood cultures.

How is infective endocarditis treated?

A multi-disciplinary approach involving microbiologists, cardiologists, neurologists, anaesthetists, surgeons, and intensivists is essential for the management of IE.

1 **Resuscitation** and supportive care
2 **Investigations**
  – TTE should be performed promptly, however the sensitivity ranges from 45–60% and the quality is not always adequate
  – TOE offers better image quality and a sensitivity of 90–100%
  – ECG
  – Full set of blood tests including inflammatory markers and renal function
  – Urinalysis
  – CXR
3 **Aggressive antimicrobial therapy**
  – Initiated after blood cultures are performed
    – At least three sets of blood cultures, taken from different sites

Table 46.2 Modified Duke criteria

Criteria	Details
Pathological criteria	**Microorganism**: demonstrated by culture or histology in a vegetation or in a vegetation that has embolised, or in a intracardiac abscess Or **Pathologic lesions**: vegetation or intracardiac abscess present confirmed by histology showing active endocarditis

Clinical criteria	Clinical criteria include:
	  i 2 major criteria
	  ii 1 major and 3 minor
	  iii 5 minor

Major criteria	**Blood culture positive for IE**
	  i Typical microorganisms consitent with IE from 2 separate blood culture
	    – *Streptococci viridans*, *Streptococcus bovis*, HACEK group, *Stapylococcus aureus*
	    Or
	    – Community- acquired enterococci, in the absence of a primary focus
	  ii Microorganism consistent with IE from persistently positive blood cultures, defined as follows:
	    – ≥2 positive cultures of blood samples drawn >12 hours apart
	    Or
	    – All of 3 or a majority of ≥4 separate cultures of blood (with first and last sample drawn at least 1 hour apart)
	  iii Single positive blood culture for *Coxiella burnetii* or antiphase I IgG antibody titre >1:800
	
	Evidence of endocardial involvement
	  i Echocardiogram positive for IE:
	    – Oscillating intracardiac mass on valve or supporting structures, in the path of regurgitant jets, or on implanted material in the absence of an alternative anatomical explanation
	    – Abscess
	    – New partial dehiscence of prosthetic valve
	  ii New valvular regurgitation

Minor criteria	i Predisposition, predisposing heart condition or intravenous drug use
	ii Fever, temperature >38°C
	iii Vascular phenomena:
	    – Major arterial emboli
	    – Septic pulmonary infarcts
	    – Mycotic aneurysm
	    – Intracranial haemorrhage

Table 46.2 (cont.)

Criteria	Details

	– Conjunctival haemorrhages
	– Janeway lesions
	iv Immunologic phenomena:
	  – Glomerulonephritis
	  – *Osler's nodes*
	  – *Roth's spots*
	  – Positive Rheumatoid Factor
	v Microbiological evidence:
	  – Positive blood culture that does not meet a major criterion
	  – Serological evidence of active infection with organism consistent with IE

- Microbiology advice should be sought in all cases
- Empirical therapy commenced and modified depending on organisms isolated from blood cultures
  - Flucloxacillin and gentamicin are used in most cases and subsequently adjusted according to microorganism sensitivity
- Prolonged treatment is required (4–6 weeks) due to high density of organisms in vegetations
4 **Cardiac surgery** is indicated in the following scenarios:
  i Acute valvular stenosis or regurgitation leading to heart failure
  ii Acute aortic or mitral regurgitation with early closure of the mitral valve
  iii Valve dehiscence
  iv Myocardial abscess or fistula
  v Fungal infection
  vi High risk of emboli (vegetations >10 mm)
  vii Persistent positive blood cultures despite treatment

What are the specific issues associated with IE secondary to intravenous drug abuse?

Infective endocarditis secondary to intravenous drug use classically (although not always) affects the right heart; patients frequently present with pneumonia and/or empyema. This is likely to be related to the predominance of tricuspid valve endocarditis in this group and secondary embolic showering into the pulmonary vasculature. Septic pulmonary embolism is the most important complication in IVDUs in contrast to systemic vascular phenomena in non-IVDUs. Symptoms of septic pulmonary embolism include chest pain, dyspnoea, cough and haemoptysis.

The predominant microorganisms isolated are *Ps. aeruginosa* and *S. aureus*. Pseudomonas has a high rate of neurological involvement, and as two distinctive features:

1 Mycotic aneurysms with a higher-than-average rate of rupture
2 Panophthalmitis

Intravenous drug users are also at risk of fungal endocarditis. This should be suspected in the presence of negative blood cultures alongside evidence of bulky vegetations on TTE/TOE, metastatic infection, perivalvular invasion, or embolisation to large blood vessels.

Who should receive antibiotic prophylaxis against bacterial endocarditis and for which procedures?

Guidance for antimicrobial prophylaxis of IE in adults and children undergoing interventional procedures was published by NICE in 2008 (CG64). There is weak evidence to support routine preoperative antibiotic prophylaxis for persons at risk of IE, hence it is no longer recommended.

However, in the case of actual infection at the operative site, antibiotic prophylaxis is still recommended in high-risk patients including:

1 Valvular heart disease
2 Previous valve replacement
3 Structural congenital heart disease, excluding repaired atrial septal defect (ASD) or ventricular septal defect (VSD) or patent ductus arteriosus

Further Reading

Li J S, Sexton D J, Mick N, et al. Proposed modifications to the Duke criteria for the diagnosis of infective endocarditis, *Clin Infect Dis* 2000; **30**: 633–638

Martinez G, Valchanov K. Infective Endocarditis. *Contin Educ Anaesth Crit Care Pain* 2012; **12**(3): 134–139

National Institute of Health and Care Excellence, 2008. Prophylaxis against infective endocarditis: antimicrobial prophylaxis against infective endocarditis in adults and children undergoing interventional procedures. Clinical guideline 64 [online]. Available at: www.nice.org.uk/Guidance/cg64 (Accessed: 2 April 2017)

Chapter 47

Inflammatory Bowel Disease and ICU

How do ulcerative colitis and Crohn's disease differ?

Inflammatory bowel disease is a chronic condition that involves inflammation of the gut. It has two main subtypes: ulcerative colitis (UC), which only affects the colon, and Crohn's disease, which can affect any part of the gut from the mouth to the anus. Both disease processes may be complicated by extra-intestinal manifestations.

Table 47.1 outlines the main differences between UC and Crohn's disease.

Table 47.1 Key differences in ulcerative colitis and Crohn's disease

	Ulcerative colitis	Crohn's disease
Disease distribution	Disease confined to the colon	Small bowel involved in 80% of cases. *Mouth to anus* distribution
Pattern of progression	Inflammation is uniform and diffuse	Patchy, discrete ulceration: *skip lesions*
Histology	Inflammation usually not transmural (limited to the mucosa and submucosa)	Transmural, granulomatous inflammation
Bleeding	Gross rectal bleeding always occurs	Gross rectal bleeding is rare
Presence of fistulae	Fistulas do not occur	Fistula and abscess development is common
Perianal disease	Perianal lesions never occur	Perianal lesions are significant
Radiographic findings	Lead-pipe colon on barium follow-through	*String sign* on barium follow-through Cobblestone mucosa
Complications	Toxic megacolon Haemorrhage Colon cancer	Fistulae Abscesses Strictures Bowel obstruction

What are the extra-intestinal manifestations of ulcerative colitis?

Eyes

- Episcleritis
- Iritis
- Conjunctivitis

Skin

- Pyoderma gangrenosum
- Erythema nodosum
- Clubbing

Musculoskeletal

- Arthritis
- Sacroileitis
- Ankylosing spondylitis

Hepatobiliary

- Primary sclerosing cholangitis
- Cholangiocarcinoma
- Gallstones

Haematological

- Thromboembolic disease

Other

- Amyloidosis

What factors impact on mortality and morbidity in the critically ill patient with IBD?

The following factors may influence the critically ill patient:

1 Disease severity
2 Immunosuppression
3 Nutritional status

Discuss the immunosuppressive agents used in the management of IBD

Immunosuppressive/disease-modifying agents used in the management of IBD are listed in Table 47.2.

Table 47.2 Immunosuppressive and anti-inflammatory agents used in the management of IBD

Drug class	Example	Complications/adverse effects
Corticosteroids	Prednisolone	Prolonged exposure increases infection risk and may result in prolonged wound healing, hyperglycaemia and adrenal insufficiency
Aminosalicyclates	Mesalazine Sulphasalazine	Serious idiosyncratic reactions (Stevens-Johnson syndrome, pancreatitis, agranulocytosis or alveolitis) are rare
Thiopurines	Azathioprine Mercaptopurine	Thiopurine-associated myelotoxicity Hepatotoxicity and pancreatitis Risk of non-melanoma skin cancer
Anti-metabolite	Methotrexate	Hepatotoxicity Pneumonitis Opportunistic infections
Calcineurin inhibitors	Ciclosporin	Renal impairment Neurotoxicity
Anti-TNF therapies	Infliximab Adalimumab	Increased risk of infections from intracellular pathogens (in particular TB) Opportunistic infections Infusion reactions

Why might patients with IBD require HDU/ICU admission?

The following indications may necessitate admission to critical care:

1 Complications specific to IBD
  i Severe exacerbations of disease
  ii Perforation
  iii Toxic megacolon
  iv Acute GI haemorrhage
  v Electrolyte imbalance
    – Hypokalaemia in particular is very common due to loss of potassium-rich faecal fluid and steroids
2 Post-operative management of both elective and emergency surgical procedures
3 Septic complications
4 Thromboembolic complications
5 Other illnesses unrelated to the IBD

What are the differential diagnoses of colitis?

Colitis describes inflammation of the colon of any aetiology. Causes include:

1 Ulcerative colitis
2 Crohn's colitis

3 Diverticular colitis
4 Radiation
5 Ischaemic colitis
6 Infective causes, e.g. *E. coli, Shigella, Salmonella, Campylobacter, C. difficile* pseudomembranous colitis
7 Drug induced
8 Typhlitis

What is severe colitis and how is it managed?

Severe colitis is characterised by:

1 >6 stools per day plus one of the following signs of systemic toxicity
2 HR >90 bpm
3 Temperature >37.8°C
4 Hb <105 g/l
5 ESR >30 mm/hour

The patient with acute colitis should be managed with an ABCDE approach, treating abnormalities as they are found. Specific management involves:

1 Initial investigations
  i Blood tests (FBC, U&E, LTFs, ESR, CRP)
  ii Autoantibodies if diagnostic uncertainty
  iii Imaging: abdominal X-ray (AXR) to exclude toxic dilatation, erect CXR if any suspicion of perforation
  iv Stool culture: MC+S; ova, cysts and parasites; *C. difficile* toxin
2 Ongoing management
  i Fluid resuscitation and electrolyte replacement +/– blood as necessary
  ii Frequent abdominal examination
  iii Stool charts
  iv Broad-spectrum antibiotics if sepsis is suspected
  v Avoid medications that reduce GI motility such as opiates
3 For severe acute ulcerative colitis also consider:
  i High dose IV steroids
  ii Pharmacological and mechanical thromboprophylaxis (increased risk of DVT in this group)
  iii Close liaison with surgical team – surgery is usually necessitated if no improvement/deterioration within 5 days of treatment

What is toxic megacolon and how is it managed?

Toxic megacolon is defined as a transverse colon diameter >5.5 cm or caecum diameter >9 cm on plain abdominal radiograph, in a patient with features of severe colitis and systemic disturbance. It is important to remember signs may be masked by steroid therapy in ulcerative colitis.

In the absence of other complications, it is reasonable to allow a trial of medical therapy for 24 hours under the close supervision of the gastroenterologist and surgical team:

1 Aggressive fluid resuscitation +/– vasopressor support
2 Broad spectrum IV antibiotics
3 Nil-by-mouth with NG tube placement for bowel decompression

Urgent surgery is indicated if:

1 The colonic diameter does not decrease within 24 hours
2 The colonic diameter increases within 24 hours
3 There is a persistent temperature/tachycardia after 24 hours of treatment.

Further Reading

Ha C, Maser E, Kornbluth A. Clinical presentation and outcomes of inflammatory bowel disease patients admitted to the intensive care unit. *J Clin Gastroenterol* 2013; **47**: 485–490

Mowat C, Cole A, Windsor A. Guidelines for the management of inflammatory bowel disease in adults. *Gut* 2011; **60**: 571–607

Chapter 48

Influenza

The influenza virus is an orthomyxovirus (Figure 48.1). The particles consist of eight strands of RNA that are protected by an M1 matrix protein. Surrounding this lies an envelope that is derived from the host cell, in which two types of glycoprotein are embedded:

1 Haemagglutinin – 16 different types: facilitates binding of the virus to host respiratory epithelial cells
2 Neuraminidase – 9 different types: allows release of new viral particles from the infected cell

It is these glycoproteins that determine the type of influenza virus (either A or B) and the subtype, e.g. H1N1, which caused the most recent pandemic in 2009. Additionally, they are the target for antiviral agents.

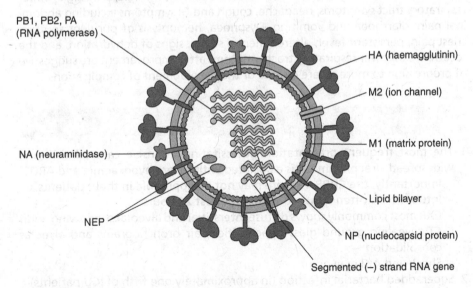

Figure 48.1 The structure of the influenza virus

What do you understand by the terms *antigenic drift* and *antigenic shift*?

Influenza A has the ability to undergo periodic changes in the antigenic characteristics of its glycoproteins. Influenza B has a lesser propensity for antigenic changes, and only drift in the haemagglutinin glycoprotein has been described.

Antigenic drift describes small genetic changes that happen continually over time as the virus replicates and produce viruses that are closely related to one another, i.e. share the same antigenic properties. An immune system with prior exposure to a similar virus will usually recognise it and respond.

Antigenic shift is an abrupt, major change that results in new haemagglutinin and/or neuraminidase producing a new influenza A subtype. People have little or no immunity against the new viral subtype, and a pandemic can result. This may also occur when a haemagglutinin/neuraminidase combination emerges from an animal population that is so different from the same subtype in humans, that most people do not have immunity to it.

How does influenza present?

The incubation period is usually between 1.5–3 days. The clinical phenotype ranges from a mild afebrile upper respiratory tract infection to fulminant viral pneumonia. Influenza most commonly presents non-specifically as a self-limiting illness in children and young adults, with fever, malaise, myalgia, arthralgia, upper respiratory tract symptoms, headache, cough and GI symptoms including abdominal pain, diarrhoea and vomiting. Dyspnoea, hemoptysis of purulent sputum, chest pain, persistent fever, altered mental status, signs of dehydration, and the recurrence of lower respiratory tract symptoms after improvement are suggestive of progression to more severe disease or the development of complications.

What complications may occur?

1 The most frequent presentation necessitating intensive care admission is widespread viral pneumonitis associated with severe hypoxaemia and ARDS
   - Importantly, the CURB 65 score may not be applicable in these patients
   - Intubation is often required within the first 24 hours
   - CXR most commonly shows diffuse interstitial and alveolar shadowing, with CT revealing ground glass opacification, air bronchograms and alveolar consolidation
   - Shock and AKI may occur
2 Superadded bacterial infection (in approximately one fifth of ICU patients)
   - Usually *S. aureus* (including MRSA), *Str. pneumoniae* or *Str. pyogenes*

3 Decompensation of pre-existing conditions, particularly severe, prolonged exacerbations of COPD and asthma
4 Neurological manifestations are less common, and include:
   - Altered mental state
   - Seizures
   - Acute or post-infectious encephalopathy
   - Encephalitis
5 Viral myocarditis is unusual but often carries a poor prognosis

Which patients are at high risk of developing severe illness or complications of influenza?

The following groups of patients were identified to be at the highest risk of complications in the 2009 pandemic:

1 Extremes of age
   - Children <5 years old; increased risk especially in those under two, with the highest rates of hospitalisation in infants <1 year-old
   - Adults ≥65 years old (highest fatality rate but lowest rate of infection)
2 Pregnant women
   - Atypical presentation may occur
   - Risk of hospitalisation increased by a factor of 4–7
   - Highest risk in third trimester
   - Increased risk of severe illness, spontaneous abortion, pre-term labour and delivery, and fetal distress
3 Those with chronic disease
   - Respiratory: asthma, COPD, CF
   - Cardiovascular: congestive cardiac failure (CCF), coronary artery disease
   - Neurological: neuromuscular, neurocognitive or seizure disorders
   - Renal disease: those on dialysis or post-transplantation
   - Cirrhotic liver disease
   - DM
4 Morbid obesity (body mass index (BMI) ≥40)
5 Immunocompromised patients (may present atypically)
   - Immunosuppression including chemotherapy and steroids
   - HIV infection
   - Organ transplant recipients
   - Malnutrition

How is influenza diagnosed?

Clinical presentation is suggestive. Detection of viral RNA by real time reverse transcriptase PCR of nasopharyngeal aspirates will provide microbiological diagnosis. There is increased yield from endotracheal or bronchoscopic samples, so

BAL is recommended in patients with a negative upper respiratory tract sample if clinical suspicion remains high.

What is the management of influenza?

Patients with influenza should be managed with an ABCDE approach, treating abnormalities as they are found. Organ support should be instituted as necessary. Specific ICU management of influenza involves:

1 Strict infection control
   - Isolate in a side room
   - Barrier nursing with strict hand hygiene
   - Aerosol-generating procedures mandate full personal protective equipment (PPE), including FFP_3 or 3M respirator masks
2 Initiate antiviral therapy with a neuraminidase inhibitor, e.g. oral oseltamivir, inhaled zanamivir
   - In the 2009 pandemic, antiviral therapy was recommended for patients with suspected or confirmed H1N1 influenza who were severely ill or who had risk factors for complications
   - There were several studies during the 2009 pandemic that suggested that early treatment of hospitalised patients with a neuraminidase inhibitor reduced disease severity and mortality
   - The 2009 strain was almost universally resistant to amantidine
3 Initiate antibiotic therapy if suspicion of superadded bacterial infection (IV beta-lactam + macrolide)
   - Stop early if there is no confirmed evidence of bacterial infection
4 There is no evidence for steroids
5 Other general ICU measures:
   - Thromboprophylaxis
   - Enteral feeding +/– acid suppression therapy
   - VAP bundle
6 Post-exposure prophylaxis is recommended for adults and children who:
   - Have been in close contact with a confirmed or suspected case of pandemic influenza
   - Are at increased risk of developing complications of influenza
   - Health care professionals

You mentioned infection control measures: Are you able to expand on this?

1 Healthcare professionals should receive yearly flu vaccinations
2 PPE and meticulous hand hygiene is necessary in any infectious disease to protect staff and reduce transmission rates:
   - Gloves
   - Gown or apron

- Goggles
- Surgical mask
3 Isolation in a side room or cohort
   - Should continue for at least 24 hours after resolution of fever, or for 7 days after the onset of the illness (whichever is longer)
   - Immunocompromised patients should remain isolated for the duration of their ICU admission
4 Aerosol-generating procedures (e.g. suctioning, chest physio, intubation, tracheostomy care, bronchoscopy and CPR) should be performed with as few staff present as possible, and all should wear full PPE including FFP_3 or 3M respirator masks
5 Care of ventilated patients:
   - Disposable circuits with a bacterial filter should be used
   - Closed circuit suction is mandatory
   - Minimise circuit breaks and wear respirator masks if breaks are necessary
   - For patients on NIV, the ventilator should only be turned on when the close-fitting mask is in place, humidification should be avoided where possible (increased risk of aerosol dispersal), and a negative pressure room is preferable
6 Differential pressure rooms
   - Negative pressure rooms (allow air to flow into, but not out of, the room) are used to isolate patients with airborne infectious diseases, e.g. influenza, measles, TB
   - Positive pressure rooms are used to isolate immunocompromised patients (positive pressure is also used in operating theatre design)

How should patients with severe hypoxic respiratory failure be managed?

In addition to the management outlined above, these patients should be intubated and ventilated as per any patient with ARDS (see page 33).

1 Appropriate level of sedation
2 Paralyse for the first 24–48 hours
3 Measure and monitor the PaO_2/FiO_2 ratio
4 Oxygenation:
   - Aim for PaO_2 8–9 kPa, titrate FiO_2 and PEEP as per ARDSNet protocol
   - Accept PaO_2 7–8 kPa if FiO_2 ≥0.8 and no evidence of organ dysfunction or cardiovascular history
5 Ventilation:
   - Tidal volume (Vt) 4–6 ml/kg
   - P_{plat} <30 cmH_2O
   - Permissive hypercapnia (aim pH >7.25, or pH >7.2 if no haemodynamic instability)
   - Consider increasing sedation or paralysing to facilitate these parameters
6 Fluid management
   - Aim neutral to negative fluid balance after initial resuscitation
   - Diuretic therapy or RRT may be required

Early referral to a respiratory centre with ECMO capability should be considered in the following circumstances:

1 Oxygenation criteria:
   - Unable to achieve PaO_2 >8kPa with FiO_2 >0.8 and/or PEEP >15 cmH_2O on days 0–2
   - Unable to maintain PaO_2 >8kPa with FiO_2 >0.8 and/or PEEP >15 cmH_2O on days 2–7
2 Ventilatory criteria:
   - Unable to maintain Vt <6 ml/kg, P_{plat} <30 cmH_2O and pH >7.25 (7.2 if haemodynamically stable) on days 0–2
   - Uncompensated respiratory acidosis with pH <7.2 despite optimal therapy for 48 hours on days 2–7
3 Respiratory complications, e.g. bronchopleural fistula
4 Cardiovascular complications, e.g. biventricular failure, moderate-severe pulmonary hypertension
5 High risk patients
6 Evolving multi-organ failure

Refractory hypoxaemia and haemodynamic instability may be a sign of PE, viral myocarditis or pulmonary hypertension with associated biventricular failure. These causes should be sought and investigated appropriately using CT, ECG and echocardiography.

During a pandemic, critical care resources will be at a premium: How would you manage this, and how would you decide who is admitted and who Is not?

In order to facilitate care of these critically ill patients, elective operating may have to be reduced, staff retrained or reallocated, and extra critical care beds created, e.g. by using theatre recovery areas. Additionally, paediatric patients may need to be accommodated in adult ICUs. An internal major incident should be declared (see page 284).

During the 2009 pandemic, the Department of Health issued guidance advising the use of the Sequential Organ Failure Assessment (SOFA) score in conjunction with inclusion and exclusion criteria as a triage tool. The guidance stated that any patient with a SOFA score >11 plus any of the exclusion criteria should not be admitted to ICU during a pandemic, and withdrawal of care considered. However, it has been shown that had this tool been used as a blanket approach to guiding ICU admission, care would have been withdrawn in a number of patients with influenza who were ventilated for short periods and went on to survive.

What is the prognosis of pandemic influenza?

The overall mortality rate in the 2009 pandemic was <0.5% (0.026% in the UK). However, between 9–31% of hospitalised patients were admitted to the ICU, and in this subset the mortality was up to 46%.

Predictors of poor outcome include:

1 Older age
2 Presence of comorbidities
3 Requirement for mechanical ventilation

Further Reading

Johnstone C, Hall A, Hart I J. Common viral illnesses in intensive care: presentation, diagnosis and management. *Contin Educ Anaesth Crit Care Pain* 2014; **14**(5): 213–219

Writing Committee of the WHO Consultation Aspects of Pandemic (H1N1) 2009 Influenza. Clinical aspects of pandemic 2009 influenza A (H1N1) virus infection. *N Engl J Med* 2010; **362**: 1708–1719

Chapter 49

Interstitial Lung Disease and Critical Care

How is interstitial lung disease classified?

Interstitial lung disease (ILD) has recently been reclassified by the American Thoracic Society/European Respiratory Society (ATS/ERS) international multidisciplinary panel (Figure 49.1). The historical gold standard histological diagnosis was abolished and there should now be close collaboration between clinician, radiologist and pathologist if necessary.

What are the common causes of interstitial lung disease?

The common causes of ILD can be grouped according to whether the upper or lower lobes are predominantly affected (Table 49.1).

Table 49.1 Common causes of ILD

Upper lobe predominant	Lower lobe predominant
C Coal-workers pneumoconiosis	C Cryptogenic fibrosing alveolitis (now idiopathic pulmonary fibrosis)
H Histiocytosis	A Asbestosis
A Allergic bronchopulmonary aspergillosis	R Rheumatoid arthritis
A Ankylosing spondylitis	D Drugs (bleomycin, methotrexate, amiodarone)
R Radiation pneumonitis	S Scleroderma
T Tuberculosis	
S Silicosis	
S Sarcoidosis	

How is idiopathic pulmonary fibrosis diagnosed?

Idiopathic pulmonary fibrosis (IPF) is essentially a diagnosis of exclusion, with a largely unknown aetiology. Early diagnosis is essential to try to prevent disease progression. It is the most common form of ILD, and is a devastating progressive

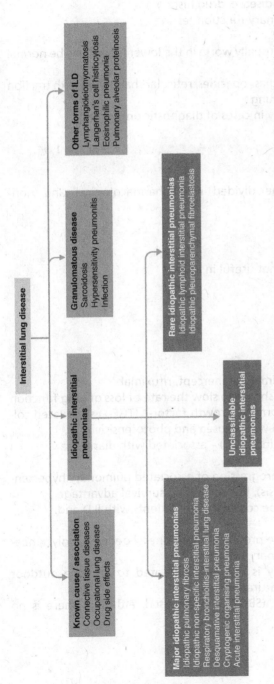

Figure 49.1 The classification of ILD, including the ATS/ERS multidisciplinary classification of idiopathic interstitial pneumonias Adapted with permission from Du Bois RM (*Nature Reviews Drug Discovery* 2010) and the American Thoracic Society (Travis WD, et al. *Am J Respir Crit Care Med* 2013). Copyright © 2017 American Thoracic Society

The following text appears within the figure:

Interstitial lung disease

Known cause / association
Connective tissue diseases
Occupational lung disease
Drug side effects

Idiopathic interstitial pneumonias

Granulomatous disease
Sarcoidosis
Hypersensitivity pneumonitis
Infection

Other forms of ILD
Lymphangioleiomyomatosis
Langerhan's cell histiocytosis
Eosinophilic pneumonia
Pulmonary alveolar proteinosis

Major idiopathic interstitial pneumonias
Idiopathic pulmonary fibrosis
Idiopathic non-specific interstitial pneumonia
Respiratory bronchiolitis-interstitial lung disease
Desquamative interstitial pneumonia
Cryptogenic organising pneumonia
Acute interstitial pneumonia

Rare idiopathic interstitial pneumonias
Idiopathic lymphoid interstitial pneumonia
Idiopathic pleuroparenchymal fibroelastosis

Unclassifiable idiopathic interstitial pneumonias

condition with no definitive treatment. It is important to differentiate IPF from other types of ILD because the mortality is significantly worse.

1 Clinical assessment
   - Full history including environmental/occupational exposure, presence of symptoms/signs of systemic disease, drug history
   - Restrictive deficit on pulmonary function testing
2 Radiological investigation
   - CXR: interstitial shadowing, usually worse in the lower lobes (may be normal early in the disease)
   - High-resolution CT: ground glass opacities, reticular shadowing with traction bronchiectasis, honeycomb lung
3 Tissue biopsy may be necessary in cases of diagnostic uncertainty

What treatment options are available for ILD?

The treatment of ILD can be divided into pharmacological and non-pharmacological therapies.

Pharmacological therapies

1 Immunosuppressive therapy (not useful in IPF)
   - Corticosteroids
   - Cyclophosphamide
   - Azathioprine
   - Mycophenylate
   - Ciclosporin
   - Methotrexate
   - Biological agents, e.g. infliximab, etanercept, rituximab
2 Antifibrotic agents have been shown to slow the rate of loss of lung function
   - Pirfenidone (inhibits transforming growth factor-β (TGF-β) stimulated collagen synthesis) – associated with nausea and photosensitivity
   - Nintedanib (tyrosine kinase inhibitor) – associated with diarrhoea
3 Oxygen therapy
   - Used to slow down rate of progression of associated pulmonary hypertension (which worsens prognosis), but confers no survival advantage
   - The BTS recommends LTOT be considered in patients with ILD and:
     i Resting PaO_2 ≤7.3 kPa
     ii Resting PaO_2 ≤8 kPa in the presence of peripheral oedema, polycythaemia or evidence of pulmonary hypertension
   - Ambulatory oxygen therapy is primarily indicated to improve outdoor mobility (i.e. those who desaturate on exercise)
   - Short-burst oxygen therapy (SBOT) may be used, although there is no evidence supporting its use

Non-pharmacological therapies

1 Pulmonary rehabilitation
   - Consists of six-week programme of exercise and education sessions
   - Patients benefit most from pulmonary rehabilitation when it is commenced early following diagnosis, although it may be undertaken at other points throughout the course of the disease
   - There is evidence that pulmonary rehabilitation improves breathlessness, exercise capacity and health-related quality of life
   - Additionally, patients are encouraged to walk or exercise where able to prevent deconditioning (breathless patients may become stuck in a vicious cycle of progressive deterioration – they don't want to exercise *because* they feel breathless)
2 Management of comorbidities
   - Gastro-oesophageal reflux is heavily implicated in progression of IPF
   - Pulmonary arterial hypertension
3 Management of acute exacerbations (see below)
4 Lung transplantation
   - Transplant is the only therapy that has been proven to extend life expectancy in patients with ILD
   - Mortality ~20% at one year and ~50% at 5 years (similar to mortality rates for patients requiring lung transplant for other indications)

How is an acute exacerbation of ILD managed?

The patient with an exacerbation of ILD should be managed with an ABCDE approach, treating abnormalities as they are found. A cause for the exacerbation should be sought, and close liaison with the respiratory team is essential.

1 Investigations
   i Blood tests (FBC, CRP, cultures, ABG)
   ii Radiology:
      - CXR (may show new infiltrates)
      - High-resolution CT (HRCT) if CXR is non-diagnostic (may show new infiltrates, evidence of infection)
      - CT pulmonary angiogram (CTPA) if PE is a possibility
   iii Echocardiography (CCF is a frequent cause of acute exacerbations of ILD, and may reveal evidence of RVF due to pulmonary hypertension which can guide therapy and aid prognostication)
   iv Bronchoscopy and BAL should be considered to confirm/rule out infection
2 Pharmacological management
   i Pulsed methylprednisolone
      - Often used in acute exacerbations of IPF
      - Single study supporting their use – others have shown a high mortality despite their use

ii Immunosuppression – no strong evidence supporting the use of ciclosporin or cyclophosphamide in acute exacerbations of ILD

3 Non-pharmacological management

i Non-invasive ventilation
- In most cases, the excessive work of breathing associated with acute exacerbations of ILD cannot be managed effectively by NIV for prolonged periods
- Current data does not support use of NIV in these patients unless a rapidly reversible cause is found

ii Invasive ventilation
- Most of the current knowledge regarding practicalities of PPV in patients with ILD has been gleaned from experience of managing patients with ARDS
- However, the pattern of lung damage in ILD is less homogenous than in ARDS, increasing the risk of VILI – high PEEP, recruitment manoeuvres and prone ventilation should be avoided
- Some studies have suggested that these patients should not be intubated unless they are eligible for lung transplantation

iii ECMO can be used as a bridge to transplantation in ILD

iv Lung transplantation
- May be expedited if the patient is already on the transplant waiting list
- May be considered for super-urgent listing if there is an acute deterioration in a patient who has not yet been assessed for transplantation

What specific considerations should be taken into account if these patients are referred to critical care?

Patients with idiopathic pulmonary fibrosis who deteriorate to the point where they need intensive care have an extremely poor prognosis: the mortality in this group is 60–90%. The cornerstones of management are good supportive care and treatment of the underlying cause. Close collaboration with the respiratory physicians is mandatory, with early discussion as to the appropriateness of escalation of therapy and cardiopulmonary resuscitation.

Further Reading

Bhatti H, Girdhar A, Usman F, et al. Approach to acute exacerbation of idiopathic pulmonary fibrosis. *Ann Thorac Med* 2013; 8: 71–77

Du Bois R M. Strategies for treating idiopathic pulmonary fibrosis. *Nature Reviews Drug Discovery* 2010; 9: 129–140

Travis W D, et al. On behalf of the ATS/ERS Committee on Idiopathic Interstitial Pneumonias. An official American Thoracic Society/European Respiratory Society statement: update of the international multidisciplinary classification of the idiopathic interstitial pneumonias. *Am J Respir Crit Care Med* 2013; **188**(6): 733–748

Chapter 50

Intracerebral Haemorrhage

What is an intracerebral haemorrhage?

Intracerebral haemorrhage is an acute extravasation of blood into the brain parenchyma. It may be classified according to cause or location. Intracerebral haemorrhage accounts for 10–30% of all strokes but is a major cause of disability and is associated with a 30-day mortality of ~40%.

What are the causes of intracerebral haemorrhage?

1 Hypertension (60–70%)
  – Most commonly involves deep brain structures (arising from the small arterial branches of large trunk vessels, which are the most prone to hypertensive damage)
  – Most common locations:
    i Caudate
    ii Thalamus
    iii Pons
    iv Cerebellum
2 Amyloidosis (15%)
3 Haemorrhage into a tumour
4 Haemorrhage into an infarct
5 Vasculitis
6 Coagulopathy (including following thrombolysis)
7 Mycotic aneurysms secondary to bacterial endocarditis

The risk factors for ICH are:

1 Hypertension
2 Amyloidosis
3 Alcohol abuse
4 Cocaine use
5 Antiplatelet or anticoagulant therapy

How should blood pressure be managed in patients with ICH?

Hypertension is common in the first 6 hours following ICH. Caution was advised historically on acute BP reduction in ICH based on the potential risk of a detrimental drop in cerebral blood flow to areas of brain in the vicinity of the ICH; however, several studies have indicated that blood pressure reduction decreases haematoma expansion, whilst not affecting perihaematoma blood flow.

NICE recommend treating a SBP >200 mmHg (CG68) in ICH. Consensus guidelines from the European Stroke Organisation in 2014 advised that intensive BP reduction is safe, and may be superior to previous targets of <180 mmHg.

The **INTERACT2** trial (NEJM, 2013) was a large multi-centre RCT studying the effect of initial intensive blood pressure reduction (targeting a SBP <140 mmHg over one hour) compared to a control target of SBP <180 mmHg on the degree of disability following ICH. There was a trend towards superiority in the intervention arm. The **ATACH-2** trial (NEJM, 2016) was designed to answer the same questions, but failed to demonstrate a difference in death or poor outcome between the intensive BP management and control groups. It was stopped early for futility.

NICE are currently reviewing Clinical Guideline 68 and the update will address appropriate BP targets in ICH.

It is important to consider reducing the rate of BP reduction if neurological deterioration occurs. Oral anti-hypertensives should be commenced before titrating IV medications down.

> **A 59-year-old gentleman on warfarin for atrial fibrillation presents to the ED with a sudden drop in GCS (E1 V1 M3). His BP is 205/110 mmHg. How would you manage this patient?**

The patient should be managed with an ABCDE approach, treating abnormalities as they are found. The history is suggestive of an anticoagulation-related ICH. Important points in this case include:

1 **Airway control and ventilatory support**
   - A GCS <8 is an indication for endotracheal intubation for airway protection
   - Ensure the ETT is taped rather than tied
   - Mechanical ventilation should be targeted to PaO_2 >10 kPa and $PaCO_2$ 4.5–5.0 kPa to minimise secondary brain injury
   - End-tidal CO_2 and ABG monitoring should be instituted rapidly to ensure ventilatory targets are met
2 **Blood pressure control/cardiovascular support**
   - IV antihypertensive therapy should be commenced aiming for a target SBP of 160–180 mmHg, e.g. labetalol, nitrates, hydralazine or SNP
   - A SBP <90 mmHg should be supported with appropriate fluid resuscitation and vasopressors or inotropes
3 **Monitor pupils** closely following sedation and ventilation

4 **Prompt imaging**
   – CT is first line to confirm the diagnosis of ICH – the cause may be suggested by the pattern of the bleed
   – CT angiography may be considered, especially in young patients with no clear risk factor for ICH
   – MRI may be useful as a follow-up to CT to detect associated vascular malformations or an underlying neoplasm
5 **Neuroprotective measures** should be instigated (normothermia, normoglycaemia, adequate cerebral venous drainage – see page 480)
6 **Haemostatic management**
   The outcome after acute ICH is worse in patients who were taking anticoagulant drugs at the time of the haemorrhage:
   – Stop the warfarin
   – Liaise with haematology
   – IV vitamin K plus prothrombin complex concentrate (PCC) or FFP is advocated in warfarin-related ICH
   – The **INCH** trial (Lancet Neurology, 2016) suggested superiority of PCC over FFP in terms of achieving an INR ≤1.2 within 3 hours of treatment and haematoma expansion. The trial was stopped after recruitment of 50 patients because of weak evidence of more pronounced haematoma expansion in the FFP group. There was no comparison of long-term clinical outcomes.
7 There is no evidence for corticosteroids in ICH

Is there any evidence for prophylactic antiepileptic therapy in ICH?

There is insufficient evidence surrounding the use of prophylactic antiepileptic treatment after ICH either for the prevention of seizures or for improvement of long-term outcome. Additionally, it is not known when, how or to whom antiepileptic drugs (AEDs) should be given to to reduce the risk of epilepsy after ICH.

What is the role of surgery in ICH?

The **STICH** trial (Lancet, 2005) was an international multi-centre RCT that looked at early surgical evacuation (within 24 hours) or conservative management in patients with ICH. There was no significant difference in primary outcome (favourable Extended Glasgow Outcome Scale (GOSE) at 6 months) or any secondary outcome including mortality. Subgroup analysis showed that patients with haematomas ≤1 cm from the cortical surface were more likely to have a favourable outcome from early surgery than those with deep haematomas.

The **STICH II** trial (Lancet, 2013) was an international multi-centre RCT based on the subgroup analysis of STICH. Participants were randomised to receive either early (within 12 hours) surgical intervention or conservative management (with delayed surgery if the deterioration occurs). There was no increase in death or disability at 6 months. Patients with a predicted poor prognosis were more likely to have a favourable outcome with early surgery than with initial conservative treatment; there was no difference in outcome in patients with a predicted good prognosis.

There have been several small trials of decompressive craniectomy in ICH that have suggested a survival benefit, but no RCTs to date.

Further Reading

National Institute for Health and Care Excellence, 2008. Stroke and transient ischaemic attack in over 16s: diagnosis and initial management. Clinical guideline CG68 [online]. Available at: www.nice.org.uk/guidance/cg68/ (Accessed: 24 March 2017)

Steiner T, Salman R A S, Beer R, et al. European Stroke Organisation (ESO) guidelines for the management of spontaneous intracerebral hemorrhage. *Int J Stroke* 2014; 9(7): 840–855

Chapter 51

Magnesium

Magnesium is the second most important intracellular cation after potassium.

Table 51.1 Magnesium homeostasis

Normal serum Mg²⁺	0.7–1.0 mmol/l
Total body magnesium	~1000 mmol
Average daily requirement	0.1 mmol/kg/day
Absorption	Small intestine (increased by PTH)
Homeostasis	Found predominantly in bone (50–60%), muscle and soft tissues 90% bound to organic matrices The kidney is the primary organ involved in magnesium homeostasis
Excretion	Only 1% of absorbed magnesium is excreted (renal and GI loss) Renal excretion is increased by: i Aldosterone (volume expanded states) ii Hypercalcaemia iii Increased urinary flow
Roles	Essential component of enzyme systems within the body E.g. ATPase is only fully active when chelated with Mg²⁺ – in hypomagnesaemia there is intracellular K⁺ depletion and renal potassium loss DNA, RNA and protein synthesis Regulation of calcium flux, acts as a natural calcium antagonist

Hypermagnesaemia

Define hypermagnesaemia

Serum magnesium >1.0 mmol/l.

What are the causes of hypermagnesaemia?

Hypermagnesaemia is almost invariably iatrogenic.

Describe some of the complications of hypermagnesaemia

Magnesium acts to antagonise the entry of calcium into cells and prevent excitation. The patient may complain of GI symptoms (nausea, vomiting), and neurological signs including weakness (that may progress to respiratory failure) and ultimately coma. There is loss of deep tendon reflexes at serum magnesium levels of 4–6 mmol/l. Cardiovascular complications of hypermagnesaemia include conduction abnormalities and cardiac arrest.

What would the ECG look like in a patient with hypermagnesaemia?

As serum Mg^{2+} rises, progressive conduction abnormalities develop:

1 Prolonged PR interval, usually with normal P wave morphology
2 Wide QRS complexes
3 High-grade AV block
4 Conduction block (bundle branch blocks, fascicular blocks)
5 Bradyarrhythmias
6 Cardiac arrest will ensue if left untreated

How do you manage hypermagnesaemia?

The management of hypermagnesaemia should follow an ABCDE approach, treating abnormalities as they are found. A neurological examination and ECG should be performed urgently to assess clinical severity. Specific management involves:

1 **Stop magnesium administration**
2 **Give calcium**
   - Antagonises the effects of the magnesium
   - 10 ml calcium chloride 10% or 30 ml calcium gluconate 10% IV over 5–10 minutes
3 **Remove magnesium from the body**
   - Diuretics
   - RRT in severe cases
4 **Monitoring**
   - Regular serum magnesium
   - Repeated examination of deep tendon reflexes to monitor clinical response to treatment
   - Continuous ECG monitoring
5 **Prevent recurrence**

Hypomagnesaemia

Define hypomagnesaemia

Serum magnesium <0.7 mmol/l.

What are the causes of hypomagnesaemia?

Hypomagnesaemia is very common in hospitalised patients and is present in up to 65% of patients in critical care. It may be acute or chronic. Causes of chronic hypomagnesaemia include dietary insufficiency and malabsorption. The causes of acute hypomagnesaemia can be classified according to the underlying mechanism (Table 51.2).

Table 51.2 The causes of hypomagnesaemia

Renal loss	Hyperaldosteronism / volume expanded states
	DM
	Hyperparathyroidism
	Hypercalcaemia
	Polyuric phase of AKI
	Drugs: Diuretics
	Aminoglycosides
	Alcohol
Altered balance	Refeeding syndrome
	Phosphate depletion
GI loss	Diarrhoea and vomiting, nasogastric suctioning
	Short bowel syndrome
	Acute pancreatitis

Tell me some of the complications of hypomagnesaemia

Hypomagnesaemia may be diagnosed incidentally on blood tests. It often coexists with other electrolyte/biochemical abnormalities (e.g. hypocalcaemia, hypokalaemia, metabolic alkalosis) which account for many of the clinical features. The absorption of calcium and magnesium are interdependent and hypomagnesaemia impairs hypocalcaemia-induced PTH release.

The patient may present with GI symptoms (nausea, vomiting, abdominal pain), neuromuscular hyperactivity (weakness, ataxia, tremor, carpopedal spasm, laryngospasm and generalised seizures) and neurological disturbance (confusion progressing eventually to coma). There may be hypertension, angina and rhythm disturbance. Additionally, there is increased potential for digoxin toxicity as with hypokalaemia.

What ECG changes would you see in a patient with low magnesium?

The primary abnormality is a prolonged QT interval (Figure 51.1). There may also be signs of hypokalaemia (prolonged PR, T wave inversion, U waves).

With worsening hypomagnesaemia there are frequent supraventricular and ventricular ectopics and supraventricular tachyarrhythmias. The ECG may degenerate into VT, polymorphic VT (torsades de pointes) and VF. Whether these changes are due to hypomagnesaemia *per se* or concurrent hypokalaemia is uncertain.

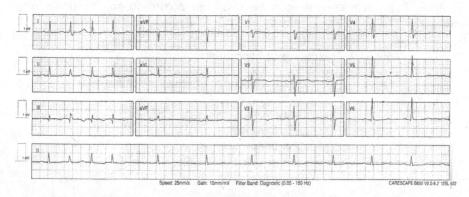

Speed: 25mm/s   Gain: 10mm/mV   Filter Band: Diagnostic (0.05 - 150 Hz)   CARESCAPE B650 V2.0.6.2 12SL v22

Figure 51.1 An ECG showing a QTc of 643 ms, T wave flattening and ventricular ectopics (serum Mg^{2+} 0.57 mmol/l and K^+ 3.2 mmol/l)
These changes resolved with correction of these electrolyte abnormalities

How would you manage hypomagnesaemia?

The management of hypomagnesaemia should follow an ABCDE approach, treating abnormalities as you find them. An ECG should be obtained urgently. The ultimate treatment is directed at the underlying cause, but it is important to actively manage the low magnesium in the meantime.

1 **Stop all magnesium-wasting drugs**
2 **Magnesium supplementation**
   – 10–20 mmol (2.5–5 g) of $MgSO_4$ should be given as a slow IV bolus over 10–15 minutes in severe and symptomatic hypomagnesaemia
   – IV magnesium may be administered peripherally in 250 ml of normal saline, concentrated via a central line with continuous ECG monitoring, or in PN
   – Oral magnesium is used for mild and asymptomatic hypomagnesaemia, but is associated with diarrhoea
   – Correct coexisting hypokalaemia

3 **Monitoring**
 - Regular serum magnesium and potassium
 - Continuous ECG monitoring
 - The magnesium infusion should be stopped if there is hypotension, brady-cardia or loss of deep tendon reflexes, or if serum Mg^{2+} >2.5 mmol/l

4 **Prevent recurrence**

How is magnesium used therapeutically in the critically ill patient?

1. *Asthma*
   The British Thoracic Society recommends that a single dose of 2 g (8 mmol) magnesium sulphate IV is given to patients with acute severe asthma who have had little or no response to initial inhaled bronchodilator therapy.

   Magnesium sulphate may improve lung function and reduce intubation rates in these patients. In addition, it may also reduce hospital admissions in adults with acute asthma who have had little or no response to standard treatment.

   The mechanism of action involves inhibition of smooth muscle contraction, mast cell degranulation and acetylcholine release from cholinergic nerve terminals.

2. *Pre-eclamsia*
   The **Magpie** trial (Lancet, 2002) supports the use of magnesium as prophylaxis and treatment of eclamptic seizures.

   4 g (16 mmol) is given IV over 5 minutes, followed by an infusion of 1 g/h for 24 hours.

   Magnesium is a CNS depressant, increases endothelial prostacyclin (prostaglandin (PG) I_2) production and causes vasodilatation. Care should be taken as it has a tocolytic effect that can prolong labour and increase maternal blood loss.

3. *Arrhythmias*
   Magnesium acts as a natural calcium antagonist, causing negative chronotropic and ionotropic effects.

4. *Treatment of vasospasm in SAH*
   The **MASH-2** trial (Lancet, 2012) showed no improvement in outcome after aneurysmal SAH. Its routine use is therefore not recommended.

Further Reading

The Magpie Trial Collaborative Group. Do women with pre-eclampsia, and their babies, benefit from magnesium sulphate? The Magpie Trial: a randomised, placebo-controlled trial. *Lancet* 2002; **359** (9321): 1877–1890

Mees S M D, Algra A, Vandertop W P et al. Magnesium for aneurysmal subarachnoid haemorrhage (MASH-2): a randomised placebo-controlled trial. *Lancet* 2012; **380**(9836): 44–49

Parikh M, Webb S T. Cations: potassium, calcium and magnesium. *Contin Educ Anaesth Crit Care Pain* 2012; **12**(4): 195–198

Chapter 52

Major Incidents

Define the term *major incident*

A major incident is any occurrence that presents a serious threat to the health of a community, disruption to a service or necessitates special arrangements by the emergency services.

Communication from ambulance control generally activates the hospital major incident plan. Once a major incident is declared, the hospital can cancel all non-urgent elective operations and expedite the discharge of medically fit patients. All personnel on the major incident call-out list are notified, given action cards and deployed to their designated location.

How are major incidents classified?

Major incidents can be either external or internal (e.g. fire, flood, power failure). External major incidents can be grouped into:

1 *Big bang* e.g. crash, explosion
2 *Rising tide* e.g. epidemic, pandemic
3 *Cloud on the horizon* e.g. potential war/conflict, nuclear disaster in France or Ireland
4 *Headline news* e.g. people panicking about Ebola or severe acute respiratory syndrome (SARS)

What is the command and control framework for major incidents?

A command and control framework for major incidents exists in the NHS. A hospital *control room* is designated, and in this room are:

Gold (strategic) *commander*	On call director
	Responsible for assessing the effect of the major incident on the trust, including financial impact, recovery phase planning and the return to normal operation

Silver (tactical) commander	Directly responsible for coordination of the major incident response
	Makes decisions about staff deployment and resource allocation, e.g. responsible for cancelling elective lists
	Delegates responsibility for running individual departments to bronze commanders
Bronze (operational) commander	Usually clinical staff, organised on departmental basis (see below)
	Not directly involved in patient care, but oversee it; responsible for coordination of patient flow, updating silver commander

What roles are assigned to clinical staff?

Each institution has their own variation on a standard major incident plan, and it is important to familiarise yourself with the one in your trust. A typical structure is:

ED Commander	This is the consultant in charge in the ED
Nurse in Charge of ED	
Triage Officer	An ED registrar or consultant, with assistance from a nurse and a clerical worker
Resus Team Leader	An ED consultant, based in resus
Theatre Commander	A senior surgeon, based in resus
Anaesthetics Commander	On call consultant anaesthetist, based in resus
ICU Commander	Nurse in charge of ICU, based on ICU
Theatre Coordinator	Coordinating nurse, based in theatres

How are patients triaged?

Triage is summarised in Table 52.1.

What are the priorities of the receiving staff in a major incident?

Damage control principles apply in the context of a major incident. This aims to prevent hypothermia, coagulopathy and acidosis (associated with increased mortality in trauma). The teams' aims should be:

1 Identify and control haemorrhage
2 Permissive hypotension

Table 52.1 Major incident triage

Priority		Suggested Location of Care
P1	Emergency, high priority for immediate life-saving care	Resus
P2	Urgent care	Majors
P3	Walking wounded	Minors
P4	Expectant – Unsurvivable injuries – Injuries so severe that their treatment would compromise the care of a large number of other injured patients	Other holding area for comfort care
P5	Dead	Mortuary

3 Transfusion of blood products based on clinical findings (not on laboratory coagulation tests) and VHAs
   – Avoid the use of clear fluids where possible
4 Temperature management (active warming of infused fluids and patients)
5 Damage control surgery (aimed at haemostasis only rather than definitive procedures)
6 A period of stabilisation in the ICU to allow for correction of acidosis, coagulopathy and hypothermia
7 Return to theatre for definitive surgery once physiology allows

What are the priorities of the consultants on ICU?

1 Assess the need for ICU beds and potential time frame
   – Liaise with Theatre and Anaesthetics Commanders
   – Liaise with nurse in charge to identify potential for increases in capacity
2 Setting up satellite ICUs
   – This involves finding appropriate locality (usually recovery or anaesthetic rooms, where staff are more familiar with caring for unwell, ventilated patients), staff and equipment
3 Assess need for extra staffing, and allocating staff appropriately
4 Discharge coordination
   – Non-clinical transfers across the critical care network (usually necessitates senior anaesthetic escort in an ambulance, and means these resources are taken away from patient care/major incident response)
   – Ward discharges
5 Ensure care of existing ICU patient cohort is not compromised
6 Coordination of ongoing care for trauma patients including ensuring completion of tertiary surveys and further surgical planning, e.g. re-look/definitive surgery and reconstruction

What happens after stand down?

Once stand down is declared, the major incident is perceived to be over and the trust can begin to formulate a plan to resume normal operation as soon as is feasible.

Ongoing care of those admitted during the major incident (and the existing patient population) is coordinated. Secondary and tertiary surveys are crucial, and more in-depth investigation may be undertaken. This will have an ongoing effect on elective work, and additional lists may be scheduled to manage the inevitable backlog.

Debriefing is important in order to allow the trust (and the wider medical population) to learn from individual cases and events. It is time consuming and may occur over a period of weeks or months. The trust resilience team should be involved in debriefing, and psychological support for staff should be widely available.

Further Reading

Johnson C, Cosgrove J F. Hospital response to a major incident: Initial considerations and longer-term effects. *BJA Educ* 2016; **16**(10): 329–333

Shirley P, Mandersloot G. Clinical review: The role of the intensive care physician in mass casualty incidents: planning, organisation and leadership. *Crit Care* 2008; **12**: 214–220

Chapter 53

Malaria

What causes malaria?

Malaria is caused by infection of blood cells by a protozoan parasite belonging to the *Plasmodium* genus.

What is the vector for the spread of malaria?

The female anopheles mosquito.

What are the different species of protozoa causing malarial infection?

Four species are classically considered to cause disease in humans (Table 53.1). A fifth, *P. knowlesi*, is now recognised as a zoonotic cause of malaria in parts of Malaysia.

Table 53.1 The different species of *Plasmodia*

Plasmodium species		Incubation period
P. falciparum	Commonest species identified Causes a more severe form of malaria	9–14 days
P. malariae	Less severe illness Causes fevers at 3-day intervals	2–4 weeks
P. ovale	Dormant parasite stage in the liver that causes relapses of infection	12–18 days
P. vivax	2nd most important causative agent of human malaria Dominant malaria species outside Africa Dormant parasite stage in the liver that causes relapses of infection	12–18 days
P. knowlesi	Parasite burden may expand rapidly resulting in severe and sometimes fatal illness (short 24-hour asexual cycle)	9–12 days

What is the pathophysiology of malaria infection?

1 Plasmodium parasites are introduced via the bite of an infected mosquito as sporozoites
2 Sporozoites are taken up by hepatocytes where they mature over 7–10 days to form schizonts
3 Schizonts rupture to release variable numbers of merozoites into the blood
4 Merozoites rapidly invade erythrocytes, forming trophozoites
5 Trophozoites then mature into schizonts over a period of 24–72 hours, depending on the species
6 The mature schizonts rupture, causing haemolysis and releasing further merozoites into the blood where they invade more erythrocytes

It is this periodic haemolysis that causes the majority of symptoms associated with malaria. Different species of malaria rupture the red blood cells at different intervals, which leads to the diagnostic cycles of fever that characterise malaria; *P. vivax*, for example, tends to produce cycles of fever every two days, whereas *P. malariae* produces fever every three.

Figure 53.1 shows the lifecycle of the malaria parasite.

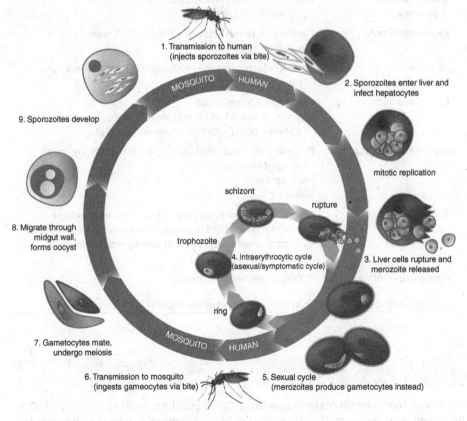

Figure 53.1 The lifecycle of the malaria parasite
Reproduced with permission from Klein EY (*Int J Antimicrob Agents* 2013)

What are the criteria for severe malaria?

Criteria for severe malaria have been defined by the WHO; those for *P. falciparum* malaria are shown in Table 53.2. The commonest reasons for admission to the ICU are cerebral malaria, ARDS and AKI.

Table 53.2 Criteria for severe malaria

Impaired consciousness	GCS <11 in adults Blantyre coma score <3 in children
Prostration	Generalised weakness such that the person is unable to sit, stand or walk without assistance
Multiple seizures	More than two episodes within 24 hours
Acidosis	Base excess >-8 mEq/l Bicarbonate <15 mmol/l or lactate >5 mmol/l
Hypoglycaemia	<2.2 mmol/l
Severe malarial anaemia	Haemoglobin concentration ≤70 g/l Haematocrit of ≤20%
Renal impairment	Plasma or serum creatinine >265 μmol/l (3 mg/dl) Blood urea >20 mmol/l
Jaundice	Plasma or serum bilirubin >50 μmol/l (3 mg/dl) with a parasite count >100 000/μl
Pulmonary oedema	Radiologically confirmed Oxygen saturation <92% on room air with a respiratory rate >30/min, often with chest indrawing and crackles
Significant bleeding	Recurrent or prolonged bleeding from the nose, gums or venepuncture sites Haematemesis Melaena
Shock	Compensated shock: capillary refill ≥3 s or temperature gradient on leg (mid to proximal limb), but no hypotension Decompensated shock: SBP <80 mmHg with evidence of impaired perfusion
Hyperparasitaemia	*P. falciparum* parasitaemia > 10%

Adapted with permission from WHO guidelines for the treatment of malaria (2015)

How do you treat severe malaria?

Mortality from severe malaria (particularly cerebral malaria) approaches 100%. However, with prompt effective antimalarial treatment and supportive care the rate falls to 10–20% overall. Management should always be discussed with a specialist.

1 **HDU/ICU admission for severe or complicated falciparum malaria**
   i Cardiac and glucose monitoring
      – Malaria is associated with hypoglycaemia, complicated by quinine-induced hyperinsulinaemia
      – Infusion of 10% dextrose may be necessary
   ii Meticulous attention to fluid balance
      – Avoid over-filling and exacerbating increased pulmonary capillary permeability
   iii Respiratory support as necessary
2 Urgent appropriate parenteral therapy with **antimalarials**
   Artesunate IV or IM is the treatment of choice for all adults and children (including infants and pregnant women) with severe malaria
   – Given for at least 24 hours and until they can tolerate oral medication
   – Should be followed by a full dose of effective oral **artemisinin-based combination therapy**
3 **Consider broad spectrum antibiotics** if evidence of shock or secondary bacterial infection. Complicating bacteraemia (*algid malaria*) should be treated appropriately.

Further Reading

Marks M, Gupta-Wright A, Doherty J, et al. Managing Malaria in the Intensive Care Unit. *Brit J Anaesth* 2014; 113(6): 910–921

World Health Organisation (WHO), 2015. *Guidelines for the Treatment of Malaria* [online]. Available at: www.who.int/malaria/publications/atoz/9789241549127/en/ (Accessed: 22 October 2016)

Chapter 54

Mental Capacity and Deprivation of Liberty in the ICU

What is capacity?

Capacity is the ability to make your own decisions. Importantly, patients may have capacity for some decisions but not others.

Are you aware of any legislation surrounding capacity?

The **Mental Capacity Act 2005** protects vulnerable adults and empowers them to make their own decisions. It applies to patients over the age of 16.

The five statutory principles of the act are:

1 A person is assumed to have capacity until proven otherwise
2 A person is not to be treated as unable to make a decision unless all practicable steps to help him/her to do so have been taken without success
3 A person is not to be treated as unable to make a decision merely because he/she makes an *unwise* decision
4 An act done, or decision made, under this Act for or on behalf of a person who lacks capacity must be done, or made, in his/her *best interests*
5 Before the act is done, or the decision is made, regard must be had to whether the purpose for which it is needed can be as effectively achieved in a way that is *least restrictive* of the person's rights and freedom of action

How do you assess capacity?

Stage 1: Is there a disorder or disability of the brain or mind?

Stage 2: Can the patient:

1 Understand the information given to him/her
2 Retain this information long enough to make a decision
3 Weigh the information in the decision-making process
4 Communicate their decision – verbal or non-verbal, interpreter etc.

What do you do if the patient does not have capacity?

If the patient is deemed not to have capacity, the principle of *best interests* is applied. This involves:

1 Ascertaining the patient's past and present wishes, including advanced decisions/directives
2 Ascertaining the beliefs and values of the patient that may influence their decision
3 Discussion with the next of kin or an *independent mental capacity advocate* (IMCA)

(Note that the doctor is not obliged to adhere to the opinions of the IMCA but should document clearly why not)

What is a deprivation of liberty safeguard and to whom is it applied?

The Mental Capacity Act was amended in 2009 to include Deprivation of Liberty Safeguard (DOLS) after a judgement by the European Court of Human Rights – *The Bournewood Judgement*. Article 5 of the Human Rights Act 1998 requires that no one should be deprived of their liberty except in certain, pre-defined, circumstances. There must also be an appropriate, legally based, procedure in place to protect the individual's rights.

The purpose of DOLS:

1 To protect vulnerable adults who lack capacity against arbitrary detention that is not in their best interests
2 Gives the person a right to challenge the confinement.

A DOLS order applies to anyone who lacks capacity to consent to detention imputable to the state (i.e. in a public sector facility) that is determined by an independent review to be in their best interests, e.g. patients with delirium, those requiring pharmacological or physical restraints, long stays and those with *red flags* (trying to leave, family conflicts etc.)

The Supreme Court judgement in March 2014 in the case of **Cheshire West** clarified an *acid test* for what constitutes deprivation of liberty. All three elements must be present for the acid test to be met:

1 The patient lacks the capacity to consent to their care/treatment arrangements
2 The patient is under continuous supervision and control
3 The patient is not free to leave.

In a landmark judgement in January 2017, the Court of Appeal in **Ferreira vs Coroner of Inner South London** ruled that any deprivation of liberty resulting from the administration of life-saving treatment to a person falls outside Article

5(1), as long as it is unavoidable as a result of circumstances beyond the control of the authorities and necessary to avert a real risk of serious injury or damage, and is kept to the minimum required for that purpose. Moreover, the Court emphasised that the *not free to leave* element of the acid test requires that the patient *wants* to leave but is being prevented by the state. This means that the acid test is not met where the reason for the patient not being able to leave is their underlying medical condition, or the essential treatment of it, rather than any restrictions imposed by the hospital.

Additionally, a DOLS order is not necessary in:

i Patients who have previously consented to this accommodation, e.g. as part of pre-operative assessment for elective surgery
ii Patients who are deeply unconscious
iii Patients who are expected to regain capacity within seven days
iv Patients who are expected to die

Why may it be appropriate to deprive a patient of their liberty?

The Mental Capacity Act DOLS code of practice highlights that deprivation of liberty is justifiable, where the person lacks capacity to consent to this:

1 If it is in their best interests to protect them from harm
2 If it is a proportional response when compared to the potential harm faced by the person
3 If there is no less restrictive alternative

How does one apply for a DOLS authorisation?

An application is made to the trust (if urgent) or to the local authority (if not urgent). Urgent authorisations can only be made where a standard authorisation has been applied for (either contemporaneously or previously) but is not yet granted. An independent assessment is then carried out (usually by a psychiatrist). Importantly, a DOLS authorisation is not transferable between institutions.

Further Reading

Crews M, Garry D, Phillips C, et al. Deprivation of liberty in the intensive care. *Journal of the Intensive Care Society* 2014; **15**(4): 320–324

Department of Health Guidance: Response to the Supreme Court Judgment/ Deprivation of Liberty Safeguards. DOH, October 2015.

Faculty of Intensive Care Medicine, 2017. ICS/FICM guidance on MCA/DoL [online]. Available at: www .ficm.ac.uk/sites/default/files/ics-ficm-post-ferreira-briefing-feb2017.pdf (Accessed: 10 February 2017)

HL vs United Kingdom ECtHR [2004] 40 EHRR 761

P vs Cheshire West and Chester Council and another [2014] UKSC 19

Chapter 55

Myasthenia Gravis

What is myasthenia gravis?

Acquired myasthenia gravis (MG) is an autoimmune condition characterised by the presence of IgG autoantibodies targeting the post-synaptic acetylcholine receptor (AChR) at the nicotinic neuromuscular junction (NMJ). These AChR antibodies reduce the number of functional receptors by blocking the attachment of acetylcholine molecules, resulting in fluctuating, fatigable weakness in characteristic muscles.

The condition commonly involves either isolated ocular dysfunction such as diplopia and ptosis, or takes a generalised form affecting bulbar function with dysarthria and dysphagia, or neck and proximal muscle weakness.

How is myasthenia gravis diagnosed?

1 Clinical features
   - Weakness of voluntary muscle that is exacerbated by repetitive exercise (fatiguable weakness) is a characteristic finding
   - In 15% of patients the disease is confined to the eyes (ocular MG): diplopia and ptosis are the most common symptoms/signs
   - The generalised form may present with, or progress to, weakness of the flexors and extensors of the neck and proximal muscles of the trunk
   - Respiratory failure (may require intubation and ventilation)
2 Electromyography
   - Diagnostic test of choice
   - A characteristic EMG pattern is seen in MG (progressively smaller action potentials with repetitive nerve stimulation)
3 Edrophonium (Tensilon) test
   - Up to 10 mg of edrophonium (a rapidly acting cholinesterase inhibitor) is administered IV
   - Patients with MG show a rapid improvement in muscle power within 10 seconds and sustained for around 5 minutes
   - This test is no longer widely available due to the risk of profound bradycardia and heart block
4 Serum autoantibodies
   - Serum AChR antibodies or anti-muscle specific kinase (MUSK) antibodies

- Not required for a diagnosis of MG, but should be sent prior to the initiation of immunotherapy (to distinguish immune from non-immune myasthenic syndromes)
- Anti-AChR antibodies are elevated in 85–90% of patients with generalised MG

How is myasthenia gravis treated?

1 Pharmacotherapy
  i Drugs inhibiting the action of the cholinesterase enzyme are first-line
    - **Pyridostigmine** acts within 30 mins and has a peak effect at 2 hours
    - It has few muscarinic side effects
    - Its effects may diminish over months and most patients then require immunosuppression
  ii Immunosuppression
    - **Corticosteroids** are used to initiate or maintain remission by reducing AChR antibodies
    - **Azathioprine** and **cyclosporin** are steroid-sparing agents, used in refractory or steroid-dependent cases
2 Surgical management – **thymectomy**
  - A thymoma is seen in up to 15% of MG patients, and thymic hyperplasia in up to 65%
  - A thymectomy is an elective procedure and should not be performed during a myasthenic crisis
  - Thymectomy does not generally lead to remission in MG (however, an RCT in 2016 did find benefit)
3 **Plasma exchange** and **IVIg** are both used in the critical care setting to treat acute exacerbations of MG

Why might a patient with myasthenia gravis require intensive care admission?

1 *Myasthenic crisis*
  - A myasthenic crisis is defined as severe respiratory muscle weakness necessitating admission to a critical care unit
  - It is characterised by:
    i FVC <1 litre
    ii Negative inspiratory force of ≤20 cmH$_2$O
    iii Need for mechanical respiratory support
  - It can occur spontaneously or be triggered by infection, treatment omission, stress or pregnancy
  - Precipitating factors should be addressed and PEx or IVIg commenced
  - Cholinesterase inhibitors are usually withdrawn until a response to treatment is seen and weaning from the ventilator is started

2 *Cholinergic crisis*
   – A cholinergic crisis results from anticholinesterase toxicity, leading to an excess of acetylcholine (ACh) which then overstimulates ACh receptors
   – Overstimulation of muscarinic AChRs results in the SLUDGE syndrome:
     Salivation
     Lacrimation
     Urination
     Defecation
     Gastrointestinal cramps
     Emesis
   – Overstimulation of the nicotinic AChRs results in involuntary twitching, fasciculations and weakness – this can be misdiagnosed as worsening of MG symptoms and wrongly treated as a myasthenic crisis
   – Cholinergic crises are rare – they can be definitively differentiated from a myasthenic crisis by using edrophonium, however this is unreliable and hazardous in this setting and is not advocated

How should a patient with a myasthenic crisis be assessed?

Monitoring respiratory muscle strength and prompt recognition of impending respiratory failure is key. The specific assessment of a myasthenic crisis involves:

1 Respiratory assessment
   i Assess VC: this should be measured every 2–4 hours
      Consider invasive ventilation if VC <**20** ml/kg
   ii Assess negative inspiratory force: consider intubation if less than **30** cmH$_2$O
      This '**20/30**' rule is probably the most helpful when making the decision of whether to intubate
   iii Hypercapnia and hypoxia are late signs of neuromuscular respiratory failure, and hence are not good indications of respiratory strength – they should not be used to determine the threshold for intubation in MG
2 Assess bulbar function
   – Severe bulbar weakness predisposes to aspiration
3 Determine the underlying trigger
   i Have a high index of suspicion for infection
   ii Review medications; take particular care to avoid medications that can exacerbate the condition

What are the potential indicators of need for ICU admission?

Admission to HDU/ICU should be considered if the following are present:

1 Rapid, shallow breathing, use of accessory muscles, paradoxical abdominal breathing
2 Baseline FVC <30 ml/kg ideal body weight
3 Inability to complete sentences

Which drugs should be used cautiously or avoided in myasthenia?

The drugs that may worsen neuromuscular transmission in MG are listed in Table 55.1.

Table 55.1 Drugs that may exacerbate myasthenia

Drug group	Examples
Antibiotics	Aminoglycosides
	Quinolones
	Macrolides
	Colistin
	Lincosamides
	Tetracyclines
	Polymyxins
	Ampicillin
Anticonvulsants	Phenytoin
	Gabapentin
Anaesthetic agents	Diazepam
	Ketamine
	Lignocaine
	Non-depolarising NMBAs
Cardiovascular drugs	Procainamide
	Quinidine
	Beta-blockers
	Calcium channel blockers
Other drugs	Acetazolamide
	Oral contraceptive pill
	Glucocorticoids
	Magnesium

What is Lambert-Eaton Myasthenic Syndrome?

Lambert-Eaton Myasthenic Syndrome (LEMS) presents with weakness that improves with repetitive stimulation of the muscle. Autoantibodies are directed at presynaptic voltage-gated calcium channels involved with neurotransmitter release. Characteristic clinical features include proximal muscle weakness, depressed tendon reflexes, post-tetanic potentiation and autonomic change.

LEMS is often a paraneoplastic disorder, usually associated with small cell lung cancer.

Further Reading

Jani-Acsadi A, Lisak R P. Myasthenic crisis: Guidelines for prevention and treatment. *J Neurol Sci* 2007; **261**(1–2): 127–133

Myasthenia Gravis Foundation of America, 2016. *Emergency Management of Myasthenia Gravis* [online]. Available at: http://myasthenia.org/HealthProfessionals/EmergencyManagement.aspx (Accessed: 27 December 2016)

Wolfe G I, Kaminski H J, Aban I B, et al. Randomised trial of thymectomy in myasthenia gravis. *N Engl J Med* 2016; **375**(6): 511–522

Chapter 56

Necrotising Fasciitis

What is necrotising fasciitis?

Necrotising Fasciitis (NF) is a fulminant bacterial infection of the deep fascia and subcutaneous fat. It is differentiated from cellulitis in that cellulitis originates at the junction of the superficial fascia and the dermis.

Causative organisms release exotoxins, endotoxins and enzymes that facilitate rapid spread of infection through the fascial planes causing extensive tissue damage. There is subsequent interruption of the microcirculation and vascular thrombosis causing local necrosis and cutaneous ischaemia. Destruction of superficial nerves causes overlying loss of sensation. NF is a rare but potentially lethal necrotising soft tissue infection, with an incidence of approximately 500 cases in the UK per year and a reported mortality of between 20 and 40%.

What types are there? What organisms cause necrotising fasciitis?

It is most commonly classified according to underlying microbial aetiology (Table 56.1).

How does necrotising fasciitis present?

The key symptom is severe pain, often out of proportion with other clinical findings, which precedes skin changes by up to 48 hours.

It is important to note that early in the pathological process, skin may look normal despite extensive underlying infection, and clinical examination may underestimate the severity of the infection. As the disease progresses, haemorrhagic bullae, ulceration and skin necrosis subsequently manifest as deeper structures become involved. Thrombosis of large numbers of dermal capillary beds must occur before these skin changes appear.

In the latter stages of the disease patients may present with fulminant sepsis, septic shock, TSS and multi-organ failure, which is associated with a high mortality.

Table 56.1 Classification of necrotising fasciitis

Type	Causative Organism(s)	Clinical Presentation
I	**Polymicrobial** Gram-positive cocci and bacilli, Gram-negative bacilli, anaerobes Usually ≥1 anaerobic species, e.g. Clostridium, Bacteroides plus ≥1 facultative anaerobic streptococci and Enterobacteriaceae, e.g. Enterobacter, E coli, Proteus	70–80% of cases Most commonly perineal (Fournier's gangrene) and trunk in immunocompromised patients Risk factors: DM, HIV, IVDU, alcohol abuse, trauma (e.g. indwelling medical devices, insect bites, chicken pox) Mortality depends on underlying comorbidities
II	**Group A Streptococcus** (GAS, Strep. pyogenes) **+/− S aureus** GAS are sequestered in macrophages and may evade antibiotic therapy even in well perfused tissue thought to be amenable to antibiotic penetration	20–30% of cases Classically occurs in extremities or trunk May be associated with toxic shock syndrome (TSS) Often occur in immunocompetent individuals +/− history of trauma Mortality >32% (especially if associated with myositis or TSS)
III	**Gram-negative monomicrobial** (typically Vibrio)	Uncommon, may be associated with water contamination Mortality 30–40% despite early diagnosis and aggressive antibiotic therapy
IV	**Fungal** (usually Candida)	Most commonly occurs in trauma patients, e.g. wounds and burns, and immunocompromised patients Mortality >47% (higher if immunocompromised)

Dermatological features of NF can be classified into three stages:

Stage 1 Erythema with tenderness extending beyond, swelling, hot skin
Stage 2 Formation of skin bullae and blisters, fluctuant skin
Stage 3 Haemorrhagic bullae, crepitus, skin necrosis and gangrene

How would you investigate this condition?

The diagnosis of NF is largely clinical, and radiological investigation should *not* delay surgical exploration and debridement. This often reveals fascial necrosis with or without myonecrosis, lack of resistance to blunt dissection, lack of bleeding and the presence of classical foul-smelling *dishwater* pus.

Investigations:

1 Blood tests
   - FBC (may detect anaemia and thrombocytopenia in severe sepsis, leucopenia or leucocytosis)
   - Biochemistry (raised CK indicates muscle involvement and may be associated with hypocalcaemia as calcium is deposited in necrotic tissue)
   - Other derangements in biochemistry may reflect multi-organ dysfunction in the context of septic shock
   - Coagulation screen (may reveal coagulopathy or DIC)
2 Microbiology
   - Blood cultures are positive in 20% of cases of type I NF and 11–60% of patients with type II NF
   - Tissue samples and aspirates should also be sent for MC+S
   - Fungal culture should be considered in high risk patients
3 Histology of samples of the advancing edge and central necrotic areas to confirm fascial involvement
4 Radiological investigation may aid diagnosis in early NF if the clinical picture is not clear
   - T2-weighted MRI imaging is probably the most useful radiological investigation and differentiates between oedematous and necrotic tissue
   - CT scans demonstrate deep fascial thickening and enhancement; fluid and gas may be seen within soft tissue planes in and around the superficial fascia
   - Ultrasonography may reveal distortion and thickening of the fascia and fluid collections

Do you know of any scoring systems for NF?

The Laboratory Risk Indicator for Necrotising Fasciitis (LRINEC) score (see Table 56.2) was designed to help distinguish NF from other soft tissue infections, mainly cellulitis. A score of >6 has a positive predictive value of 92% and a negative predictive value of 96%. A score of 8 is strongly predictive of NF, with a positive predictive value of 93.4%.

How do you manage necrotising fasciitis?

Necrotising fasciitis should be managed with an ABCDE approach, treating abnormalities as they are found. The mainstays of treatment are:

1 **Resuscitation and supportive care** with ICU admission
2 **Early surgical exploration and debridement**
   - Delayed/inadequate debridement increases mortality
   - Repeated 're-look' surgical debridement is necessary at regular intervals until the process stops
3 **Empirical aggressive broad-spectrum antimicrobial therapy**
   - Usually extended spectrum beta lactam + clindamycin (clindamycin is used to switch off toxin production)

Table 56.2 Laboratory Risk Indicator for Necrotising Fasciitis score

Variable		Score
CRP	<150	0
	≥150	4
WCC (cells/mm³)	<15	0
	15–25	1
	>25	2
Hb (g/l)	>13.5	0
	11–13.5	1
	<11	2
Na⁺ (mmol/l)	≥135	0
	<135	2
Cr (μmol/l)	≤141	0
	>141	2
Glucose (mmol/l)	≤10	0
	>10	1

Reproduced with permission from Wong CH, et al. (*Crit Care Med* 2004)

- Benzylpenicillin + clindamycin if Gram-positive organism suspected
- Add ceftriaxone or ciprofloxacin if mixed Gram-positive and Gram-negative infection suspected
- Consider MRSA cover with a glycopeptide if indicated

4 **IVIg**
- Indicated in critically ill patients with Streptococcal or Staphylococcal NF

5 **HBOT** may be used to switch off toxin production in Clostridial infection, but evidence in non-Clostridial NF is weak

You mentioned IVIg: How does that work in this situation?

Intravenous immunoglobulin works in four ways:

1 Induces antibodies against exotoxin
2 Neutralises superantigens
3 Inhibits the membrane attack complex (C5b-9) and complement activation
4 Facilitates opsonisation of GAS organisms

Further Reading

Davoudian P, Flint N J. Necrotising fasciitis. *Contin Educ Anaesth Crit Care Pain* 2012; **12**(5): 245–250

Wong C H, Khin L W, Heng K S, et al. The LRINEC (Laboratory Risk Indicator for Necrotizing Fasciitis) score: a tool for distinguishing necrotizing fasciitis from other soft tissue infections. *Crit Care Med* 2004; **32**: 1535–1541

Chapter 57

Non-Invasive Ventilation

What is non-invasive ventilation?

The BTS defines NIV as *the provision of ventilatory support using a mask or similar device via the patient's upper airway*. This is in comparison to invasive techniques that traverse the upper airway into the chest and lower airway.

The mode most commonly used for NIV is bi-level, pressure-targeted ventilation (pressure support ventilation). Target pressures are set for inspiration (inspiratory positive airway pressure, IPAP) and expiration (expiratory positive airway pressure, EPAP). The difference between the two is the level of ventilatory assistance or pressure support. Volume-targeted non-invasive ventilators are rarely employed in the UK (outside specialist centres).

NIV augments tidal volume by sensing inspiratory effort and providing a set level of pressure support to the patient. The pressure returns to the preset EPAP level when the flow stops. NIV thus has several effects:

1 Increase in functional residual capacity (FRC), improved alveolar ventilation and recruitment
2 Decreased work of breathing (proportional to the amount of inspiratory pressure that is set)
3 Delivery of high FiO_2 (closed system with no rebreathing)

What interfaces are available for delivering NIV?

1 Face mask
   - A range of shapes and sizes are available to accommodate the natural diversity of the face
   - Pressure areas (especially bridge of nose) can be problematic in dependent patients
   - A mask that covers the whole face (excluding the ears) is available when leak is excessive or when nasal ulceration develops
2 Helmet
   - Triggering is ineffective
   - Noise caused by turbulence within the helmet can be an issue
   - Inability to provide humidified gases (due to *rain-out* within the helmet)
3 Nasal mask/nasal pillows
   - Useful in patients who cannot tolerate a face mask due to claustrophobia
   - Mouth leak limits effectiveness

What are the advantages of NIV compared with conventional ventilation with an ETT?

1 Reduced incidence of VAP
2 Avoidance of complications associated with invasive airways
3 Avoidance of requirement for induction/sedation for ETT tolerance
4 Potentially reduced ICU/hospital LOS (as demonstrated by some studies)

What are the indications and contraindications for NIV?

The BTS released updated guidelines on the use of NIV in 2016. Figure 57.1 depicts a general summary for providing NIV in the acute clinical situation.

Research has shown clear benefit for NIV in acute exacerbations of COPD in terms of reducing ICU admissions, need for tracheal intubation and overall mortality (see page 133). A second group of patients who have shown significant benefit from NIV over invasive ventilation are those with neutropenia. Similarly, there is good evidence to show that CPAP improves outcomes in patients with cardiogenic pulmonary oedema.

Further indications for NIV include:

1 Prevention of re-intubation after weaning from conventional ventilation **Jaber, et al (JAMA, 2016)** showed that the use of NIV reduced the need for re-intubation within 7 days in hypoxaemic respiratory failure after abdominal surgery compared to standard oxygen therapy
2 As a weaning tool in resolving respiratory failure

What are the advantages and disadvantages of delivering oxygen via high-flow nasal cannulae?

Advantages

1 Can generate FiO_2 of 1.0 and PEEP ≤ 7.4 cmH_2O at 60 l/min
2 More comfortable
3 Improved compliance compared to face mask

Disadvantages

1 Variable PEEP
   – PEEP drops to ~2 cmH_2O when the patient's mouth is open
2 Complications include:
   i Epistaxis, local trauma
   ii Blocked cannulae due to secretions
   iii Gastric distension

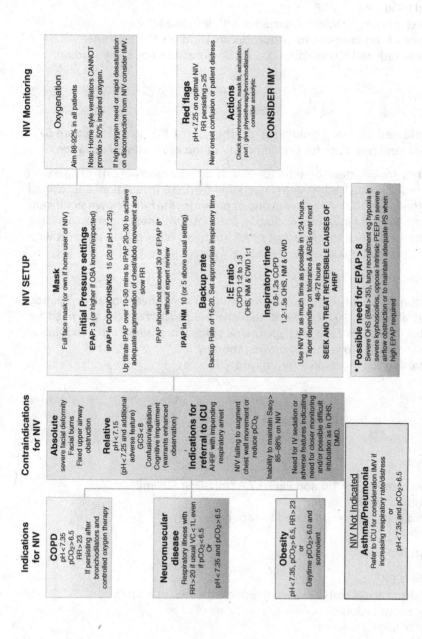

Figure 57.1 Summary for providing acute non-invasive ventilation
Reproduced with kind permission from the British Thoracic Society (*Thorax* 2016)
IMV – invasive mechanical ventilation; AHRF – acute hypercapnic respiratory failure; OHS – obesity hypoventilation syndrome; DMD – Duchenne muscular dystrophy; KS – kyphoscholiosis; NM – neuromuscular; CWD – chest wall disease

What is the evidence for high-flow nasal oxygen in the ICU?

The small, multicentre **FLORALI** trial (NEJM, 2015), demonstrated that high-flow oxygen via nasal cannula reduced 90-day mortality compared with standard oxygen therapy and NIV. No difference in intubation rates was seen between the three groups of patients with acute hypoxaemic respiratory failure.

A recent RCT by **Hernández, et al** (JAMA, 2016) demonstrated that the use of high-flow nasal oxygen reduced the incidence of re-intubation in patients that were deemed low risk for requiring re-intubation following a period of at least 12 hours of mechanical ventilation.

Further Reading

British Thoracic Society Standards of Care Committee. Non-invasive ventilation in acute respiratory failure. *Thorax* 2002; **57**: 192–211

Davidson A C, Banham S, Elliott M, et al. BTS/ICS guideline for the ventilatory management of acute hypercapnic respiratory failure in adults. *Thorax* 2016; **71**: ii1–ii35

Chapter 58

Nosocomial Infection and Ventilator-Associated Pneumonia

Define *nosocomial infection*

Infection that is diagnosed 48–72 hours after admission to hospital.

Why is nosocomial infection particularly problematic in intensive care patients?

The **EPIC** study (JAMA, 1995) revealed that 21% of patients admitted to the ICU have at least one ICU-acquired infection. The **EPIC II** study (JAMA, 2009) revealed the predominant sites of infection to be:

1 Respiratory tract (63.5%)
2 Abdominal (19.6%)
3 Bacteraemia (15.1%)
4 Urinary tract (14.3%)

Critically ill patients are at particular risk of infection because their natural defences are compromised:

1 Skin is breached by intravascular devices, surgical incisions or trauma
2 Loss of cough reflex and respiratory tract protection with endotracheal intubation and sedation
3 Urethral catheterisation causes inflammation and stagnation of urine, predisposing to UTI
4 Gut mucosal injury and ischaemia predisposes to bacterial translocation
5 Bacteria from the GI tract may gain access to the respiratory tract due to NG tube insertion, ileus and drug therapy to suppress gastric acid production
6 Malnutrition, acute and chronic disease, and immunosuppressive drugs (e.g. steroids, etomidate) depress native immune function
7 Insertion of foreign material/prostheses may encourage the formation of biofilms
8 Courses of broad-spectrum antibiotics produce alterations in protective commensal flora

Hospital-acquired infections are more likely to be caused by resistant organisms than community-acquired infections, and therefore may be more difficult to treat.

When would you treat bacteriuria in ICU patients?

Nearly all patients on the ICU will have a urinary catheter, and the likelihood of colonisation increases with duration of catheterisation. Asymptomatic bacteriuria should *not* be treated. If infection is suspected, a urine sample should be sent for MC+S. Symptomatic patients should receive antibiotic treatment as per local microbiological guidelines. Empirical therapy that covers *Enterobacteriaceae,* including ESBL, is usually necessary. The threshold for treatment is often lower in immunocompromised patients.

What is a catheter-related bloodstream infection and how common is it?

Catheter-related bloodstream infection (CRBSI) refers to nosocomial infection related to the presence of an indwelling vascular device. Soon after insertion, both the inner and outer surfaces of the catheter become coated with fibrin, and bacteria from the skin or from a contaminated catheter port can colonise this fibrin sheath. Common causative organisms include coagulase-negative Staphylococci, *S. aureus*, Gram-negative organisms (*Enterococci, E. coli, Klebsiella*) and, importantly although less commonly, *Candida* species.

The rate of CRBSI is approximately 0.8% with arterial lines and 4% with central lines.

How is CRBSI managed?

Blood cultures should be taken peripherally and from all indwelling catheters before initiating antimicrobial therapy. Empirical agents should include an anti-staphylococcal drug, e.g. flucloxacillin, or a glycopeptide if MRSA is suspected. Whether or not removal of the catheter is necessary depends on the causative pathogen:

- Coagulase-negative staphylococcal infection can be treated with a seven-day course of glycopeptide in 80% of cases, therefore these agents may be chosen if line insertion is difficult in a particular patient
- Infection with *S. aureus* or *Candida* is an absolute indication for intravascular catheter removal/replacement (delayed removal is associated with increased mortality), and a longer course of antimicrobials is often necessary to reduce complications related to pathogenic seeding of other tissues

Do you know of any care bundles that are used to help prevent CRBSIs?

The international *Matching Michigan* programme is based on work by **Pronovost, et al** (BMJ, 2010), which resulted in a significant and sustained reduction in CRBSIs. The care bundle includes five elements:

1 Hand hygiene
2 Strict asepsis with full barrier precautions
3 Use of 2% chlorhexidine in 70% alcohol for skin preparation
4 Avoidance of the femoral route
5 Daily review, with removal of catheters as soon as they were no longer needed

What is ventilator-associated pneumonia?

Ventilator-associated pneumonia is pneumonia that occurs 48–72 hours after endotracheal intubation. It is characterised by the presence of a new or progressive infiltrate, signs of systemic infection (fever, altered white blood cell count), changes in sputum characteristics, and detection of a causative agent.

VAP can be further classified as early onset (within 4 days) or late onset (after 4 days) after intubation:

Early onset VAP

Classically associated with community acquired, antibiotic-sensitive bacteria:

1 *Streptococcus pneumoniae*
2 *Haemophilus influenzae*
3 MSSA
4 Antibiotic-sensitive Gram-negative bacteria (*Escherichia coli, Klebsiella pneumonia, Enterobacter* species, *Proteus* species and *Serratia marcescens*)

Late onset VAP

Associated with multi-drug resistant organisms:

1 MRSA
2 *Acinetobacter*
3 *Pseudomonas*
4. ESBL-producing bacteria

VAP is estimated to occur in 9–27% of all mechanically ventilated patients and contributes to approximately half of the cases of hospital-acquired pneumonia.

What are the risk factors for VAP?

The following are risk factors for the development of VAP:

1 Severe burns
2 Acute or chronic respiratory pathology
3 Supine body position
4 Enteral nutrition
5 Excessive sedation
6 Smoking

How is VAP diagnosed?

There is no universally accepted, gold-standard criteria for VAP diagnosis. Several clinical methods have been described: one of the best-known methods is the Clinical Pulmonary Infection Score (CPIS, Table 58.1), proposed by Pugin, et al. in 1991. The CPIS has been criticised for the potential for inter-observer variability, and there has also been debate with regard to its diagnostic validity.

Table 58.1 CPIS for the diagnosis of VAP

Sign	Score 0	1	2
Temperature (°C)	36.5–38.4	38.5–38.9	<36 or >39
Leucocytes in blood ($\times 10^9$/l)	4–11	<4 or >11	>500 band forms
PaO_2/FiO_2 (mmHg)	>240 or ARDS		<240 and no ARDS
CXR	No infiltrate	Diffuse or patchy infiltrates	Localised infiltrate
Tracheal secretions (subjective visual scale)	None	Non-purulent	Purulent
Culture of tracheal aspirate	No or mild growth	Moderate or florid growth	Moderate or florid growth *and* pathogen consistent with gram stain

Scoring range is between 0 and 12; a score >6 shows good correlation with the presence of VAP

What is the management of VAP?

A high index of suspicion should be maintained, according to your institution's criteria of choice. VAP should be managed with an ABCDE approach, treating abnormalities as they are found. Specific interventions include:

1 Administration of **appropriate antimicrobials** based on timing, MRSA status, presence of immunosuppression etc.
   - If there is a high clinical suspicion, start antibiotics promptly but ideally obtain microbiological samples first
2 Take **appropriate samples** for Gram stain and culture:
   - Endotracheal aspirate: easiest to obtain, does not require provider involvement
   - BAL: requires bronchoscopic guidance

  – Mini-BAL: performed without bronchoscopic guidance
  – Protected specimen brush: utilises a brush at the tip of the catheter which is rubbed against the bronchial wall
3 **Rationalise antibiotic therapy** based on the pathogen identified
4 Ensure **lung-protective ventilatory settings** to minimise further VILI

How can VAP be prevented?

There are three potential ways of preventing VAP:

1 Reduce colonisation of the gastrointestinal tract and oropharynx by Gram-negative organisms
2 Prevent aspiration
3 Limit the duration of mechanical ventilation

The Institute of Healthcare Improvement proposed a five-element *ventilator bundle* including three interventions targeting VAP and two aimed at preventing stress ulceration and venous thromboembolism (VTE):

1 Head-up (>30°)
2 Oral decontamination (with chlorhexidine)
3 Daily sedation holds (i.e. aiming to decrease the duration of ventilation)
4 Thromboprophylaxis
5 Gastric ulcer prophylaxis

Other suggested measures include:

1 Subglottic suction
2 Silver-coated endotracheal tube
3 Maintaining cuff pressures at an adequate level (~20 cmH$_2$O) with regular checks
4 Modified cuff with fewer, narrower longitudinal folds when inflated
5 Prophylactic probiotics
6 Minimise re-intubation
7 Early removal of invasive devices

Further Reading

American Thoracic Society, Infectious Diseases Society of America: Guidelines for the management of adults with hospital-acquired, ventilator-associated, and healthcare-associated pneumonia. *Am J Respir Crit Care Med* 2005; **171**: 388–416

Kalanuria A, Ziai W. Ventilator-associated pneumonia in the ICU. *Critical Care* 2014; **18**: 208

Pronovost P J, Goeschel C A, Colantuoni E, et al. Sustaining reductions in catheter related bloodstream infections in Michigan intensive care units: observational study. *Br Med J* 2010; **340**: 309–314

Pugin J, Auckenthaler R, Mili N, et al. Diagnosis of ventilator-associated pneumonia by bacteriologic analysis of bronchoscopic and nonbronchoscopic "blind" bronchoalveolar lavage fluid. *American Rev Respir Dis* 1991; **143**: 1121–1129

Vincent J L, Rello J, Marshall J, et al. International study of the prevalence and outcomes of infection in intensive care units. *J Am Med Assoc* 2009; **302**(21): 2323–2329

Chapter 59

Novel Anticoagulants

Can you tell me about novel anticoagulant agents?

Novel anticoagulants (NOACs) are a group of new drugs whose mechanism of action do not rely on vitamin K-dependent pathways. They show more predicable activity, require less monitoring and have a more rapid onset compared with conventional anticoagulation with coumarins. There are several subtypes:

1 Direct thrombin inhibitors, e.g. dabigatran (oral, bd)
   - Uses:
     i Equivalent to LMWH for thromboprophylaxis after primary total hip replacement (THR) and total knee replacement (TKR)
     ii Equivalent to warfarin for treatment of DVT
     iii Superior to warfarin for prophylaxis of stroke in AF
   - Bioavailability is variable: enteric-coated capsule (if broken, 10 times drug dose released)
   - Compliance is poor due to tablet size
   - New reversal agent: monoclonal antibody to immediately reverse action, Idacaruzumab
2 Direct factor Xa inhibitors, e.g. rivaroxaban, apixaban (oral)
   - Uses:
     i Superior to LMWH in thromboprophylaxis after primary THR and TKR
     ii Treatment of VTE
     iii Prevention of thromboembolic complications in AF
   - Half-life not prolonged provided creatinine clearance >50 ml/min
3 Indirect factor Xa inhibitors, e.g. fondaparinux (subcutaneous)
   - Synthetic heparin pentasaccharide, acts via antithrombin III to inhibit factor Xa
   - Uses:
     i Non-ST-elevation MI (NSTEMI) and unstable ACS in patients with high risk of bleeding (unless PCI planned within 24 hours)
     ii Thromboprophylaxis in medical patients, and post THR and TKR
     iii Treatment of VTE
   - Longer half-life
   - Renal clearance

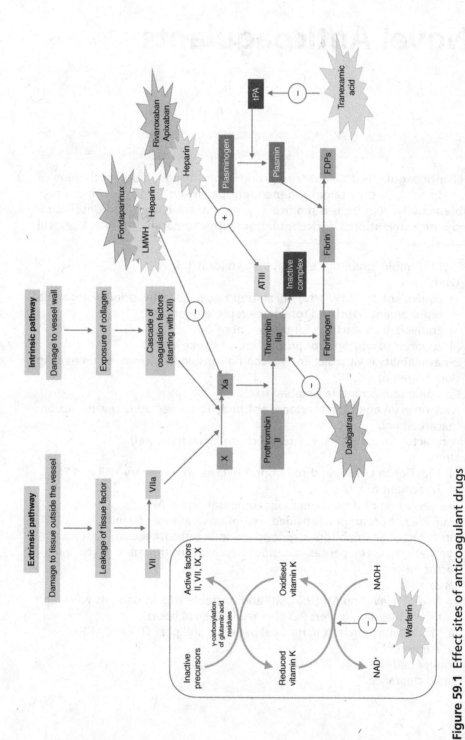

Figure 59.1 Effect sites of anticoagulant drugs

ATIII – antithrombin III; NAD⁺ – nicotinamide adenine dinucleotide; NADH – reduced nicotinamide adenine dinucleotide; tPA – tissue plasminogen activator

What are the indications for their use?

NICE have approved dabigatran, rivaroxaban and apixaban for the treatment and prophylaxis of:

1 The thromboembolic complications of non-valvular AF
2 Venous thromboembolism
3 VTE after elective hip or knee replacement

Additionally, rivaroxaban is licensed for use in the prevention of adverse outcomes (MI or stroke) after acute management of ACS with raised cardiac enzymes.

What are the advantages and disadvantages of their use compared to warfarin?

These are summarised in Table 59.1.

Table 59.1 Advantages and disadvantages of NOACs

Advantages	Disadvantages
Rapid onset	No specific antidote
Short half lives	No widely available or reliable measure of activity
Similar/improved efficacy	Limited experience (have only been around <10 years)
Fewer interactions with drugs and food compared to warfarin	Effect of renal impairment on pharmacokinetics
No need for monitoring	
No need for bridging with heparin	
Fixed dosing	
Fewer complications, e.g. ICH, vs warfarin	

How do you monitor their effects?

They have no reliable effect on standard coagulation tests (vs warfarin and PT/INR). It is possible to measure serum levels of some NOACs.

A 72-year-old lady who is taking rivaroxaban for AF is admitted to the ED with a significant UGI bleed. You are called to assess her. Explain how you would manage this patient.

The management of this patient should follow an ABCDE approach, treating abnormalities as they are found. Specific management includes:

1 Give 100% O_2
2 Treat the catastrophic haemorrhage
   – Source control – stop the bleeding
   – Large bore IV access/trauma line
   – Blood tests (FBC, haemocue, clotting, U+Es, LFTs, crossmatch, blood gas)
   – Consider near-patient VHAs
   – Activate major haemorrhage protocol
   – Give blood and FFP 1:1
   – Consider platelets and cryoprecipitate or fibrinogen concentrate
   – Give 1 g tranexamic acid over 10 minutes then consider infusion
3 Discuss with haematology – likely will require prothrombin complex concentrate and vitamin K +/– recombinant activated factor VII (rFVIIa), although there is no evidence for latter

Recently there has been development of Andexanet (an antidote to the direct Xa inhibitors). There have been good results from phase II studies, and a phase III trial is awaited.

Further Reading

Levy J H, Faraoni D, Spring J L, et al. Managing new oral anticoagulants in the perioperative and intensive care unit setting. *Anesthesiology* 2013; **118**: 1466–1474

National Institute of Health and Care Excellence, 2016. Anticoagulants, including non-vitamin K antagonist oral anticoagulants (NOACs). Key therapeutic topic (KTT16) [online]. Available at: www.nice.org.uk/advice/ktt16 (Accessed: 10 February 2017)

Siegal D M, Crowther M A. Acute management of bleeding in patients on novel oral anticoagulants. *Eur Heart J* 2013; **34**: 489–500

Chapter 60

Nutrition in the ICU

Why is nutrition important in critically ill patients?

Malnutrition is present in ~50% of patients admitted to the ICU and is associated with a poorer outcome:

1 Altered immunity with increased susceptibility to infection
2 Prolonged mechanical ventilation
3 Increased LOS

It is difficult to recognise due to confounding factors such as obesity and peripheral oedema. Of interest, a BMI of 25–35 is associated with the lowest mortality rate in observational data.

How should the nutritional status of critically ill patients be assessed?

Assessing nutritional status in critically ill patients is difficult, but a number of methods can be employed to evaluate it:

1 Laboratory markers and anthropometric assessment
   - Traditional markers of nutritional status (albumin and anthropometry) are inaccurate in critical illness because of fluid resuscitation and the acute phase response
2 Clinical information, including:
   i Recent weight loss
   ii Comorbid illness
   iii Severity of illness
   iv GI dysfunction

How are the total energy requirements of a critically ill patient calculated?

The energy requirements of critically ill patients continue to be debated and will vary significantly between individuals. Energy requirement can be measured/estimated using the following methods:

1 Indirect calorimetry

2 Through use of a nutritional index such as the Harris-Benedict and Schofield index

3 Estimation based on IBW (+ 20% in obesity): *25–30 kcal/kg/day*

Exceptions include patients with burns, multiple trauma and necrotising pancreatitis who are likely to have higher requirements.

The **TICACOS** trial (Intensive Care Med, 2011) aimed to identify whether targeting energy intake to indirect calorimetry measurements was associated with lower mortality, ICU stay or ventilation in comparison with using 25 kcal/kg/day. The indirect calorimetry group received more calories during their ICU stay. There was increased duration of ventilation and length of ICU stay in this group but a trend towards reduced mortality.

The **EDEN** trial (JAMA, 2012) was designed to assess whether trophic feeding (about 25% of the target) for the first 6 days may alter overall length of ventilation. Patients who were assigned to the approach that allowed underfeeding received fewer calories but had outcomes that were at least as good as those that received full feeding.

How much protein does a critically ill patient require?

Protein catabolism is increased in critically ill patients. For most of these patients, protein requirements are proportionately higher than energy requirements and are subsequently not easily met by provision of routine enteral formulations.

Weight-based calculations can be used to monitor adequacy of protein provision. Typically, 1.2–2 g/kg/day is required to show benefit. Nitrogen balance studies are desirable to assess needs.

A patient who has a negative nitrogen balance is excreting more nitrogen than they consume and are catabolising muscle. A positive nitrogen balance indicates that patients are excreting less nitrogen than they consume and hence are incorporating nitrogen into newly formed protein. This is the goal of nutritional support.

Nitrogen balance can be calculated using the following formula:

$$\text{Nitrogen balance} = \frac{\text{Total protein intake}}{6.25}\text{(g)} - [\text{UUN} + 4\text{ g}]$$

Where 6.25 = grams of protein per gram of nitrogen, UUN = grams of nitrogen excreted in the urine over a 24-hour period, 4 g = amount nitrogen lost each day as insensible losses via the skin and GI tract

The open abdomen represents a significant source of protein/nitrogen loss in the critically ill. Although a direct measurement of abdominal fluid protein loss would be preferable, an estimate of 2 g of nitrogen per litre of abdominal fluid output should be included in the nitrogen balance calculations of such patients.

Carbohydrate should constitute 60% of the non-protein calories and lipid 40%.

What are the daily requirements of water and electrolytes?

This is detailed in Table 60.1.

Table 60.1 Daily requirement of water and electrolytes

Electrolytes	Daily requirement (per kg per day)
Water	30 ml
Sodium	1–2 mmol
Potassium	0.8–1.2 mmol
Calcium	0.1 mmol
Magnesium	0.1 mmol
Phosphorus	0.4 mmol

What do you know about immunonutrition?

Certain nutrients appear to modulate the immune and inflammatory response.

1 *Glutamine*
   - Amino acid that facilitates nitrogen transport and reduces protein catabolism alongside preserving intestinal permeability and function
   - It has been suggested as a beneficial supplement particularly in patients with burns and trauma
   - The **REDOXS** trial (NEJM, 2013) showed that the early administration of glutamine in critically ill patients with multi-organ failure was harmful (increased in-hospital and 6-month mortality)
2 *Arginine*
   - Amino acid that improves macrophage and natural killer cell cytotoxicity
   - Causes harm in patients with severe sepsis
3 *Omega-3-polyunsaturated fatty acids*
   - Omega-3 oils have many anti-inflammatory properties
   - The **OMEGA** trial (JAMA, 2011) was stopped for futility as the patients given omega-3 fatty acids had fewer ventilator-free days and longer ICU stays

What routes are available for nutrition provision and what are their advantages and disadvantages?

Nutrition can be delivered by both enteral (NG, nasojejunal (NJ), percutaneous endoscopic gastrostomy (PEG)) and parenteral routes. The advantages and disadvantages of both routes are shown in Table 60.2.

Route of feeding is a controversial topic. Unless an absolute contraindication to enteral feeding exists, e.g. ischaemic bowel or bowel obstruction, enteral

Table 60.2 Advantages and disadvantages of parenteral and enteral routes of feeding

	Enteral	Parenteral

Advantages	Physiological
	Cheaper
	No central line required
	Maintains GI tract integrity
	  – Maintains structure
	  – Encourages perfusion and
	    motility
	  – Reduces ulceration
	Reduces bacterial translocation
	Promotes immune function
	  – Mucosa-associated lymphoid
	    tissue
	  – IgA and hormone production
		Does not require functional GI
		  tract
		Can be started early hence no
		  delay in caloric intake
		Fewer interruptions

Disadvantages	Dependent on functioning GI tract
	Diarrhoea
	NG tube malposition
	Independent risk factor for VAP
	  (microaspiration; decreased
	  with postpyloric feeding)
	Sinusitis with NG tube
	Metabolic derangement:
	  electrolytes, hyperglycaemia,
	  re-feeding syndrome
		Non-physiological
		Hyperosmolar and irritant –
		  requires central access (and
		  the associated risk of
		  complications)
		Higher risk of systemic infection
		Expensive
		Hypercholesterolaemia
		PN is a lipid emulsion (usually)
		  and may cause intrahepatic
		  cholestasis and fatty liver

nutrition (EN) should be initiated preferentially. The nasogastric route is most commonly used, but impaired gastric emptying can limit infusion rates. Current practice generally focuses on optimising oral/enteral nutrition, avoiding forced starvation if at all possible and the judicious use of supplemental PN.

The **CALORIES** trial (NEJM, 2014) was designed to evaluate route of early nutritional support. It concluded that among adults with an unplanned ICU admission (in whom early nutritional support could be provided through either the parenteral or the enteral route), there was no significant difference in mortality at 30 days in those fed enterally versus parenterally.

What measures can be employed to improve the delivery of enteral nutrition, when enteral nutrition is inadequate?

The following interventions can be employed to improve/optimise the delivery of enteral nutrition:

1 Prokinetics: erythromycin and metoclopramide may increase gastric emptying
2 Post-pyloric feeding: the small bowel can be fed directly via surgical jejunostomy or NJ tubes

When should feeding be initiated in a critically ill patient?

Enteral feeding should be initiated within 24–48 hours in the critically ill patient who is unable to maintain volitional intake. Feeding should be commenced after initial resuscitation when haemodynamic support is stable, to limit stress placed on both cardiovascular and splanchnic systems. The presence of bowel sounds and the passage of flatus are not necessary before initiation of EN.

If enteral feeding is failing, it can be supplemented with PN. Guidelines differ on optimal timing for this:

1 European (ESPEN) guidelines suggest starting PN after 24–24 hours if the patient cannot tolerate EN
2 American and Canadian (ASPEN) guidelines have advised considering supplemental PN after 7–10 days if unable to meet >60% of energy or protein requirements by the enteral route alone

The **EPaNIC** trial (NEJM, 2011) compared outcomes of critically ill patients at risk of malnutrition in whom PN was started on either day 3 or day 8. Late initiation was associated with an increased survival on ICU, and shortened durations of mechanical ventilation and RRT.

What are the components of PN?

Standard formulations of PN are available in combination bags. Most formulations contain around 40% of non-protein calories as lipid and 60% as carbohydrate. Amino acids, vitamins (vitamin B_1, folate, fat-soluble vitamins (A, D, E, K), water soluble B vitamins, vitamin C) and trace elements (zinc, copper, selenium) are added. The electrolyte concentration can be altered depending on clinical circumstances as well as additional vitamins and trace elements as required.

What is the appropriate glycaemic target for non-diabetic critically ill patients?

The **NICE-SUGAR** trial (NEJM, 2009) was a multi-centre RCT that evaluated the effect of tight glycaemic control compared to conventional glucose control on a number of clinical outcomes. The 90-day mortality was significantly higher in the tight glycaemic control group. Severe hypoglycaemic events were also more common in this group. This study contradicted and overrode the trend towards intensive glycemic control that had resulted following earlier single-centre trials.

Although there is currently no consensus for glucose targets in the medical literature, a range of 4–10 mmol/l is strongly suggested for the majority of ICU patients. An intravenous insulin infusion is used following a standard protocol when spontaneous food intake is not possible. Avoidance of hypoglycaemia is of the utmost importance. Glucose measurements should be performed on arterial samples (rather than venous or capillary), using laboratory or blood gas analysers rather than point-of-care glucose meters.

What is refeeding syndrome? Can you outline the pathophysiology?

Refeeding syndrome is a clinical condition that results from reinstitution of nutrition to patients who have been starved. Chronic malnutrition leads to protein catabolism with total body phosphate depletion despite normal serum phosphate. The sudden introduction of carbohydrates leads to an anabolic state, unmasking total body phosphate depletion and leading to a precipitous drop in serum phosphate. The release of insulin results in marked uptake of phosphate, potassium and magnesium into cells. Figure 60.1 illustrates the pathophysiology.

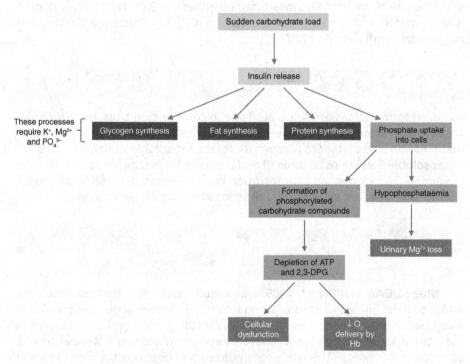

Figure 60.1 The pathophysiology of refeeding syndrome
2,3-DPG – 2,3-diphosphoglycerate

Refeeding syndrome may manifest as severe electrolyte derangement and fluid shifts associated with metabolic abnormalities and abnormal glucose metabolism. Hypophosphataemia, hypomagnesaemia and hypocalcaemia are typical. Thiamine deficiency can also occur, leading to Wernicke's encephalopathy.

Table 60.3 highlights the clinical features of refeeding syndrome.

Table 60.3 Clinical features of refeeding syndrome

Cardiovascular	Arrhythmias Congestive cardiac failure
Gastrointestinal	Constipation Vomiting Anorexia
Respiratory	Respiratory muscle weakness Ventilator dependency
Musculoskeletal	Weakness Osteomalacia
Neurological	Ataxia Delirium Coma Central pontine myelinosis Korsakoff's syndrome or Wernicke's encephalopathy
Metabolic	Infections

What are the risk factors for refeeding syndrome?

All malnourished patients are at risk of re-feeding syndrome. The NICE criteria for determining people at high risk of developing refeeding problems are shown in Table 60.4.

Table 60.4 NICE criteria for determining people at high risk of refeeding syndrome

Patient has one or more of:	Patient has two of more of:
BMI <16 kg/m^2	BMI <18.5 kg/m^2
Unintentional weight loss >15% within last 3–6 months	Unintentional weight loss >10% within last 3–6 months
Little of no nutritional intake for >10 days	Little or no nutritional intake for >5 days
Low levels of potassium, magnesium and phosphate prior to feeding	A history of alcohol abuse or drugs including insulin, chemotherapy, antacids or diuretics

Specific risk factors can be divided into the following three categories:

1 Decreased intake
   – Eating disorders
   – Alcoholism
   – Depression
   – Postoperative phase with prolonged nil-by-mouth
   – Chronic malnutrition
2 Decreased absorption
   – Malabsorptive syndromes (IBD, CF, chronic pancreatitis, short bowel syndrome)
3 Increased catabolism
   – Inflammatory processes
   – Malignancy

How is refeeding syndrome managed?

The general principles regarding the prevention and management of refeeding syndrome are as follows:

1 Recognise patients at risk
2 Adequate electrolyte supplementation
   i Provide adequate electrolyte, vitamin and trace element supplementation
   ii Pabrinex should be administered (one pair) for three days followed by thiamine 200–300 mg daily and vitamin B co-strong 1–2 tablets tds
3 Avoid fluid overload
4 Cautious carbohydrate administration
   The prescription for people at high risk of refeeding syndrome should consider:
   i Starting nutritional support at a maximum of 10 kcal/kg/day, increasing levels slowly to meet full needs by day 4–7
   ii Using 5 kcal/kg/day in extreme cases (BMI <14 kg/m^2)
5 Investigations
   i Daily phosphate, potassium, magnesium, calcium monitoring
   ii Check thiamine
   iii Monitor blood sugar

Can you describe the deficiency syndromes that develop from low levels of vitamins, minerals and trace elements?

Failing to include essential components of nutrition, whether administered via EN or PN, can result in severe complications. Table 60.5 outlines essential vitamins, minerals and trace elements and the complications/syndromes associated with deficiency.

Table 60.5 Vitamins and trace elements with associated deficiency syndromes

Vitamin/ element	Main functions	Deficiency symptoms/syndromes
Vitamin A	i Maintenance of the immune system ii Vision iii Growth and development	Night blindness Xerophthalmia
Thiamine (vitamin B1)	i Coenzyme in metabolism and ATP production ii Cardiac and nerve function	Dry beri-beri – Wasting and partial paralysis resulting from damaged peripheral nerves – Sensory ataxia Wet beri-beri – High output cardiac failure – Peripheral oedema Wernicke's encephalopathy – Ataxia – Ophthalmoplegia – Confusion Korsakoff's syndrome – Severe memory impairment
Riboflavin (vitamin B2)	i Antioxidant ii Red blood cell production iii Metabolism, energy production and growth	Ariboflavinosis – Stomatitis including red painful tongue with sore throat – Chapped and fissured lips – Angular stomatitis
Niacin (vitamin B3)	i Metabolism and energy production ii Skin formation iii CNS function	Pellagra – Diarrhoea – Dermatitis – Dementia
Folate (vitamin B9)	i CNS function ii Mental and emotional health iii DNA and RNA production iv Red blood cell production	Glossitis, diarrhoea, depression, confusion, anaemia Foetal neural tube defects
Vitamin B12 (cobalamin)	i Production of DNA and RNA ii Red blood cell production iii CNS health	Pernicious anaemia Subacute combined degeneration of the spinal cord
Vitamin C	i Collagen production ii Wound healing iii Repairing and maintaining teeth and bone	Weakness, weight loss, general aches and pains Scurvy results from long-term deficiency

Table 60.5 (cont.)

Vitamin/ element	Main functions	Deficiency symptoms/syndromes
Vitamin D	i Calcium absorption; bone strength and health ii Immune system regulation	Rickets Osteomalacia
Vitamin E	Antioxidant and free-radical scavenging	Dysarthria Loss of deep tendon reflexes Spinocerebellar ataxia and myopathies Anaemia Retinopathy
Vitamin K	i Coagulation ii Bone metabolism	Hypocoagulable states
Selenium	Necessary for the conversion of T4 into T3	Hypothroidism (extreme fatigue, cognitive slowing) Kashin-Beck disease (along with iodine deficiency) – osteochondropathy
Zinc	i Hormone production ii Immune system function iii Growth and mental health	Diarrhoea Acne or skin rashes Attention and motor disorders
Copper	i Metabolic functions (incorporated into metalloenzymes) ii Iron transportation iii Antioxidant and free-radical scavenging iv Maintenance of bone, connective tissue, cardiac function	Myelodysplasia Anaemia Leukopaenia/ neutropaenia
Manganese	i Bone production ii Skin integrity iii Blood sugar control iv Protection against free-radical damage	Bone demineralization and malformation Altered carbohydrate and fat metabolism Impaired glucose tolerance

Further Reading

Casaer M P, Van den Berghe G. Nutrition in the acute phase of critical illness. *N Eng J Med* 2014; **370** (13): 1227–1236

Harvey S E, et al for the CALORIES Trial Investigators. Trial of the route of early nutritional support in critically ill adults. *N Engl J Med* 2014; **371**: 1673–1684

Ichai C, Preiser J C. International recommendations for glucose control in adult non diabetic critically ill patients. *Critical Care* 2010; **14**(5): R166

National Institute of Health and Care Excellence, 2006. Nutrition support for adults: oral nutrition support, enteral tube feeding and parenteral nutrition. Clinical guideline CG32 [online]. Available at: www.nice.org.uk/guidance/cg32 (accessed: 1st May 2017)

Chapter 61

Percutaneous Tracheostomy

What are the indications for performing a tracheostomy?

The indications can be divided into four categories:

1 Airway-related, e.g. upper airway obstruction (burns, oropharyngotracheal trauma, extrinsic compression from haematoma etc.)
2 Secretion management and airway protection, e.g. brainstem pathology, motor neurone disease, following TBI
3 To facilitate weaning from mechanical ventilation
4 Prolonged/lifelong mechanical ventilation, e.g. high cervical cord injury

What are the advantages of tracheostomy insertion in critically ill patients?

1 Reduction in laryngeal trauma
   – Prolonged translaryngeal intubation is associated with laryngeal injury such as pressure necrosis and mucosal abrasions, e.g. during movement or coughing
2 Reduced sedation requirement (better tolerated than ETT)
3 Facilitation of gradual weaning from mechanical ventilation (reduced work of breathing, less dead space)
4 Improved oral hygiene
5 Allows rehabilitation, e.g. improved mobility, speaking, oral intake
6 Improved communication (written or spoken)
7 Reduced LOS in ICU

When should tracheostomies be performed during an admission?

There is a paucity of evidence to support either early or late tracheostomy. A Cochrane review in 2012 failed to provide a consensus.

The British **TracMan** study (JAMA, 2013) compared the effect of early (within four days of admission) or late (on/after day 10) tracheostomy on 30-day mortality in intubated and ventilated patients who were expected to require at least seven further days of ventilation. There was no difference in mortality at any point over the two-year follow-up. There was a non-significant trend towards shorter duration of mechanical ventilation with early tracheostomy, and there were significantly fewer days of sedation administration in survivors in the early group. Only 43% of the patients in the late group went on to receive a tracheostomy (many were not intubated at this point) and the authors recommend waiting until two weeks for this reason. Additionally, there was a 6.3% complication rate for the tracheostomies that were performed. Importantly, patients with potential indications for early tracheostomy (airway obstruction, neurological illness, TBI) were excluded.

The timing of tracheostomy should therefore be decided on a case-by-case basis and the risk of unnecessary procedures (with their inherent complications) balanced with that of prolonged endotracheal intubation and sedation.

What are the complications associated with tracheostomies?

The complications can be categorised according to when they occur in relation to the insertion (Table 61.1).

What are the potential contraindications to percutaneous tracheostomy?

General contraindications to tracheostomy include:

1 Patient refusal
2 Patients unlikely to require >2 weeks' invasive ventilation
3 Patients unlikely to survive >48 hours

Potential contraindications specifically to a percutaneous approach include:

1 Emergency airway access
2 Anatomy-related
    i Morbid obesity
    ii Reduced neck movement
    iii Potential or confirmed cervical spine injury
    iv Aberrant vessels
    v Abnormal thyroid or tracheal anatomy
    vi Previous tracheostomy
3 Significant respiratory support
    i PEEP >10 cmH$_2$O
    ii FiO$_2$ >0.6
4 Coagulopathy
    i PT or APTT >1.5 times upper limit of normal
    ii Platelets <50 x 10^9/l
5 Active local infection

Table 61.1 Complications of tracheostomies

Immediate	Early/intermediate	Late

Hypoxia due to failure of ventilation during the procedure	Infection
	  i Tracheostomy site cellulitis
	  ii Tracheitis
	  iii VAP
		Bleeding
		  i Granulation tissue
		  ii Tracheo-innominate fistula

Position-related
  i Pre-tracheal insertion
  ii Endobronchial
  iii Oesophageal (tracheal transfixion)
  iv Tip abutting tracheal wall
	Erosion-related
	  i Tracheal wall ulceration
	  ii Tracheo-innominate fistula (see page 368)
	  iii Tracheo-oesophageal fistula
		Tracheal injury/dysfunction
		  i Vocal cord dysfunction
		  ii Tracheal stenosis
		  iii Tracheomalacia
		  iv Failure of closure of stoma

Injury to local structures
  i Vascular injury
  ii Haemorrhage, haematoma
  iii Airway injury (cartilage fracture, tracheal laceration)
  iv Thyroid injury
  v Recurrent laryngeal nerve injury
	Tube occlusion (mucus plugs, blood clots)	Psychological impact including that related to the scar

Air-related
  i Surgical emphysema
  ii Pneumothorax, pneumomediastinum
  iii Air embolism
	Tube displacement
	  i Accidental decannulation (if occurs early, resiting may be difficult without tracheal dilators)
	  ii Malposition (kinking, twisting)	

Equipment-related
  i Incorrect tube/size
  ii Equipment malfunction
	Dysphagia related to presence of tracheostomy tube	

What is the management of accidental decannulation?

The patient should be managed with an ABCDE approach. The first consideration should be whether they have a patent upper airway, as this will determine whether they are potentially intubatable via the oral route. The specific management of the dislodged or obstructed tracheostomy should follow the National Tracheostomy Safety Project (NTSP) guidance (Figure 61.1).

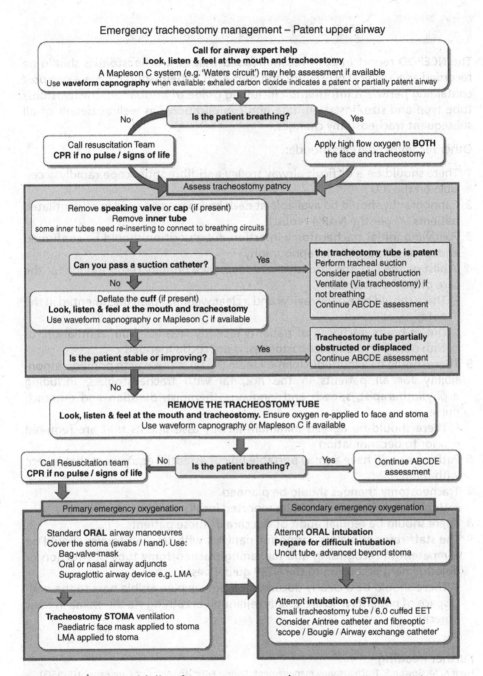

Figure 61.1 NTSP guideline for emergency tracheostomy management
Reproduced with permission from McGrath BA, et al. (*Anaesthesia* 2012)

How should patients with tracheostomies be cared for?

The NCEPOD report in 2014 recommended that all tracheostomies should be recorded as a surgical procedure and that each patient should have a *passport* containing pertinent information including grade of intubation, tracheostomy tube type and size, insertion date and complications, as well as details of all subsequent tracheostomy changes.

Other recommendations include:

1 There should be a difficult airway trolley and fibreoptic scope rapidly accessible on the ICU
2 Capnography should be available at each bedspace and used in *all* ventilated patients (as per the NAP 4 report)
3 Following initial tracheostomy insertion, tube position should be confirmed endoscopically and with capnography
4 Whilst on the ICU, the intensive care team take primary responsibility for the care of tracheostomies
    - There should be a daily review and a clear weaning plan documented in the notes
    - Out-of-hours discharge of patients recently weaned from ventilation, or with newly formed tracheostomies, is not recommended
5 There should be a multi-disciplinary team (MDT) in place with primary responsibility for all patients in the hospital with tracheostomies, including a physiotherapist, speech and language therapist, dietitian and outreach nurse
    - There should be agreed minimum airway assessments that are required prior to decannulation
6 Patients should have a small portable box of essential equipment that is kept with them
7 Tracheostomy changes should be planned
    - Unplanned changes should be reported locally as a critical incident
8 There should be regular audit of the care of these patients
9 The staff responsible for caring for patients with tracheostomies should be competent in recognising and managing tracheostomy tube obstruction or dislodgement according to the NTSP guidelines
    - There should be a clearly documented airway plan visible next to the bedspace of patients who are totally reliant on breathing via the stoma in their neck

Further Reading

Hunt K, McGowan S. Tracheostomy management. *Contin Educ Anaesth Crit Care Pain* 2015; **15**(3): 149–153

McGrath B A, Bates L, Atkinson D, Moore J A. Multidisciplinary guidelines for the management of tracheostomy and laryngectomy airway emergencies. *Anaesthesia* 2012; **67**: 1025–1041

National Confidential Enquiry into Patient Outcome and Death (NCEPOD, 2014). Tracheostomy care: On the right trach? [online] Available at: www.ncepod.org.uk/2014tc.html (Accessed: 4 May 2017)

Chapter 62

Pharmacokinetics in the Critically Ill Patient

What is the difference between pharmacokinetics and pharmacodynamics?

Pharmacokinetics describes the relationship between the dose administered and the changes in drug concentration in the body over time, i.e. the effect that the body has on the drug.

Pharmacodynamics describes the relationship between drug concentration and its pharmacological effect at the target site, i.e. the effect the drug has on the body.

What are the processes that influence the concentration of a drug within the body?

Absorption

The rate and extent of drug absorption after its administration via a particular route depends on:
  i Patient factors
     – Malabsorption, e.g. coeliac disease, ileus
  ii Drug factors
     – Pharmaceutical preparation: smaller particle size allows faster absorption of oral drugs
     – Physicochemical interactions: the presence of other drugs/food may inactivate or bind orally administered drug, e.g. milk and tetracyclines
     – First-pass metabolism (FPM): this occurs within the gut wall or liver and reduces the bioavailability of orally administered drugs
       – FPM depends on the metabolic capacity of particular enzyme pathways and protein binding, e.g. a highly bound drug with a low metabolic capacity, such as phenytoin, will have a narrow therapeutic window because small alterations in protein binding will not be accommodated by an increase in metabolism as the pathway is almost completely saturated
  iii Route of administration
     – Sublingual route avoids hepatic first pass metabolism
     – Intramuscular administration avoids problems associated with oral route – onset is more rapid and bioavailability approaches 100%, but the rate of absorption depends on local blood flow

- Can therefore be unpredictable, with delayed absorption being a risk if the drug is administered when muscle perfusion is poor, e.g. shocked state
- Subcutaneous administration can be used for depot injections, but delayed absorption is a risk as with IM administration
- Inhalational administration may be used for local or systemic effect: droplets <1 μm diameter can reach the alveoli, and hence the systemic circulation

Distribution

The volume of distribution (Vd) is the theoretical volume into which a drug is distributed, and relates the plasma concentration to the administered dose. It depends on regional blood flow and factors that influence the passage of drug across the cell membrane:
  i *Molecular size*
     Graham's law states that the rate of diffusion is inversely proportional to the square root of molecular size
 ii *Concentration gradient*
     Fick's law states that the rate of diffusion is directly proportional to the concentration gradient across the membrane
iii *Ionisation*
     - The lipophilicity of the cell membrane only permits the passage of the unionised fraction of drug
     - Degree of ionisation of a drug depends upon its dissociation constant (pK_a) and the pH of the solution in which it is dissolved
 iv *Lipid solubility*
     This is independent of pK_a and may affect absorption
     - Highly lipid-soluble fentanyl may be used effectively as a transdermal patch
     - Morphine is less lipid-soluble than diamorphine so is more likely to spread cranially when administered intrathecally and produce respiratory depression
  v *Protein binding*
     Only the unbound fraction of drug in the plasma is free to cross the cell membrane, so if a drug is highly protein-bound (i.e. >90%) small changes in the bound fraction will produces large changes in the amount of unbound drug (may be compensated for by increased metabolism unless enzyme pathways are close to fully saturated)
 vi Presence of *facilitated diffusion or active transport* mechanisms

Metabolism

In general, the process of metabolism produces a more polar (water soluble) molecule that can be excreted in bile or urine. Active metabolites may result from this process, e.g. morphine-6-glucuronide (13 times more potent than morphine). There are two phases of drug metabolism:
  i *Phase I* (non-synthetic) reactions:
     - Oxidation
     - Reduction
     - Hydrolysis

Most occur in the liver (but also in the lung, GI mucosa, kidney and brain) and are carried out by the cytochrome P450 system (which is subject to genetic polymorphism). Phase I metabolism relates to mitochondrial monoamine oxidase (catecholamines), alcohol dehydrogenase (ethanol), plasma esterases (remifentanil, suxamethonium, atracurium), ACE.

ii *Phase II* reactions increase the water solubility of the drug and occur mainly in the liver
  - Glucuronidation, e.g. propofol, morphine
  - Sulphation, e.g. quinol metabolite of propofol
  - Acetylation, e.g. isoniazid
  - Methylation, e.g. catecholamines

Excretion

This refers to the processes of removal of drug from the body and mainly occurs via the urine and bile, hence may be affected by renal or liver failure. The relative role of each route depends on molecular weight (molecules >30 kDa are not filtered by the kidney) and structure of the drug (highly charged molecules may be excreted unchanged in the urine). *Elimination* is the processes of removal of drug from the plasma and includes distribution, metabolism and excretion.

How might the absorption of drugs be altered in critically ill patients?

The effects of critical illness on drug absorption are outlined in Table 62.1.

Table 62.1 Effects of critical illness on drug absorption

Delayed GI absorption	Delayed gastric emptying
	Prolonged transit time, e.g. ileus
	Altered gastric pH, e.g. with PPi/H_2RA therapy
	Reduced GI perfusion and venous drainage
Impaired GI absorption	Fast transit time, e.g. diarrhoea, prokinetic use
	Vomiting
	Bacterial overgrowth
	Villous atrophy
	Interaction with enteral nutrition
Unpredictable absorption of IM or subcutaneous drugs	

How can drug distribution be affected in critical illness?

The Vd is commonly increased due to an increase in total body water, which can result in underdosing. Additionally, plasma proteins, particularly albumin, are reduced in stress states. This produces decreased protein binding and increased free drug fraction. In turn, this may result either in increased clearance, or toxicity (particularly if a drug's metabolic pathway is close to saturation).

How may metabolism of drugs be altered in critically ill patients?

The effects of critical illness on drug metabolism are shown in Table 62.2.

Table 62.2 Effects of critical illness on drug metabolism

Reduced hepatic metabolism	Reduced hepatic blood flow due to local hypoperfusion or systemic, e.g. shock / low-flow states, vasopressor use Direct hepatic injury due to mediators released in response to illness Ischaemia (affects cyP450 system) Hypothermia (affects cyP450 system) Drug-induced cyP450 inhibition (see Table 62.3) may reduce clearance of drug
Increased hepatic metabolism	Increased basal metabolic rate, e.g. hyperthermia Drug-induced cyP450 induction (see Table 62.3) may increase clearance of drug
Reduced spontaneous degradation	Hoffmann degradation of atracurium reduced by acidosis and hypothermia
Reduced tissue metabolism	Reduced perfusion of kidneys, brain, lungs etc. due to shock / hypothermia
Reduced plasma metabolism	E.g. plasma cholinesterase deficiency in acute/chronic hepatic failure

Table 62.3 CyP450 induction and inhibition

CyP450 inducers	CyP450 inhibitors
P Phenytoin	A Amiodarone
C Carbemazepine	O Omeprazole
B Barbiturates	D Disulfiram
R Rifampicin	E Erythromycin
A Alcohol abuse	V Valproate
S Sulphonylureas	I Isoniazid
S Smoking	C Ciprofloxacin, cimetidine
	E Ethanol intoxication
	S Sulphonamides

How might drug excretion be affected in critical illness?

The effects of critical illness on drug excretion are outlined in Table 62.4.

Table 62.4 Effects of critical illness on drug elimination

Reduced urinary clearance	Reduced renal blood flow due to local hypoperfusion or systemic, e.g. shock/low-flow states, vasopressor use
	Reduced glomerular flow rate (GFR) – in general, renal drug clearance is proportional to GFR
	Inhibition of tubular secretion
	Direct renal injury, e.g. acute tubular necrosis (ATN)
Increased urinary clearance	High cardiac output states, e.g. sepsis, trauma, burns
Effect of RRT	Variable Drugs with a high molecular weight, increased protein binding and large Vd are less likely to be removed by RRT
Reduced biliary clearance	Biliary stasis
	Recirculation due to increased GI transit time

Further Reading

Blot S I, Pea F, Lipman J. The effect of pathophysiology on pharmacokinetics in the critically ill patient – concepts appraised by the example of antimicrobial agents. *Adv Drug Deliv Rev* 2014; **77**: 3–11

Peck T, Hill S, Williams M. Drug passage across the cell membrane. In: *Pharmacology for Anaesthesia and Intensive Care*. Cambridge University Press, 2014; 1–8

Peck T, Hill S, Williams M. Absorption, distribution, metabolism, excretion. In: *Pharmacology for Anaesthesia and Intensive Care*. Cambridge University Press, 2014; 9–24

Smith B S, Yogaratnam D, Levasseur-Franklin K E, et al. Introduction to drug pharmacokinetics in the critically ill patient. *Chest* 2012; **141**(5): 1327–1336

Chapter 63

Phosphate

Phosphate is the most abundant anion in the human body and comprises almost 1% of total body weight. It is predominantly intracellular, where its concentration is 100-fold that in the plasma.

Table 63.1 Phosphate homeostasis

Normal serum PO_4^{3-}	0.85–1.4 mmol/l
Total body phosphate	~700 g
Average daily requirement	20 mg/kg/day of phosphorus
Absorption	Small intestine (increased by 1,25-dihydroxyvitamin D3)
Homeostasis	85% in bone (complexed with calcium), 14% in the soft tissues and 1% in the extracellular fluid The kidney is the primary organ involved in phosphate homeostasis PTH causes phosphate resorption from bone and decreases reabsorption in the PCT
Excretion	85–90% of filtered phosphate is reabsorbed in the PCT Renal excretion is influenced by: i PTH (increased) ii Calcitonin (increased) iii Magnesium (increased) iv Vitamin D3 (decreased) v Bicarbonate (increased) vi Sodium reabsorption (decreased excretion, PO_4^{3-} is co-transported with Na^+ in the PCT)
Roles	Energy production (ATP) Membrane function (phospholipid bilayer) RBC function (2,3-DPG) Phosphorylation Buffer Bone mineralisation

Hyperphosphataemia

Define hyperphosphataemia

Serum phosphate >1.4 mmol/l.

What are the causes of hyperphosphataemia?

The causes of hyperphosphataemia can be classified according to the underling mechanism (Table 63.2).

Table 63.2 The causes of hyperphosphataemia

Reduced excretion	Renal failure (by far the most common cause) Hypoparathyroidism Hypomagnesaemia Bisphosphonate use
Exogenous load	Enteral, parenteral, enemas; intentional vs accidental Vitamin D intoxication
Increased production/release	Rhabdomyolysis Tumour lysis syndrome Malignant hyperpyrexia Haemolysis Acidosis

Tell me some of the complications of hyperphosphataemia

Phosphate forms a complex with calcium and may therefore precipitate hypocalcaemia and tetany if the rate of rise is rapid. There may be nephrocalcinosis, renal calculi and ectopic calcification in tissues.

How do you manage hyperphosphataemia?

The management of hyperphosphataemia should follow an ABCDE approach, treating abnormalities as they are found. The specific management is as follows:

1 **Stop phosphate administration**
2 **Give aluminium hydroxide** – used as a binding agent
  – Magnesium and calcium are also used
  – Aluminium toxicity is a risk
3 **Remove phosphate from the body**
  – Volume repletion and loop diuretics
  – RRT in severe cases
4 **Monitoring**
  – Regular serum phosphate and calcium
5 **Prevent recurrence**

It is important to be aware that during recovery the serum calcium may rise due to mobilisation of abnormal soft tissue calcium-phosphate deposits.

Hypophosphataemia

Define hypophosphataemia

Serum phosphate <0.85 mmol/l.

What are the causes of hypophosphataemia?

Hypophosphataemia is very common in hospitalised patients, and is present in up to 25% of high risk patients. Hypophosphataemia results from internal redistribution, increased renal excretion and reduced GI absorption (see Table 63.3).

Table 63.3 The causes of hypophosphataemia

Renal loss	Hyperaldosteronism/volume expanded states
	Hyperparathyroidism
	Vitamin D deficiency (causes hypocalcaemia and secondary hyperparathyroidism)
	Renal tubular acidosis (RTA)
	Alcoholism
	Acetazolamide therapy
Altered balance These conditions stimulate glycolysis, which leads to phosphorylation of glucose compounds and intracellular shift of phosphate	Refeeding syndrome
	Respiratory alkalosis (may precipitate clinical hypophosphataemia in a phosphate deplete patient)
	Recovery from DKA
	Sepsis
	Effects of hormones: Insulin
	Glucagon
	Cortisol
	Adrenaline
GI loss	Antacid abuse
	Vitamin D deficiency
	Chronic diarrhoea

Tell me some of the complications of hypophosphataemia

Mild hypophosphataemia may be diagnosed incidentally on blood tests. Clinical features are usually only seen once the plasma phosphate has dropped below 0.3 mmol/l. It often coexists with other electrolyte abnormalities (e.g. hypokalaemia, hypomagnesaemia due to increased urinary magnesium loss), which may contribute to the clinical presentation.

The patient may present with neuromuscular disturbance (proximal myopathy, weakness that may eventually progress to respiratory failure) and symptoms of smooth muscle dysfunction (dysphagia, ileus). Rhabdomyolysis may complicate severe cases, and phosphate release from necrotic skeletal muscle may mask the causative electrolyte disturbance. Additionally, there may be symptoms of acute cardiomyopathy.

How would you manage hypophosphataemia?

The management of severe symptomatic hypophosphataemia should follow an ABCDE approach, treating abnormalities as you find them. The ultimate treatment is directed at the underlying cause, but it is important to actively manage the low phosphate in the meantime.

1 **Stop all phosphate-wasting drugs**
2 **Phosphate supplementation**
   - Indicated if serum phosphate <0.32 mmol/l, clinical evidence of hypophosphataemia or risk factors for phosphate depletion, e.g. alcoholism, malnutrition and refeeding
   - The safest mode of replacement is oral: 1–3 g/day is usually enough
   - 10 mmol of phosphate (as potassium diphosphate) can be given IV over one hour and repeated as needed
   - Phosphate Polyfusor® contains PO_4^{3-} 100 mmol, K^+ 19 mmol and Na^+ 81 mmol in 500 ml
   - Correct co-existing electrolyte disturbances
3 **Monitoring**
   - Regular serum phosphate and calcium (there is a risk of hypocalcaemia with IV phosphate replacement)
4 **Prevent recurrence**

Further Reading

Penido M G, Alon U S. Phosphate homeostasis and its role in bone health. *Pediatr Nephrol* 2012; **27**(11): 2039–2048

Weisinger J R, Bellorín-Font E. Magnesium and phosphorus. *Lancet* 1998; **352**(9125): 391–396

Chapter 64

Plasmapheresis and Plasma Exchange

What is the difference between plasmapheresis and plasma exchange?

Plasmapheresis is a procedure where plasma is separated from other components of the blood and the plasma is removed without the use of replacement solution.

Plasma exchange is plasmapheresis followed by replacement with FFP or albumin.

What physical processes are involved in plasmapheresis?

The two main processes used are centrifugation and filtration. These are compared in Table 64.1.

Table 64.1 The processes used in plasmapheresis

	Centrifugation	Filtration
Description	Takes advantage of the specific gravities of the four major blood components and separates them into layers	Utilises a semi-permeable membrane Utilises differences in particle size to filter plasma from the cellular components of blood
Advantages	No limit to the size of molecules being removed	Can be performed on ICU
Disadvantages	Difficult to perform on ICU (commonly performed by blood bank)	Size of molecule removed is limited by pore size

Are you aware of how the indications for therapeutic plasmapheresis are categorised?

Indications for therapeutic plasmapheresis are categorised according to the American Society for Apheresis (ASFA) 2013 categories (Table 64.2).

Table 64.2 Indications for therapeutic apheresis (ASFA 2013 categories)

Category	Description	Example
I	First line therapy, either as primary stand-alone treatment or in conjunction with other modes of treatment	Guillian-Barré syndrome as first-line stand-alone treatment
II	Disorders for which apheresis is accepted as second-line therapy, either as a stand-alone treatment or in conjunction with other modes of treatment	Stand-alone secondary treatment for acute disseminated encephalomyelitis (ADEM) after failure of high-dose IV corticosteroid therapy
III	Optimum role of apheresis therapy is not established	Patients with sepsis and multi-organ failure or thyroid storm
IV	Disorders in which published evidence suggests apheresis would be ineffective or harmful	PEx for active rheumatoid arthritis

What are the indications for therapeutic plasma exchange?

Plasma exchange should only be carried out in conditions for which there are good evidence of its benefit. Indications for therapeutic plasma exchange can be classified according to speciality (Table 64.3).

Table 64.3 Indications for therapeutic plasma exchange

Speciality	Disorder	Evidence category
Neurology	AIDP (Guillian-Barré syndrome)	1
	Acute disseminated encephalomyelitis (ADEM)	2
	Chronic inflammatory demyelinating polyradiculoneuropathy	1
	Myasthenia gravis	1
	LEMS	2
	Multiple sclerosis	2
Renal	Granulomatosis with polyangiitis (previously Wegener's)	1
	Goodpasture's (anti-glomerular basement membrane disease)	1
	Antibody-mediated renal transplant rejection	1
	Myeloma cast nephropathy	2
Haematology	TTP	1
	Atypical HUS	1
	Sickle cell disease resulting in acute stroke	1

Table 64.3 (cont.)

Speciality	Disorder	Evidence category
Metabolic	Wilson's disease (fulminant)	1
	Familial hypercholesterolaemia	1
Immunology	Severe systemic lupus erythematosus	2
	Catastrophic antiphospholipid syndrome	2

How much plasma is removed with each treatment?

Typically, 30–40 ml/kg of plasma (1–1.5 plasma volumes) is removed at each procedure.

One plasma volume exchange removes approximately 66% of an intravascular component and a two-plasma volume exchange removes approximately 85%.

What replacement solutions are used in plasma exchange?

Replacement fluid is usually isotonic 4.5 or 5.0% human albumin solution. Exchange with FFP is reserved for the replacement of ADAMTS13 (in TTP) or to replace clotting factors.

What are the complications of plasma exchange?

Line related:

1 Infection
2 Misplacement
3 Pneumothorax
4 Bleeding
5 Arrhythmia

Procedure specific:

1 Hypotension
2 Hypothermia
3 Transfusion reactions (particularly with FFP)
4 Thrombocytopenia
5 Hypofibrinogenaemia
6 Hypocalcaemia

Further Reading
Szczepiorkowski Z M, Winters J L, Bandarenko N, et al. Guidelines on the use of therapeutic apheresis in clinical practice – evidence-based approach from the American Society of Apheresis. *J Clin Apher* 2010; **25**: 83–177

Chapter 65

Pleural Effusions

What is a pleural effusion?

A pleural effusion is an abnormal collection of fluid in the pleural space. They are traditionally divided into:

1 *Transudates*
   - Typically result from a systemic process that produces alterations in Starlings forces, leading to increased net filtration of pleural fluid
   - Effusions are usually bilateral
2 *Exudates*
   - Usually due to a local inflammatory process that increases capillary permeability to proteins and other cells, resulting in effusion formation

What is the differential diagnosis of a unilateral pleural effusion?

A unilateral pleural effusion is more likely to be an exudate. The causes of pleural effusion are listed in Table 65.1.

Table 65.1 Causes of pleural effusions

	Common Causes	Less Common Causes
Exudate	Parapneumonic	Pancreatitis
	Malignancy	TB
	PE	Pericarditis
	Subphrenic abscess	Chylothorax
	Autoimmune, e.g. SLE,	Haemothorax
	rheumatoid	Oesophageal rupture
Transudate (often bilateral)	Left ventricular failure	Myxoedema
	Portal hypertension	Sarcoidosis
	Hypoalbuminaemia	Meig's syndrome (triad of ascites, right
	Peritoneal dialysis	sided effusion and benign ovarian
		tumour)

What is the most common cause of pleural effusion in the UK?

Parapneumonic effusion.

What can be measured in pleural fluid and how does this relate to diagnosis?

The commonly performed tests include:

1 Gram stain and MC+S (parapneumonic effusions)
2 Acid-fast bacilli and TB culture
3 Cytology (looking for malignant cells)
4 Biochemistry
  i Protein level
    – Classically, a pleural fluid protein >30 g/l indicates an exudate
    – This is not accurate when the serum protein level is abnormal
  ii LDH
    – High levels may suggest empyema, or effusion due to malignancy or rheumatoid disease
  iii Glucose
    – Usually similar to that of the serum
    – Low pleural fluid glucose levels are seen in TB, empyema, pleural malignancy and rheumatoid
  iv Amylase (elevated in pancreatitis or oesophageal perforation)
  v pH
    – Normal pH of pleural fluid is ~7.62
    – pH <7.2 suggests infection and is an indication for drainage; it is associated with a poor outcome in patients with parapneumonic effusion
  vi Triglycerides and cholesterol (to distinguish a chylothorax)

Light's criteria (Table 65.2) are then employed using the protein and LDH levels to determine the presence of an exudative effusion. Exudative effusions meet at least one of these criteria; transudates meet none. The criteria have a sensitivity of 98% and a specificity of 83%.

Table 65.2 Light's criteria for the presence of an exudate

Ratio of pleural fluid:serum protein > 0.5
Ratio of pleural fluid:serum LDH >0.6
Pleural fluid LDH > $^2/_3$ upper limit of normal for serum LDH
Additional criteria if results equivocal: Serum albumin – pleural fluid albumin <12 g/l

What other investigations would you perform if you suspected a pleural effusion?

1 Erect CXR
   - Blunting of the costophrenic angle may be the only sign of an effusion
   - A large effusion may cause a *white-out*
   - There is homogenous opacification with the absence of air bronchograms with mediastinal shift away from the affected side
2 Chest ultrasound (used for diagnosis and to aid drainage)
   - Seen as an anechoic layer between the parietal pleura and the lung
   - The lung edge is often seen billowing in the fluid (*tentacle sign*)
   - Septae, loculations and complex effusions can also be visualised
3 CT chest (+ abdomen and pelvis if indicated)
   - May be used to delineate more complex effusions
   - Can be useful in differentiating potential aetiologies, particularly in malignancy

How would you manage a patient with a pleural effusion?

The management of a patient with a pleural effusion should follow an ABCDE approach, treating abnormalities as they are found. Specific management of the effusion depends on:

1 The size of the effusion
2 Whether there is evidence of respiratory compromise
3 Whether there is a suspected infection or haemothorax

A flowchart of suggested management is shown in Figure 65.1.

What is an empyema?

An empyema is a collection of pus within the pleural space. It is most commonly associated with pneumonia, but may complicate penetrating chest trauma, oesophageal rupture or follow lung or chest wall surgery. A large bore chest drain is often advocated in these patients as the narrow-bore drains are prone to blockage, and regular flushing with saline or fibrinolytics such as urokinase may be required.

You insert a chest drain and frank blood Is drained. What should you do?

Haemothorax is usually as a result of thoracic trauma, but may also be iatrogenic. The patient should be resuscitated as required, and a large bore chest drain inserted to facilitate drainage of blood and clot. If the haemorrhage is

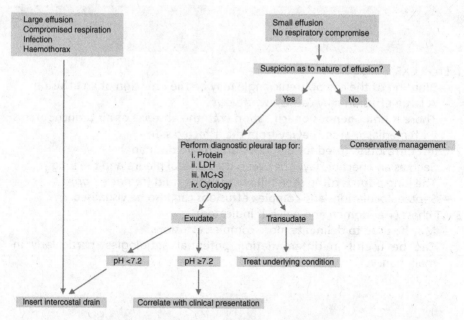

Figure 65.1 Management of pleural effusion
Adapted with permission from Paramasivam E, Bodenham A. (*Contin Educ Anaesth Crit Care Pain* 2007)

significant blood products may be required. Initial drainage of 1500 ml of blood or continued drainage of ≥200 ml/hour are indications for surgical intervention, and the case should be discussed with a cardiothoracic surgeon as a matter of urgency. Video-assisted thoroscopic surgery (VATS) or an open procedure may then be considered depending on the clinical situation.

How would your management differ in a patient with a chylothorax?

Chylothorax (collection of lymphatic fluid in the chest) is unusual and results from iatrogenic or traumatic injury to the major thoracic lymphatics. The fluid has a characteristic milky appearance and is positive for triglycerides and chylomicrons on biochemical examination. The patient will lose considerable amounts of fat, fat-soluble vitamins, protein and electrolytes into the effusion, which will require drainage. Parenteral nutrition should be instituted to reduce chyle production and ensure nutrition.

Further Reading

British Thoracic Society. BTS pleural disease guideline 2010. *Thorax* 2010; **65**(suppl ii)

Paramasivam E, Bodenham A. Pleural fluid collections in critically ill patients. *Contin Educ Anaesth Crit Care Pain* 2007; **7**(1): 10–14

Chapter 66

Potassium

Potassium is the major intracellular cation.

Table 66.1 Potassium homeostasis

Normal serum K$^+$	3.5–5.0 mmol/l
Total body potassium	50 mmol/kg
Average daily requirement	0.8–1.2 mmol/kg/day
Absorption	Small intestine
Homeostasis	Na$^+$/K$^+$ ATPase controls potassium entry into cells and is regulated by: i Aldosterone ii Insulin iii Osmolality iv β-adrenoceptor stimulation
Excretion	90% of absorbed potassium is renally excreted, influenced by: i Aldosterone and sodium reabsorption ii β-adrenoceptor stimulation iii Insulin iv Bicarbonate v Urinary flow
Roles	Regulation of acid-base balance Maintenance of the resting membrane potential of excitable tissues Cardiac and skeletal muscle contraction Nerve conduction Tubuloglomerular function

Hyperkalaemia

Define hyperkalaemia

Serum potassium >5.5 mmol/l.

It may be further subcategorised into mild (5.5–5.9 mmol/l), moderate (6.0–6.4 mmol/l) and severe (>6.5 mmol/l).

What are the causes of hyperkalaemia?

The causes of hyperkalaemia can be classified according to the underlying mechanism (Table 66.2).

Table 66.2 The causes of hyperkalaemia

Impaired renal excretion	Addison's disease
	AKI, CKD
	Drugs: Potassium-sparing diuretics
	Aldosterone antagonists
	ACEIs, ARBs
Altered balance	Acidosis
	Insulin deficiency, including DKA
	Hyperosmolality
	Haemolysis
	Tissue injury (rhabdomyolysis, tumour lysis syndrome, malignant hyperpyrexia)
	Drugs: Suxamethonium
	Digoxin toxicity
	Betablockers
Increased intake	Intentional vs accidental
	Enteral vs parenteral
	Transfusion

Discuss the complications of hyperkalaemia

The patient may complain of GI symptoms (nausea, vomiting), paraesthesiae and weakness.

Complications are primarily cardiovascular; hypotension and fatal arrhythmias can occur. Arrhythmias are related to the *rate of rise* of serum K^+ rather than the absolute value.

What would the ECG look like in a patient with hyperkalaemia?

The earliest noticeable change (K^+ >5.5 mmol/l) is peaked T waves (repolarisation abnormality).

At higher K^+ (>6.5 mmol/l) there is progressive atrial compromise:

1 Wide, flat P wave
2 Prolonged PR interval
3 Eventual disappearance of P waves

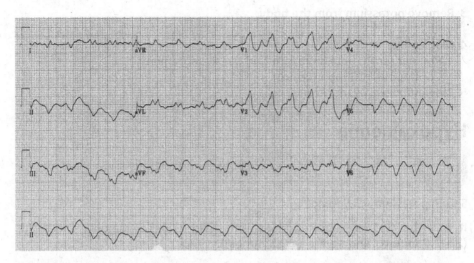

Figure 66.1 The ECG in hyperkalaemia (absent P waves, broad QRS complexes with peculiar morphology and peaked T waves)

As serum potassium rises >7.0 mmol/l conduction abnormalities and bradycardia develop:

1 Wide QRS complexes with bizarre morphology (Figure 66.1)
2 High-grade AV block with the development of slow junctional and ventricular escape rhythms
3 Conduction block (bundle branch blocks, fascicular blocks)
4 Bradyarrhythmias
5 Sine wave (a pre-terminal rhythm)

Cardiac arrest will ensue if left untreated and may be due to pulseless electrical activity (PEA), asystole or VF.

How do you manage hyperkalaemia?

The management of hyperkalaemia should follow an ABCDE approach, treating abnormalities as they are found. An ECG should be obtained urgently. The ultimate treatment is directed at the underlying cause, but it is important to actively manage the potassium in the meantime. This is achieved by following the UK Renal Association's approach:

1 **Protect the myocardium** – calcium increases cardiac conduction velocity and contractility in patients with ECG changes
   – Give 10 ml calcium chloride 10% or 30 ml calcium gluconate 10% IV over 5–10 minutes
2 **Move the potassium intracellularly** – this is a short-term temporising measure whilst the underlying cause is treated
   – Give 10 units of Actrapid insulin in 50 ml 50% glucose over 15–20 minutes
   – Nebulised salbutamol increases the efficacy of the insulin-glucose infusion

3 **Remove potassium from the body**
   – RRT
4 **Monitoring**
   – Regular serum potassium or blood gas measurements
   – Continuous ECG monitoring
5 **Prevention** – prevent recurrence

Hypokalaemia

Define hypokalaemia

Serum potassium <3.5 mmol/l.

It may be further subcategorised into mild (3.0–3.5 mmol/l), moderate (2.5–2.9 mmol/l) and severe (< 2.5 mmol/l).

What are the causes of hypokalaemia?

Hypokalaemia may be acute or chronic. Causes of chronic hypokalaemia include dietary insufficiency, malabsorption and endocrine disorders. The causes of acute hypokalaemia can be classified according to the underlying mechanism (Table 66.3).

Table 66.3 The causes of hypokalaemia

Renal loss	Hyperaldosteronism
	Cushing's syndrome
	RTA
	Diuretic phase of AKI
	Hypomagnesaemia
	Drugs: Diuretics including acetazolamide
	Carbapenems
	Corticosteroids
Altered balance	Alkalosis
	Refeeding syndrome
	Hypothermia
	Hypothyroidism
	Drugs: Insulin
	Catecholamines
	Phosphodiesterase inhibitors
GI loss	Diarrhoea and vomiting
	Fistulae
	Ureterosigmoidostomy

Tell me some of the complications of hypokalaemia.

Hypokalaemia may be an incidental finding on a blood test, with no concomitant signs or symptoms. In more severe hypokalaemia the patient may present with GI symptoms (nausea, vomiting, constipation and ileus) or neuromuscular disturbances (weakness, cramps, ascending paralysis that may progress to ventilatory failure, and hypo- or areflexia). Cardiovascular effects include hypertension (due to sodium retention) and dysrhythmias. There is often a compensatory alkalosis as the body exchanges H^+ ions for K^+ ions (there is renal hydrogen ion loss and bicarbonate reabsorption).

What ECG changes would you see in a patient with low potassium?

Changes begin to appear when K^+ <2.7 mmol/l:

1 Tall, wide P waves
2 Prolonged PR interval
3 T wave flattening and inversion
4 ST depression
5 U waves (a small deflection immediately following the T wave, usually in the same direction as the T wave)
6 Apparent long QT interval (fusion of T and U waves, i.e. long QU interval)

With worsening hypokalaemia there are frequent supraventricular and ventricular ectopics, and supraventricular tachyarrhythmias. The ECG may degenerate into VT, torsades de pointes (Figure 66.2) and VF.

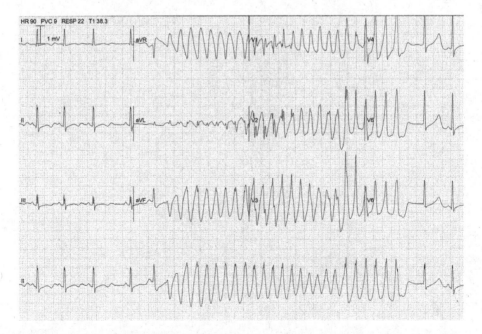

Figure 66.2 The ECG in hypokalaemia (tall P waves, T wave inversion, U waves, long QU interval, degeneration into polymorphic VT)

How would you manage hypokalaemia?

The management of hypokalaemia should follow an ABCDE approach, treating abnormalities as they are found. An ECG should be obtained urgently. The ultimate treatment is directed at the underlying cause, but it is important to actively manage the potassium in the meantime.

1 **Stop all potassium-wasting drugs**
2 **Potassium supplementation** – the maximum safe rate of replacement is 40 mmol/hour
   - Oral potassium is suitable for mild and asymptomatic hypokalaemia
   - IV potassium may be administered with maintenance IV fluids, concentrated via a central line with continuous ECG monitoring, or in PN
   - If renal impairment is present, halve the initial replacement therapy
   - Correct coexisting hypomagnesaemia
3 **Monitoring**
   - Regular serum potassium or blood gas measurements
   - Continuous ECG monitoring
2 **Prevention** – prevent recurrence

Further Reading
Parikh M, Webb S T. Cations: potassium, calcium and magnesium. *Contin Educ Anaesth Crit Care Pain* 2012; **12**(4): 195–198

Chapter 67

Pre-Eclampsia and HELLP Syndrome

Can you define *pre-eclampsia*?

Pre-eclampsia (PET) is pregnancy-induced hypertension (>140/90 mmHg) presenting after 20 weeks' gestation in the presence of proteinuria ($\geq$0.3 g/day), with or without peripheral oedema.

What is the pathophysiology?

The pathophysiology is yet to be fully elucidated, but is thought to be due to abnormal placentation:

- Impaired maternal spiral artery relaxation with failure of trophoblastic invasion results in placental hypoperfusion and ischaemia
- This causes widespread maternal endothelial dysfunction with excess thromboxane A_2 (TXA_2) and deficient prostacyclin, causing platelet aggregation and vasoconstriction

How does pre-eclampsia present?

Cardiovascular

- Vasoconstriction causes *hypertension* with reduced plasma volume

Neurological

- Headache, visual disturbance, irritability (due to cerebral hypoperfusion and oedema)

Renal

- *Proteinuria*, reduced GFR leads to AKI and hyperuricaemia
- Renal blood flow (RBF) is maintained due to activation of the RAA system

Gastrointestinal

- Nausea and vomiting, epigastric pain (due to stretching of liver capsule), transaminitis

Haematological

- Decrease plasma oncotic pressure leads to *oedema* formation
- Platelet aggregation causes microthrombi
- There is haemoconcentration (due to reduced plasma volume) and coagulopathy

How do you diagnose pre-eclampsia?

The NICE definition of severe pre-eclampsia is the presence of severe hypertension (>160/110 mmHg) with symptoms and/or biochemical or haematological derangement. The clinical features of severe pre-eclampsia are summarised in Table 67.1.

Table 67.1 The features of severe pre-eclampsia

Neurological	Severe headache Visual disturbance Clonus Papilloedema Seizures (= eclampsia)
GI	Epigastric pain Vomiting RUQ tenderness
Haematological	Plt <100 x 10^9/l
Biochemical	ALT/AST ≥70 IU/l
HELLP Syndrome	Haemolysis Elevated liver enzymes Low platelets

How is pre-eclampsia managed?

Mild disease may be managed with oral antihypertensives such as labetalol or nifedipine. Severe disease necessitates close monitoring, preferably in an HDU environment with MDT input and IV antihypertensive therapy. Pre-eclampsia should be managed with an ABCDE approach, treating abnormalities as they are found. The specific management of pre-eclampsia is:

1 Oral antihypertensives
   - Nifedipine
   - Labetolol

2 **Intravenous antihypertensive therapy,** aiming BP <150/80–100 mmHg:
   - Labetalol – bolus and/or infusion
   - Hydralazine – bolus and/or infusion
3 **Magnesium sulphate**
   - Used in severe pre-eclampsia (specific criteria) and eclampsia
   - The **Magpie** trial (2002) showed that magnesium therapy halved the risk of eclamptic seizures in mothers with pre-eclampsia (see page 283)
   - 4 g bolus over 5 minutes followed by an infusion of 1 g/hour for 24 hours
   - Aim for serum Mg^{2+} 2–3 mmol/l (there is loss of deep tendon reflexes at Mg^{2+} 4–6 mmol/l)
4 **Restrictive fluid management**
   - Patients are at risk of pulmonary oedema (leaky capillaries, low oncotic pressure due to renal protein wasting)
   - Follow protocol on each labour ward, usually use 0.5 ml/kg/hour, target urine output 0.5 ml/kg/hour
5 The definitive treatment of pre-eclampsia is **delivery of the placenta** (and baby!)
   - Steroids should be given to aid maturation of the fetal lungs before 34 weeks' gestation (delivery is then ideally delayed for 48 hours for maximum benefit)

What are the complications of pre-eclampsia?

The complications of pre-eclampsia can be divided into maternal and fetal.

Maternal

1 Eclampsia
2 Renal failure
3 VTE (due to intravascular volume depletion, renal loss of antithrombin III)
4 HELLP syndrome
5 Intracranial haemorrhage
6 Acute fatty liver of pregnancy – contentious, but thought to be part of the spectrum
7 Placental abruption

Fetal

1 Utero-placental insufficiency and intra-uterine growth retardation (IUGR)
2 Pre-term delivery
3 Fetal death

What is HELLP syndrome?

HELLP syndrome is a triad of:

1 **Haemolysis**

2 **Elevated liver enzymes**
3 **Low platelets**

It is considered to represent the extreme end of the pre-eclampsia spectrum of disease, although this is controversial. It complicates 0.1–0.6% of all pregnancies and 4–12% of cases of pre-eclampsia. The associated maternal mortality is 24% (ICH is the most common finding at post-mortem examination), and morbidity is significant (DIC in 20%, abruption in 16%, AKI in 7%, pulmonary oedema in 6%).

It presents with:

- Malaise (90%)
- Epigastric/RUQ pain (90%)
- Nausea and vomiting (50%)
- Headache (up to 68%)
- Visual disturbance (10–20%)
- Jaundice (5%)

The disease can be classified using the Mississippi Classification according to severity on the basis of platelet count, ALT/AST and LDH levels (Table 67.2).

Table 67.2 The Mississippi Classification of HELLP syndrome

	Mild	Moderate	Severe
Platelets (x 10⁹/l)	100–150	50–100	<50
ALT or AST (IU/l)	≥40	≥70	≥70
LDH (IU/l)	≥600	≥600	≥600
Incidence of bleeding	No increased risk	8%	13%

Am J Obstet Gynecol 1991; 164: 1500–1513

The management involves admission to HDU, treatment of hypertension and seizure prophylaxis, repletion of blood products as indicated, and cautious IV fluid therapy. Delivery of the fetus arranged as soon and as safely as possible; collaboration with obstetric, anaesthetic and haematology colleagues is essential. There has been no convincing evidence that the use of steroids is beneficial to maternal outcome in HELLP syndrome, and current guidelines do not recommend their use.

Further Reading

Hart E, Coley S. The diagnosis and management of pre-eclampsia. *British Journal of Anaesthesia: CEPD Reviews* 2003; **3**(2): 38–42

National Institute for Health and Care Excellence, 2010. Hypertension in pregnancy: diagnosis and management. Clinical guideline (CG107) [online]. Available at: www.nice.org.uk/guidance/cg107 (Accessed: 6 November 2016)

Chapter 68

Pseudo-Obstruction and Ileus

What do you understand by the terms *ileus* and *pseudo-obstruction*?

The term *ileus* is used to describe marked intestinal dilatation resulting from partial or complete non-mechanical obstruction of the small and/or large intestine.

Pseudo-obstruction (also known as paralytic ileus) is a more specific term describing a clinical picture suggestive of mechanical obstruction of the colon, again in the absence of any evidence of bowel obstruction.

Pseudo-obstruction syndromes can be divided into acute and chronic forms. In acute colonic pseudo-obstruction (*Ogilvie syndrome*), the colon may become massively dilated risking perforation without urgent decompression. In the case of perforation, mortality approaches 50%.

What are the clinical features of ileus?

1 Abdominal distension and pain
2 Constipation
3 Nausea and vomiting
4 Scanty or absent bowel sounds
5 X-ray reveals gaseous distention of isolated segments of intestine

What are the differential diagnoses of pseudo-obstruction/paralytic ileus?

Differential diagnoses include:

1 Mechanical obstruction
2 Megacolon due to *Clostridium difficile*

What are the risk factors for ileus and how can it be prevented?

The most common cause for ileus is following abdominal surgery. In this post-operative state, inhibition of small-bowel motility is transient. The stomach usually recovers within 24–48 hours. Colonic function may take up to 48–72 hours to return. Prolonged post-operative ileus can be found in 10–25% of patients that have undergone major abdominal surgery.

Postoperative ileus is multi-factorial in aetiology. Risk factors include:

1 Opioid use
2 Intra-operative blood loss
3 Prolonged surgical time
4 Intestinal resection

Other risk factors for ileus include:

1 Electrolyte imbalance/biochemical disturbance
2 Mechanical ventilation
3 Increased intracranial or intra-abdominal pressure
4 Sedation
5 Sepsis
6 Volume overload
7 Hypotension

Preventative strategies involve:

1 Early mobilisation
2 Post-operative patient positioning
3 Minimise enterostatic drug use, e.g. opiates, catecholamines, sedatives
4 Correct conditions impairing motility, e.g. hyperglycaemia, hypokalaemia
5 Reduced handling of the bowel during surgery
6 Chewing gum therapy (shown to reduce the incidence of post-operative ileus following open gastrointestinal surgery)

What is the management of ileus/pseudo-obstruction?

1 **Exclusion of precipitating pathology or alternate diagnosis**
   i Rule out mechanical obstruction with contrast-enhanced CT as necessary
   ii Consider other intra-abdominal pathology, e.g. haematoma, fluid collections
   iii Diligent treatment of underlying condition
2 **Resuscitation and optimisation of physiology**
   i Optimise oxygenation and minimise vasopressors/inotropes
   ii Avoid excessive IV fluid (to minimise bowel oedema)
   iii Regular evaluation and correction of electrolytes and acid-base disturbance
3 **Specific interventions**
   i Nasogastric decompression
      – Evidence does not support routine NG insertion
      – Used in patients with nausea or vomiting as prominent features
   ii Pharmacotherapy
      – Prokinetic agents, e.g. metoclopramide, erythromycin
        – Stimulates the upper GI tract (stomach and small bowel)
        – Have not been shown to reduce ileus in clinical trials

- Neostigmine
  - Stimulates small bowel and colonic motility
  - Has a dramatic effect on colonic pseudo-obstruction
  - Widespread use is limited by antimuscarinic side effects
- Peripherally-acting μ-opioid receptor antagonists (data in critical illness are lacking)

iii Nutritional support
  - Avoid prolonged starvation
  - Low rate trophic NG feed can be considered (10–20 ml/hr)
  - PN should be considered for those unable to tolerate adequate oral intake due to prolonged post-operative ileus for more than 7 days

iv Review of analgesic prescription
  - Weaning of opioids and substitution with regular paracetamol, NSAIDs (if not contraindicated) +/- regular or prn tramadol
  - Minimise anticholinergic use

v Regular ambulation

vi Surgical decompression
  - In the presence of an ileus in the context of abdominal compartment syndrome

4 Specific management of pseudo-obstruction

The above points should all be considered, alongside:

i Rectal tube/colonoscopic decompression
  - May be necessary when conservative management fails

ii Consider neostigmine infusion if no resolution occurs within 48 hours
  - Profound bradycardia and heart block my result

iii Surgical intervention
  - In cases of actual or imminent perforation or in patients who are unresponsive to maximal non-surgical measures

Further Reading

Recommendations of the ESICM working group on abdominal problems. Gastrointestinal function in intensive care patients: terminology, definitions and management. *Intensive Care Med* 2012; **38**: 384–394

Vather R, Bissett I. Management of prolonged postoperative ileus: Evidence-based recommendations. *ANZ J Surg* 2013; **83**: 319–324

Chapter 69

Puerperal Sepsis

What is sepsis in the puerperium?

Puerperal sepsis is defined as maternal sepsis that develops at any point from delivery of the placenta up to six weeks postnatally. The commonest site of infection in the UK is the genital tract, particularly the uterus (endometritis); however, sepsis originating from outside the genital tract in this period is also a significant cause of morbidity and mortality.

As a result of a number of factors including increased awareness and advances in medical management, the mortality rate related to genital tract sepsis decreased in the UK from 0.63 per 100 000 maternities in 2009–2011 to 0.29 deaths per 100 000 maternities in 2011–2013 (as per Mothers and Babies: Reducing Risk through Audits and Confidential Enquiries across the UK [MBRRACE-UK]).

What are the causes of fever outside the genital tract in the puerperal period?

1 Urinary tract infection and acute pyelonephritis
2 Skin and soft tissue infection (e.g. Caesarean section scar)
3 Mastitis or breast abscess
4 Pneumonia
5 Gastroenteritis
6 Pharyngitis
7 Infection related to regional anaesthesia (e.g. epidural abscess)
8 DVT

How does puerperal sepsis present and what are the risk factors for sepsis in the puerperium?

Symptoms and signs may be less distinctive than in the non-pregnant population and are not necessarily present in all patients; a high index of suspicion is therefore required (Table 69.1). Disease progression may be rapid; abdominal pain and tenderness not relieved by usual analgesia should prompt urgent medical review.

Table 69.1 Symptoms and signs of puerperal sepsis

Symptoms	Signs
Fever	Tender uterus
Chills and general malaise	Subinvolution of the uterus
Lower abdominal pain	Shock
Light vaginal bleeding	
Purulent, foul-smelling lochia	
Diarrhoea, vomiting	

Multiple risk factors for sepsis in the puerperium have been identified by the Confidential Enquiry into Maternal Death:

1 Obesity
2 Impaired glucose tolerance/DM
3 Immunocompromise
4 Anaemia
5 Vaginal discharge
6 History of pelvic infection
7 Cervical cerclage
8 Prolonged rupture of membranes
9 Vaginal trauma, Caesarian section, wound haematoma
10 Retained products of conception
11 Group A streptococcus in close contacts
12 Black/minority group ethic origin

How do you investigate puerperal sepsis?

1 Frequent observations using a modified early obstetric early warning score (MEOWS) chart
2 Blood tests
   – FBC, U+Es, LFTs, CRP, clotting screen
   – Cultures
   – Serum lactate
3 Imaging
   – CXR
   – Pelvic ultrasound (or pelvic CT if abscess is suspected)
4 Other microbiological samples taken should be guided by clinical suspicion of the focus of infection and include:
   – Urine
   – High vaginal swab
   – Placental swab
   – Sputum
   – CSF
   – Wound swabs

5 A woman with symptoms of pharyngitis/tonsillitis should have a throat swab taken (given the risk of community-acquired group A streptococcal infection)
6 Rapid MRSA screening if maternal status unknown

What are the specific concerns in puerperal patients?

Sepsis in the puerperium remains an important cause of maternal death in the UK. Symptoms of sepsis may be non-specific and severe sepsis can progress at an alarming rate.

What do you understand by the term *red flag sepsis*?

This is a concept developed in the Centre for Maternal and Child Enquiries (CMACE) report published in 2014, highlighting parameters that should raise concern in obstetric patients with infection:

1 RR >25 per minute
2 SpO_2 <91%
3 HR >130 bpm
4 SBP <90 mmHg
5 Anything other than *alert* on the AVPU scale
6 Serum lactate >2 mmol/l

What organisms are commonly involved?

1 Streptococci (particularly Group A streptococcus (*Str. pyogenes*))
2 *Staphylococcus aureus*
3 *Escherichia coli*
4 *Clostridium welchii*
5 *Morganella morganii*
6 Chlamydia
7 *Neisseria gonorrhoeae*

Gram-negative bacteria producing ESBL are an increasingly common cause of drug resistant urinary tract infections.

Bacteria may be either endogenous, i.e. bacteria which normally live in the vagina and rectum without causing harm (e.g. some types of streptococci and staphylococci, *E. coli, Clostridium welchii*), or exogenous, i.e. bacteria which are introduced into the vagina from the outside (e.g. streptococci, staphylococci, *Clostridium tetani*).

What is the management of puerperal sepsis?

Management should take an ABCDE approach and follow surviving sepsis guidelines with immediate administration of appropriate locally guided antibiotics. If genital tract sepsis is suspected, the prompt administration of broad-spectrum antibiotics may be life-saving. Intravenous fluid boluses will be required and the development of septic shock will necessitate vasopressor use.

Multidisciplinary team work is essential; a senior obstetrician should be involved in consultation with an intensivist, anaesthetist and microbiologist or infectious disease physician.

Appropriate source control should be carried out as soon as possible (e.g. return to theatre to remove retained products of conception).

The *Sepsis Six* was developed by **Daniels, et al** (BMJ, 2011) as an aide memoire, and incorporates:

1 Administer oxygen to aim SpO_2 >94%
2 Blood cultures (before antimicrobial therapy)
3 Empiric broad spectrum antibiotics
4 Serum lactate level
5 IV fluid resuscitation
6 Urine output measurement

Table 69.2 Most common causes of maternal mortality (CMACE 2014, for the 2009–2012 triennia)

Rank	Direct causes	Indirect causes
1	VTE	'Other' – Influenza – Non-genital tract sepsis
2	Genital tract sepsis	Cardiac disease
3	Bleeding	Indirect neurological causes – Epilepsy – Intracerebral haemorrhage – Stroke
4	Pregnancy-induced hypertension/pre-eclampsia	Psychiatric illness
5	AFE	

Further Reading

Centre for Maternal and Child Enquiries (CMACE). Saving Mothers' Lives: reviewing maternal deaths to make motherhood safer: 2006–08. The eighth report on confidential enquiries into maternal deaths in the United Kingdom. *Br J Obstet Gynaec* 2011; **118** Suppl 1: 1–203

Daniels R, Nutbeam T, McNamara G, et al. The sepsis six and the severe sepsis resuscitation bundle: a prospective observational cohort study. *Emerg Med J* 2011; **28**(6): 507–512

MBRRACE-UK, 2015. Saving lives improving mothers' care – Surveillance of maternal deaths in the UK 2011–13 and lessons learned to inform maternity care from the UK and Ireland confidential enquiries into maternal deaths and morbidity 2009–13 [online]. Available at: www.npeu.ox.ac.uk/downloads/files/mbrrace-uk/reports/ (Accessed: 30 October 2016)

Royal College of Obstetricians and Gynaecologists, 2012. *Bacterial Sepsis following Pregnancy* [online]. Available at: https://www.rcog.org.uk/en/guidelines-research-services/guidelines/gtg64b/ (Accessed: 30 October 2016)

Chapter 70

Pulmonary Haemorrhage and Haemoptysis

What is diffuse alveolar haemorrhage and how does it present?

Diffuse alveolar haemorrhage (DAH) is a life-threatening disorder referring to bleeding originating in the pulmonary microvasculature (as opposed to the bronchial circulation or the lung parenchyma itself). The patient will usually present with a cough, fever, symptoms relating to hypoxaemia and diffuse pulmonary infiltrates on CXR. Haemoptysis may or may not be present. Clinical examination will often reveal crackles on auscultation of the chest; other features may be present that allude to a potential aetiology, e.g. nasal polyps, oral ulceration.

What are the causes of diffuse alveolar haemorrhage?

There are three histological patterns of DAH (Table 70.1).

Table 70.1 Causes of diffuse alveolar haemorrhage

Vasculitis/capillaritis	Granulomatosis with polyangiitis (previously Wegener's granulomatosis) (c-ANCA) Goodpasture's syndrome (anti-GBM antibodies) Henoch-Schönlein purpura Connective tissue disease, e.g. SLE (ANA, anti-dsDNA, anti-ENA)
Pulmonary haemorrhage without vascular inflammation ('bland' pulmonary haemorrhage)	Coagulopathy Cardiovascular pathology, e.g. mitral stenosis or regurgitation, CCF Pulmonary hypertension Infective endocarditis Drugs, e.g. anticoagulants, antiplatelet agents, thrombolytic therapy, amiodarone, bleomycin, methotrexate, nitrofurantoin Toxins, e.g. crack cocaine smoking
Alveolar bleeding due to other underlying process	PE Diffuse alveolar damage, i.e. ARDS Infection, e.g. pneumonia, aspergillosis Malignancy Sarcoidosis High altitude pulmonary oedema

What investigations may be useful in a patient presenting with suspected pulmonary haemorrhage?

1 Blood tests
   - FBC, clotting screen, group and save
   - ESR, CRP, vasculitis screen
   - U+Es
2 Urinalysis (protein, blood and casts may be seen in glomerulonephritis)
3 Imaging
   - CXR: Patchy alveolar opacification
   - CT: Patchy consolidation or ground glass shadowing
4 Bronchoscopy (BAL for cytology and MC+S; may permit visualisation of pathology +/– therapeutic intervention)
5 Spirometry (although patients are often too unwell for this)
   - Increased diffusing capacity of the lungs for carbon monoxide (DLCO)
   - May reveal a restrictive pattern

What is the management of pulmonary haemorrhage?

Pulmonary haemorrhage should be managed with an ABCDE approach, treating abnormalities as they are found. Specific management should include an MDT approach (liaison with respiratory, rheumatology and potentially renal physicians) in addition to the following medical treatments:

1 **Correct hypoxaemia** using supplemental oxygen +/– ventilation
2 Anaemia is not unusual and **transfusion** may be necessary
3 **Source control**
   i Stop all potentially offending drugs
   ii Bronchoscopy
      - Diagnosis is established when sequential BAL samples from the same location are progressively more haemorrhagic
      - Samples should be sent for bacterial, viral and fungal studies
      - May be used to diagnose and treat bronchial bleeding
   iii Tranexamic acid
4 **Steroids**, e.g. pulsed methylprednisolone
5 Consider **cyclophosphamide** or **PEx** for autoimmune conditions, e.g. Goodpasture's syndrome, granulomatosis with polyangiitis (Wegener's granulomatosis)

What is the definition of massive haemoptysis and from where does it usually originate?

There is no agreed definition for massive haemoptysis in terms of blood volume, but it is often used to refer to haemoptysis of sufficient volume to cause impaired gas exchange or circulatory compromise, the former being much more common.

Haemoptysis usually originates from the bronchial circulation.

What are the causes of haemoptysis?

1 Bronchogenic carcinoma
2 Inflammatory disorders, e.g. chronic bronchitis, infections (including fungal, aspergillosis), vasculitides, bronchiectasis including CF, TB
3 PE
4 Coagulopathy
5 Iatrogenic
6 Broncho-vascular fistulae and vascular malformations (rare)
7 Tracheo-innominate fistula (TIF)

Can you tell me about trachea-innominate fistulae?

This is a rare cause of massive haemoptysis in the ICU and is almost invariably fatal without prompt management.

The innominate (brachiocephalic) artery lies anterior to the 6–9th tracheal rings. A low-lying tracheostomy balloon can cause pressure necrosis of the anterior tracheal and posterior arterial walls with disastrous consequences. A torrential bleed may occur any time from one week-post tracheostomy insertion, and is often preceded by a sentinel bleed from or around the tracheostomy tube.

Specific immediate management involves either:

1 Removing the tracheostomy and applying digital compression to the artery anteriorly on to the posterior surface of the manubrium (will require alternative definitive airway)
2 Leaving the tracheostomy in situ and overinflating the cuff to tamponade the haemorrhage

Distal airway soiling should be controlled by either:

1 Removing the tracheostomy and inserting a cuffed ETT through the stoma
2 Leaving the tracheostomy in situ and inserting a small cuffed ETT through the tracheostomy tube

In either scenario, the cuff should be positioned so that it lies distal to the fistula but proximal to the carina.

Figure 70.1 illustrates the stepwise management of TIF.

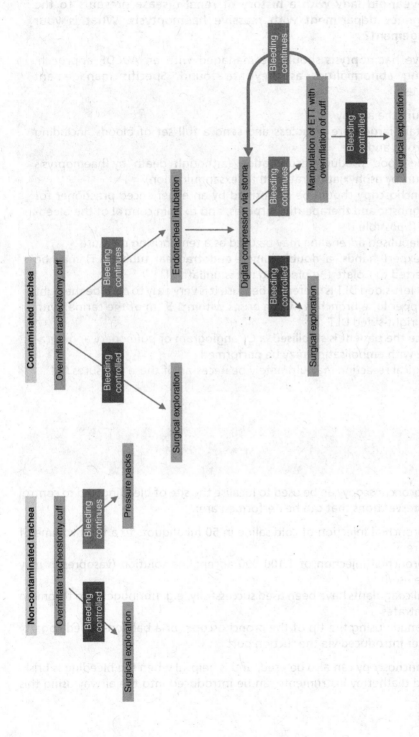

Figure 70.1 The management of a tracheo-innominate fistula
Reproduced with permission from Grant CA, et al. (*Br J Anaesth* 2006)

A 56-year-old lady with a history of renal disease presents to the emergency department with massive haemoptysis. What is your management?

Massive haemoptysis should be managed with an ABCDE approach, treating abnormalities as they are found. Specific management involves:

1 Secure the airway
2 Obtain **large bore IV access** and send a full set of bloods, including a group and save
3 Fluid/blood product **resuscitation** (although death by haemoptysis occurs by asphyxiation rather than exsanguination)
4 **Bronchoscopy** should be performed by an experienced practioner for diagnostic and therapeutic purposes, and to gain control of the bleeding if possible
   – Nebulised adrenaline may be used as a temporising measure
5 In expert hands, a **double-lumen endotracheal tube** (DLT) may be inserted to isolate the bleeding if it is unilateral
   – A left-sided DLT is preferred because it is very easy to occlude the right upper lobe bronchus (which arises within 1.5 cm of the carina) with a right-sided DLT
6 Once the patient is stabilised, a CT angiogram or pulmonary angiography with embolisation may be performed
7 Surgical resection may ultimately be necessary if these measures fail

Which interventions can you perform during bronchoscopy?

Flexible bronchoscopy can be used to localise the site of bleeding and to control it. The interventions that can be performed are:

1 Endobronchial injection of cold saline in 50 ml aliquots to a total volume of one litre
2 Endobronchial injection of 1:100 000 adrenaline solution (vasopressin may also be used)
3 Topical coagulants have been used successfully, e.g. fibrinogen and thrombin concentrates
4 Tamponade using the tip of the bronchoscope, or a balloon-tipped Fogarty catheter introduced via the suction port

Rigid bronchoscopy can also be used, and is helpful when the bleeding is brisk. Laser and diathermy instruments can be introduced into the airway using this method.

Further Reading

Grant C A, Dempsey G, Harrison J, Jones T. Tracheo-innominate artery fistula after percutaneous tracheostomy: Three case reports and a clinical review. *Brit J Anaesth* 2006; **96**(1): 127–31

Lara A R, Schwarz M I. Diffuse alveolar haemorrhage. *Chest* 2010; **137**(5): 1164–1171

Chapter 71

Pulmonary Hypertension

Define *pulmonary hypertension*

Pulmonary arterial hypertension is defined as a mean pulmonary artery pressure (MPAP) of ≥25 mmHg at rest, or ≥30 mmHg with exercise. Pulmonary venous hypertension is defined as an elevated PCWP ≥18 mmHg.

What are the causes of pulmonary hypertension?

The causes of pulmonary hypertension can be subdivided according to the World Symposium on Pulmonary Hypertension (WSPH) classification (Table 71.1).

Alternatively, pulmonary hypertension may be classified according to the primary location of the pathological process (see Table 71.2).

Describe the pathophysiology of pulmonary hypertension

Pulmonary hypertension occurs due to one of three underlying processes:

1 *Increased flow*
  i Left-to-right shunting in congenital heart disease
  ii Back-up of flow due to LV dysfunction or valvular heart disease leading to raised venous pressure and eventually raised arterial pressure
  This results in vascular smooth muscle remodelling, capillary congestion causing lymphatic distension, and subsequent compensatory pulmonary arterial hypertension to drive flow forward.

2 *Pulmonary arterial vasoconstriction*
  i Endothelial dysfunction
    – In idiopathic PAH, endothelial dysfunction leads to reduced production of endothelium-derived vasodilators, e.g. nitric oxide
    – There is intimal proliferation and medial hypertrophy leading to fibrosis, which then promotes platelet aggregation and thrombosis
  ii Hypoxic pulmonary vasoconstriction (HPVC)
    – This is a physiological response and occurs chronically in lung disease
    – Mechanically induced stress due to lung hyperinflation can cause further capillary destruction

Table 71.1 Classification of pulmonary hypertension (5th WSPH, 2013)

Group		Subcategory
I	**Pulmonary arterial hypertension (PAH)** Includes all causes that lead to structural narrowing of the vessels	1.1 Idiopathic PAH 1.2 Heritable PAH 1.3 Drug and toxin induced PAH 1.4 PAH secondary to collagen vascular disease, portal hypertension, HIV, congenital heart disease and schistosomiasis 1′ Pulmonary veno-occlusive disease and/or pulmonary capillary haemangiomatosis 1″ Persistent pulmonary hypertension of the newborn
II	**Pulmonary hypertension secondary to left-sided heart disease**	2.1 LV systolic dysfunction 2.2 LV diastolic dysfunction 2.3 Valvular disease 2.4 Congenital/acquired left heart inflow/outflow tract obstruction and congenital cardiomyopathies
III	**Pulmonary hypertension related to lung disease or hypoxaemia**	3.1 COPD 3.2 Interstitial lung disease 3.3 Other pulmonary diseases with mixed restrictive and obstructive pattern 3.4 Sleep-related breathing disorders 3.5 Alveolar hypoventilation disorders, e.g. obesity, neuromuscular weakness, kyphoscoliosis 3.6 Chronic exposure to high altitude 3.7 Developmental lung disease
IV	**Pulmonary hypertension secondary to chronic thromboembolic disease**	
V	**Pulmonary hypertension due to multifactorial mechanisms**	5.1 Haematological disorders: sickle cell disease 5.2 Systemic disorders: sarcoidosis, pulmonary histiocytosis, lymphangioleiomyomatosis 5.3 Metabolic disorders: glycogen storage disorders, Gaucher's disease 5.4 Other: fibrosing mediastinitis, tumoural calcinosis, renal failure

Reproduced with permission from Simonneau G, et al. (*J Am Coll Cardiol* 2013)

3 *Small pulmonary vessel structural change or destruction*
   i Pulmonary veno-occlusive disease involves widespread vascular obstruction, commonly in the post-capillary venules
   ii Pulmonary capillary haemangiomatosis involves obstruction of the alveolar capillary bed
   iii Chronic thromboembolic disease causes mechanical obstruction and increased arterial resistance to flow

Table 71.2 Alternative classification of pulmonary hypertension

Category	Primary Vessels Involved	Additional Radiographic Findings	Examples
Pre-capillary	Arterial	Peripheral pruning of pulmonary vasculature Mosaic attenuation (heterogeneous lung opacification, representing differential parenchymal perfusion)	Idiopathic PAH Familial PAH Drug-related Left to right intra-cardiac shunt
Lung-related	Arterial	Parenchymal lung disease	COPD Interstitial lung disease Obstructive sleep apnoea
Post-capillary	Venous	Evidence of pulmonary venous hypertension: – Ground glass opacities – Septal lines – Pleural effusion	LVF LV inflow or outflow obstruction Pulmonary veno-occlusive disease

What might the ECG show in a patient with pulmonary hypertension?

The ECG is likely to show signs of RVH (Figure 71.1).

1 P pulmonale, particularly in leads II and V1 (represents right atrial enlargement)
   – P wave amplitude >2.5 mm in inferior leads and >1.5 mm in V1 and V2
2 Right axis deviation
3 Tall R wave in V1 and V2
4 RBBB
5 RV strain pattern: ST depression and T wave inversion in V1-V3 and the inferior leads

What is cor pulmonale?

Cor pulmonale is defined as acute or chronic pressure overload of the right ventricle in response to pulmonary hypertension. The pathophysiology is shown in Figure 71.2.

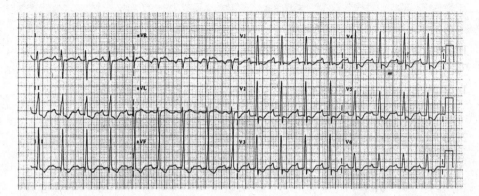

Figure 71.1 ECG changes in pulmonary hypertension (P pulmonale, RVH, RV strain pattern)
Reproduced with permission from British Cardiac Society Guidelines and Medical Practice Committee (*Heart* 2001)

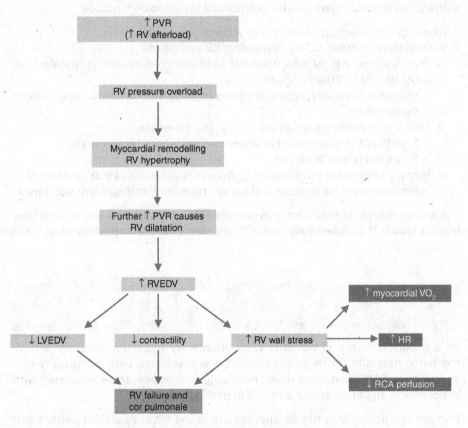

Figure 71.2 The pathophysiology of cor pulmonale
RVEDV – right ventricular end-diastolic volume; LVEDV – left ventricular end-diastolic volume; RCA – right coronary artery

How is pulmonary hypertension managed in the ICU?

The management of chronic pulmonary hypertension is primarily directed at managing the underlying cause:

1 **LTOT** for advanced COPD
   - Improves survival in patients with hypoxaemia
   - Oxygen reduces HPVC, improving RV stroke volume and CO
2 **NIV** may be beneficial in exacerbations of COPD or in obstructive sleep apnoea (OSA)
   - No data exist on outcome benefit in acute cor pulmonale
   - Corrects hypoxaemia and acidosis, thus offloads the RV by reducing PA pressure
3 **Pulmonary endarterectomy** for pulmonary veno-occlusive disease
   - 5–10% operative mortality compared to <10% five-year survival in untreated disease
4 **Anticoagulation** in chronic thromboembolic pulmonary hypertension

Subsequent medical therapies for pulmonary hypertension include:

1 **Diuretics** to manage RV failure and volume overload
2 **Vasodilators** improve CO by decreasing RV afterload
   i Prostacyclins, e.g. IV epoprostenol (administered centrally), inhaled iloprost (prostacyclin analogue)
      - Improves haemodynamics, symptomatology and outcome in pulmonary hypertension
   ii Endothelin-receptor antagonists, e.g. oral bosentan
      - Significant improvement in symptoms and short-term outcomes
      - Side effects may limit use
   iii Phosphodiesterase inhibitors, e.g. IV or oral sildenafil (a PDE_5 inhibitor)
      - Improve exercise capacity but no improvement in long-term outcomes

The management of pulmonary hypertension and associated acute right ventricular failure is outlined fully in the 'Right Heart Failure' topic (see page 390).

Would you admit a patient with severe pulmonary hypertension to critical care?

As a group, critically ill patients with pulmonary hypertension have a high mortality: necessity for inotropic support was associated with a mortality rate approaching 50% in one case series. Poor outcomes appear to be associated with hypotension, hyponatraemia and AKI in particular.

Invasive ventilation may not be appropriate in the critically ill PAH patient, but as always this should be addressed on a case-by-case basis. For example, a newly diagnosed treatment-naïve patient with pulmonary hypertension may be a candidate for aggressive therapy including consideration for lung transplantation. Conversely, the patient with progressive end-stage disease in whom super-urgent transplantation is not an option is unlikely to benefit from critical care.

Further Reading

British Cardiac Society Guidelines and Medical Practice Committee, and approved by the British Thoracic Society and the British Society of Rheumatology. Recommendations on the management of pulmonary hypertension in clinical practice. *Heart* 2001; **86**: i1–i13

Condliffe R, Kiely DG. Critical care management of pulmonary hypertension [online]. *BJA Educ* 2017. Available at: https://academic.oup.com/bjaed/article/3044180/ (Accessed: 15 May 2017)

Elliot C A, Kiely D G. Pulmonary hypertension. *Contin Educ Anaesth Crit Care Pain* 2006; **6**(1): 17–22

Simonneau G, Gatzoulis M A, Adatia I, et al. Updated clinical classification of pulmonary hypertension. *J Am Coll Cardiol* 2013; **62**(25) Suppl D: 34–41

Chapter 72

Rehabilitation After ICU

Why is rehabilitation after critical illness important?

1 Regaining (reasonable, if not premorbid level) quality of life (QoL) following critical illness is of paramount importance to the majority of patients and their relatives, often over mortality
2 To reduce the economic burden
   - Ongoing medical and psychological issues may require further input in the community, including nursing and social care
   - Loss of earnings for the patient
   - Family members often provide the majority of care, which may impact on their own ability to generate income
   - Subsequent benefit requirement

Why do patients need rehabilitation after a critical illness?

Physical problems and weakness may persist for months or years following critical illness. This has a significant impact on the patient's ability to self-care and return to work: one study found that 25% of patients needed assistance with activities of daily living at 6 months and 22% at one year. The psychological consequences of critical illness are also very important. They can affect the patient's relationships, ability to return to their normal activities and reintegration into the community.

What are the ongoing issues in a patient rehabilitating from critical illness?

1 Physical
   i Weakness (most common symptom), stiffness, paraesthesiae
   ii Postural hypotension (as a result of being bed-bound for protracted periods)
   iii Reduced cardiopulmonary reserve
   iv Incontinence, sexual dysfunction
   v Communication problems, changes in vision, hearing or speech

vi Iatrogenic problems, e.g. tracheal stenosis, scarring (from NG tubes, ETT ties, tracheostomy stomas, following high-dose vasopressor therapy), compression neuropraxia

vii Worsening of premorbid conditions

2 Psychological

   i Anxiety

   ii Depression

   iii Guilt related to their relatives' experience of their critical illness

   iv Emotional distress resulting from scarring or significant changes to their appearance, e.g. weight loss, hair loss, skin changes

   v Post-traumatic stress disorder

   vi Sleep disturbance

     – Often persists post-discharge

     – May relate to the illness itself, the use of opioids and sedatives, or related to the ICU environment (the lack of a proper day and night, the constant noise and disturbance for interventions or observations on the ICU)

     – Nightmares, often persecutory in nature

     – Disturbance to normal circadian rhythm

   vii Cognitive and behavioural dysfunction

     – Poor memory, which compounds anxiety and distress

     – Reduced attention span

     – Confusion

     – Difficulty sequencing

     – Apathy

     – Disinhibition

3 Nutritional

   i Poor appetite

   ii Alterations in sense of smell or taste are common, but usually resolve quickly

   iii Swallowing difficulties

   iv Fatigue and apathy contribute to malnutrition

4 Chronic pain

5 Drug withdrawal following prolonged or repeated administration of narcotic or sedative agents

Additionally, ongoing organ support (either on the ward or in the community) may be required, for example:

– Tracheostomy care/complications (see 'Percutaneous Tracheostomy' topic)
– RRT
– Nutritional support
– VADs

How is rehabilitation delivered?

NICE has provided guidance on rehabilitation following ICU admission (CG83). They key points are highlighted below:

1 Early intervention is key to preventing physical and psychological complications
2 A comprehensive assessment should be performed to identify rehab needs if the patient is at risk of significant adverse consequences of their critical illness, in conjunction with the patient's relatives. This should:
   – Identify pre-existing physical and psychological impairment, as well as that acquired whilst in ICU
     – Set short-term goals (i.e. before the patient leaves hospital)
     – Set medium-term goals (i.e. to help the patient return to normal activities, if possible)
     – This assessment should be repeated once the patient has been discharged to the ward
3 The patient and their family should be *debriefed* by staff involved in their care regarding the nature of the illness and interventions they underwent, residual problems they have or disability they may experience on discharge, and also address any nightmares or abnormal perceptions related to their ICU admission
   – Ideally this should occur more than once to aid understanding
4 There should be clear communication regarding the expected recovery time, and advice regarding their convalescence and rehabilitation
5 Rehabilitation should begin on the ICU as early as possible by considering these points:
   – Prevention of potential complications, e.g. minimising the use of NMBAs and steroids to reduce the incidence of ICUAW, minimise the use of benzodiazepines to reduce the incidence of delirium
   – Physiotherapy
   – Nutritional support
   – Individualised, structured rehabilitation plan with regular reviews and follow-up
6 Input from various allied health professionals is key to rehabilitation:
   – Physiotherapy
   – Occupational therapy
   – Dietetics
   – Clinical psychology
7 There should be follow-up for at least 6 months post-ICU stay, addressing medical, physical and psychological problems
   – It is important to remember that patients may need considerable support and guidance once they are discharged from the ICU to be able to continue participating in their rehab, e.g. they may lack the determination required to exercise

How do we know if it has worked?

1 *Health-related Quality of Life (HRQoL) assessment tools*
   Several quality-of-life measures can be applied to assess outcomes in patients following critical illness. Two of the most commonly used questionnaires are:

 i *Short Form-36* (SF-36)
   Reliably measures health-related QoL following ICU admission
   Questions cover:
   – Physical functioning
   – Whether they are able to fulfil their desired physical and emotional role
   – General health
   – Vitality
   – Social functioning
   – Mental health
 ii *EuroQol-5-Dimension* (EQ-5D)
   Questions cover:
   – Mobility
   – Self-care
   – Usual activities
   – Pain and discomfort
   – Anxiety and depression

Results from such assessment tools may not be entirely accurate as patients may be lost to follow up, there may be recall bias regarding their premorbid QoL, and patients' perception of their ill health may improve with time. Additionally, patients who respond to their post-ICU questionnaire may be self-selecting, and not representative of the whole cohort.

2 *Follow-up clinics*
  NICE advised the implementation of multidisciplinary follow-up clinics in their guidance in 2009: They are increasingly commonplace, but their format is not standardised. Uptake by patients is only modest (between 50–60%); the reasons most cited for non-attendance are being too unwell or, paradoxically, too well to attend
  Figure 72.1 illustrates the role of the ICU follow-up clinic.

Is there any evidence for ICU follow-up clinics?

Not at present: in 2009, the **PRaCTICaL** study concluded that the nurse led follow-up clinic did not provide significant benefits. There was no evidence of such clinics being effective (or cost effective) in improving patients' quality of life in the year after discharge from ICU.

What is PTSD and how do we minimise it?

Post-traumatic stress disorder occurs in 9–27% of ICU survivors. It is a severe anxiety disorder centred around the recurrent re-living of a triggering traumatic event that persists for over a month and impairs social function. There is a classical triad of symptom complexes:

1 Intrusive unpleasant and unsettling flashbacks associated with emotional upset

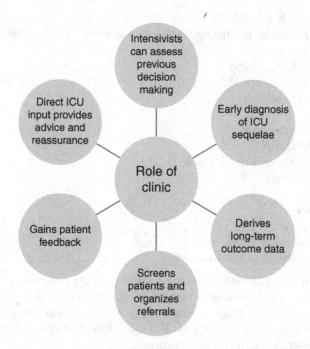

Figure 72.1 The role of the ICU clinic
© *Oxford Textbook of Critical Care 2016* (2nd ed.) by permission of Oxford University Press

2 Subsequent avoidance of situations and stimuli associated with the trigger
3 Increased level of alertness, e.g. hypervigilance, irritability; or chronic anxiety state with flattened affect

Risk factors include:

1 Previous psychological condition prior to ICU admission
2 Increased duration of sedation and mechanical ventilation
3 Benzodiazepine use
4 Delirium
5 ARDS
6 Sepsis

It has been demonstrated that patients who have factual memories are less likely to develop PTSD. To that end, attendance in ICU follow-up clinics and visits to the unit may help them address their flashbacks and formulate a more coherent timeline of their ICU admission. The use of retrospective diaries has been suggested, which can direct discussion. It may also be helpful for relatives to keep a diary that the patient can read once they are recovering.

Is there any evidence for diary keeping whilst on the ICU?

A diary written in lay terms by the healthcare professionals caring for the patient, with contributions from relatives if they choose and accompanied by photographs, has been shown to significantly reduce the incidence of new PTSD.

Further Reading

Cuthbertson B H, Rattray J, Campbell M K et al. The PRaCTICaL study of nurse led, intensive care follow-up programmes for improving long term outcomes from critical illness: A pragmatic randomised controlled trial. *Brit Med J* 2009; **339**: b3723

Das P, Waldmann C. The ICU Survivor Clinic. In: Webb A, Angus D, Finfer S, Gattinoni L, Singer M, eds. *Oxford Textbook of Critical Care* (2nd ed). Oxford: Oxford University Press, 2016

Griffiths R, Jones C. Recovery from intensive care. *Brit Med J* 1999; **319**(7207): 427–429

Griffiths J A, Gager M, Waldmann C. Follow-up after intensive care. *Contin Educ Anaesth Crit Care Pain* 2004; 4(6): 202–205

National Institute for Health and Care Excellence, 2009. Rehabilitation after critical illness in adults. Clinical guideline (CG83) [online]. Available at: www.nice.org.uk/guidance/cg83 (Accessed: 25 February 2017)

Chapter 73

Rhabdomyolysis

What are the causes of rhabdomyolysis?

The causes of rhabdomyolysis can be divided into traumatic and non-traumatic causes.

Traumatic causes:

1 Trauma, especially crush injuries
2 Excessive muscle strain, e.g. exercise, seizures, tetanus
3 Electrical current

Non-traumatic causes:

1 Congenital myopathies
2 Endocrinopathies, e.g. hypothyroidism, DKA (electrolyte abnormalities)
3 Drugs and toxins, e.g. statins, cocaine, MDMA, amphetamines, carbon monoxide poisoning
4 Hyperthermia, e.g. exercise, sepsis, NMS, MH
5 Occlusion or hypoperfusion of vasculature
6 Infections, e.g. cellulitis, necrotising fasciitis
7 Electrolyte abnormalities, e.g. hyperosmotic conditions, hypokalaemia, hypophosphatemia, hypo/hypernatraemia
8 Autoimmune disease, e.g. dermatomyositis, polymyositis

What is the mechanism behind the condition?

Muscle ischaemia, damage and eventual necrosis lead to rhabdomyolysis. There is ATP depletion due to increased muscle activity and/or failure of oxygen delivery to the myocyte. This then disrupts cellular transport mechanisms (Na^+/K^+ ATPase pump, active transport of calcium into the sarcoplasmic reticulum) and electrolyte balance. A rise in intracellular calcium levels results in hyperactivity of proteases, producing free radicals that degrade the myofilaments and damage the cell membrane. This leads to leakage of cell contents (potassium, phosphate, urate, CK and myoglobin) into the plasma. This process is summarised in Figure 73.1.

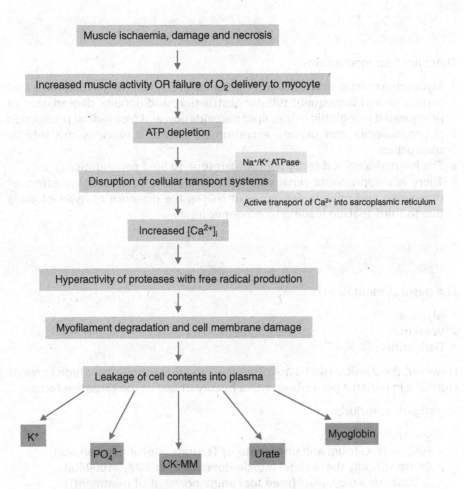

Figure 73.1 The pathophysiology of rhabdomyolysis

What are the complications of rhabdomyolysis?

1 Electrolyte abnormalities
   i Hyperkalaemia, which may be life-threatening
   ii Hypocalcaemia occurs as calcium is chelated with phosphate and deposited in necrotic tissue (rarely symptomatic)
      − Treat this cautiously as the patient will usually have rebound hypercalcaemia on recovery
   iii Hyperphosphataemia
2 Hyperuricaemia
3 Hypovolaemia due to *third-spacing* particularly at the site of muscle injury
4 AKI − occurs in up to 65% of patients
5 Compartment syndrome
6 DIC

What are the mechanisms of AKI?

There are four mechanisms:

1 Myoglobin combines with Tamm-Horsfall protein, resulting in insoluble cast formation and subsequent tubular obstruction; additionally, degradation of precipitated myoglobin causes lipid peroxidation and free radical production
2 Hyperuricaemia and urinary excretion of uric acid worsens the tubular obstruction
3 The haem moiety is directly nephrotoxic (due to lipid peroxidation)
4 There is inappropriate renal vasoconstriction (due to scavenging effect of myoglobin and relative deficiency of NO) in the presence of hypovolaemia due to third-spacing leading to ischaemic injury

How is rhabdomyolysis diagnosed?

The classic presentation is:

1 Myalgia
2 Weakness
3 Dark urine

However, the classical triad is not often seen and there should be a high index of suspicion in patients presenting with a history of any of the causative factors.

Investigations include:

1 Blood tests:
    – FBC, U+Es, calcium and phosphate, LFTs, urate, clotting screen, ABG
    – CK (specifically the skeletal muscle isoenzyme, CKMM) >1000 IU/l
        – Establish a peak level (used for commencement of treatment)
        – AKI is associated with peak levels of >5000 IU/l
2 Urine
    – Microscopy (looking for casts)
    – Myoglobin level
3 ECG (looking for signs of hyperkalaemia)
4 Radiology targeted at any area of injury

How is it managed?

The management of rhabdomyolysis should follow an ABCDE approach, treating abnormalities as they are found. Specific management includes:

1 Administer 100% oxygen
2 Insert two large bore cannulae and commence large volume **IV crystalloid resuscitation**
    – Target urine output 2–3 ml/kg/hour (i.e. aim for high output, and match with high input)

- Compound sodium lactate may aid in urinary alkalinisation, but contains potassium so should be used with caution
- Normal saline may contribute to hyperchloraemic acidosis
3 Management of life-threatening hyperkalaemia
- Insulin and glucose infusion, salbutamol, calcium chloride/gluconate
4 Sodium bicarbonate (1.26%)
- Alkalinises the urine, increasing the solubility of myoglobin and reducing its direct tubular toxicity
- Aim for urinary pH >6.5 (if urine is already alkaline, bicarbonate is not necessary)
5 **Mannitol**
- There is no evidence that mannitol is any better than crystalloid
- Theoretical benefits:
  i Flushes nephrotoxic agents through the tubules
  ii Extracts fluid that has accumulated in injured muscle
  iii Acts as a free radical scavenger
6 Consider **diuretics** once patient is volume replete and urine is clear
7 **Fasciotomies and debridement** may be necessary for source control
8 **RRT** may be required

Are there any drugs that should be avoided in patients with rhabdomyolysis?

Suxamethonium should be avoided as it may worsen the hyperkalaemia and precipitate arrhythmias or cardiac arrest. Additionally, statins should be avoided in view of their association with rhabdomyolysis.

Further Reading

Bosch X, Poch E, Grau J M. Rhabdomyolysis and acute kidney injury. *N Engl J Med* 2009; **361**: 62–72

Williams J, Thorpe C. Rhabdomyolysis. *Contin Educ Anaesth Crit Care Pain* 2014; **14**(4): 163–166

Chapter 74

Right Heart Failure

Why is right ventricular failure important?

Right ventricular failure is as common as isolated LV failure, but carries a worse prognosis. The condition is less well-understood and is often poorly managed as a result.

Describe the pathophysiology of right ventricular failure

The thin-walled right ventricle can accommodate increases in preload relatively easily, but tolerates increases in afterload poorly. A sudden rise in PVR increases the right ventricular end-diastolic pressure (RVEDP), increasing RV work. The raised RVEDP in turn results in a reduction in coronary perfusion. The flow profile then begins to mirror that seen in the LV, i.e. occurring predominantly during diastole. The RV rapidly dilates in an effort to maintain stroke volume. The crescentic shape is lost and the interventricular septum bulges into the LV cavity. As a result, LV filling (and thus stroke volume) is reduced. This phenomenon is known as *ventricular interdependence*. This results in systemic hypoperfusion and a further reduction in coronary perfusion. Unless the RV is offloaded, a vicious cycle ensues leading to circulatory failure and death.

The pathophysiology of RVF is illustrated in Figure 74.1.

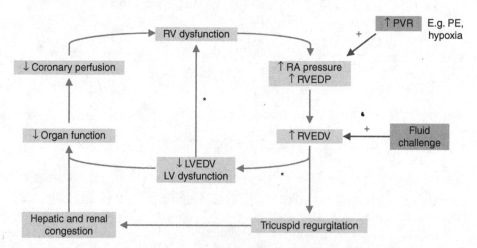

Figure 74.1 The pathophysiology of right ventricular failure
* represents ventricular interdependence

What are the causes of right ventricular failure?

The causes of RVF may be classified physiologically into RVF associated with normal or increased afterload, or that associated with volume overload (Table 74.1).

Table 74.1 The causes of right ventricular failure

Intrinsic RV failure (normal afterload)	RV infarction Cardiomyopathy
RV failure with increased afterload	Pulmonary embolus Pulmonary hypertension (e.g. mitral valve disease, congenital heart disease, interstitial lung disease, ARDS, COPD, OSA) Other causes of increased pulmonary vascular resistance (e.g. hypoxia, hypercapnia, acidosis, noradrenaline, protamine) LVAD implantation
RV failure with volume overload	LV failure Left to right intracardiac shunting (e.g. ASD, VSD)

How is RV failure diagnosed?

Right ventricular failure should be considered in high-risk groups of patients, i.e. those with pre-existing pulmonary hypertension or other predisposing conditions.

The patient may exhibit signs of RVF including peripheral oedema, raised JVP, tender hepatomegaly, a pansystolic tricuspid regurgitation (TR) murmur, third heart sound/gallop rhythm or loud P_2 due to raised pulmonary arterial pressure. The CVP will be high, and there may be giant V waves in the presence of TR.

Investigations include:

1 Blood tests including cardiac enzymes and BNP level
2 12 lead ECG
   – There may be right axis deviation, RBBB, RV strain pattern (ST depression and T wave inversion in V1-3 and the inferior leads) or evidence of a PE, e.g. $S_1Q_3T_3$
   – The ECG may also be normal
3 CXR
   – A PE may present with PA dilatation or oligaemia of the affected lung (*Westermark's sign*)
   – Cardiomegaly may or may not be present
4. Echocardiography (preferably TOE)
   – Will reveal a dilated, poorly functioning ventricle

- May show hypertrophy or TR, or demonstrate septal bulging into the LV cavity
- RV hypokinesia with apical sparing *(McConnell's sign)* may suggest a PE

How would you manage a patient with right ventricular failure?

The patient with RVF should be managed with an ABCDE approach, treating abnormalities as they are found. Specific management is as follows:

1 **Optimise volume status**
   - This depends on the afterload: If PVR is high, offload with diuretics
   - Guide with CVP, SvO_2 and lactate
   - TOE is useful – particularly repeated assessment to guide intervention
   - Consider inserting a PAC
2 **Reduce PVR**
   i Administer oxygen (to reduce hypoxic pulmonary vasoconstriction)
   ii Correct pH and pCO_2 (acidosis and hypercapnia both increase PVR)
   iii Optimise lung volume (PVR is minimal at FRC, and increases at volumes above and below this value)
   iv Consider pulmonary vasodilators, e.g. inhaled nitric oxide (no proven mortality benefit), nebulised or IV prostacyclin, IV sildenafil (PDE_5 inhibitor)
      Note that IV prostacyclin will worsen V/Q matching (increases shunt) and may cause hypotension and flushing
   v Treat intercurrent illness, e.g. sepsis
3 **Improve RV function**
   i Modifying ventilator settings may offload the RV
      - Avoid excessively high intrathoracic pressures (reduce venous return, increase afterload)
      - Limit mean airway pressure (avoid excessive PEEP, limit inspiratory pressures)
   ii Maintain right coronary artery perfusion (ensure DBP>RVEDP)
      - May need to add vasopressor
      - Low dose vasopressin has a better PVR profile than noradrenaline
   iii Add an inotrope if tricuspid annular plane systolic excursion (TAPSE) <16 mm
      - Try to avoid adrenaline (increases PVR)
      - Dobutamine increases CO (β_1) and causes pulmonary vasodilatation (β_2)
      - Low dose dopamine has β_1 activity, and D_1 activity causes vasodilatation
      - PDE_3 inhibitors such as milrinone cause inodilation (increase contractility and cause systemic and pulmonary vasodilatation)
4 **Treat coexisting LVF**
5 If none of the above have been successful, the decision is then whether to provide mechanical support (ECMO, VAD, biventricular pacing), to consider referral for super-urgent cardiac transplant, or to palliate

Further Reading

De Asua I, Rosenberg A. On the right side of the heart: Medical and mechanical support of the failing right ventricle. *Journal of the Intensive Care Society* 2017; **18**(2): 113–120

Kevin L G, Barnard M. Right ventricular failure. *Contin Educ Anaesth Crit Care Pain* 2007; 7(3): 89–94

Chapter 75

Scoring Systems

What are the features of an ideal scoring system?

1 *Valid*, i.e. should have been developed in a similar population
2 *Simple* to use
3 Shows *discrimination* – the ability of model to distinguish survivors from non-survivors based on predicted mortality
   - This is represented by plotting sensitivity against specificity to produce a receiver-operating characteristic curve
   - The area under this curve (AUROC) is calculated to represent discrimination
   - The closer the number is to 1, the better the discrimination (should be at least 0.7)
   - AUROC of 0.5 means that the scoring system is no better than a coin toss
4 *Calibrated* – represents the degree of accuracy, i.e. predicted vs observed mortality
5 Good *uniformity of fit* – reflects models performance in patient subgroups e.g. location prior to ICU, elective/emergency admissions, physiological derangement

What are scoring systems used for?

1 To assess the performance of the ICU
2 To assess the patient's risk of death
3 To compare or match populations for clinical studies
4 To facilitate audit
5 To tailor treatment

What scoring systems are you aware of?

Scoring systems used on the ICU may be divided into:

1 Illness severity scoring systems (Table 75.1)
2 Disease specific scoring systems (see Table 75.2 for examples)

Table 75.1 Illness severity scoring systems

Scoring System	Calculation	Notes

APACHE II Score (Acute Physiology and Chronic Health Evaluation) Worst score in first 24 hours after ICU admission Maximum score = 71	**Age** (score = 0 if ≤44 years-old, score = 6 if ≥75 years-old)
	
	 Acute physiology score — Each scores 0–4
	 – Physiological – Biochemical
	    i Temperature i pH
	    ii HR ii Na$^+$
	    iii MAP iii K$^+$
	    iv PaO$_2$/FiO$_2$ ratio iv Creatinine
	    v RR v Haematocrit
	    vi GCS vi WCC
	
	 Chronic disease
	 – Cirrhosis
	 – NYHA stage 4 heart failure
	 – Chronic respiratory disease
	 – Dialysis-dependent CKD
	 – Immunosuppression
		AUROC 0.85
		 Maximum score = 71
		 Score of 25 represents a predicted mortality of 50%
		 Score of >35 represents a predicted mortality of 80%

SAPS II (Simplified Acute Physiology Score) Worst score in first 24 hours after ICU admission	**Age**
	
	 Physiology score
	 – Physiological – Biochemical
	    i Temperature i Na$^+$
	    ii HR ii K$^+$
	    iii MAP iii Urea
	    iv PaO$_2$/FiO$_2$ ratio iv Bicarbonate
	    v GCS v Bilirubin
	    vi Urine output vi WCC
	
	 Chronic disease
	 – Metastatic cancer
	 – Haematological malignancy
	 – AIDS
	
	 Type of admission
	 – Elective surgical
	 – Emergency surgical
	 – Medical
		AUROC 0.86
		 SAPS III adjusts for geographic variation

MPM II (Mortality Prediction Model) Compares score at admission against that at 24 hours	Computes calculated risk of mortality during hospital admission by logistic regression Measures 16 variables at admission and a further 13 at 24 hours Each variable is either present (score = 1) or absent (score = 0)	AUROC 0.84 Can be repeated daily Allows probability of in-hospital death to be calculated (rather than a score)

Table 75.1 (cont.)

Scoring System	Calculation	Notes
SOFA Score (Sequential Organ Failure Assessment) Repetitive scoring system	Each organ system is scored from 0–4 based on degree of derangement (either positive or negative) from baseline **Respiratory** – PaO_2/FiO_2 ratio, mechanical ventilation **Cardiovascular** – MAP, inotrope/vasopressor requirement **Neurological** – GCS **Renal** – creatinine, urine output **Gastrointestinal** – bilirubin **Haematological** – platelet count	Initially developed for scoring of patients with sepsis Allows repeated scoring at 48-hour intervals to observe trends Average value used to predict mortality (rapid worsening of SOFA score suggests poor prognosis)
MODS (Multiple Organ Dysfunction Score) Repetitive scoring system	Each organ system is scored from 0–4 based on degree of derangement (either positive or negative) from baseline **Respiratory** – PaO_2/FiO_2 ratio **Cardiovascular** – pressure-adjusted HR **Neurological** – GCS **Renal** – creatinine **Gastrointestinal** – bilirubin **Haematological** – platelet count	Allows repeated scoring to observe trends
ICNARC Score (Intensive Care National Audit and Research Centre) Calculated with data from first 24 hours of admission to critical care	**Age** **Acute physiology score** similar to APACHE II **Reason for admission** including body system affected, surgical/medical **CPR** prior to admission **Type of admission** – elective/emergency	
POSSUM Score		Discussed in 'High Risk Surgical Patient' (see page 218)
Therapeutic Intervention Score (TISS) Assessment of	**Basic activities** e.g. standard monitoring, drain care **Ventilatory support** e.g. mechanical ventilation, care of artificial airway **Cardiovascular support** e.g. >1 vasoactive	Daily data collected from each patient on 28 possible interventions Mainly used to assess

Table 75.1 (cont.)

Scoring System	Calculation	Notes
nursing workload	drug infusion, arterial line **Neurological support** e.g. ICP monitoring **Renal support** e.g. RRT, urine output measurement **Metabolic support** e.g. enteral feeding, treatment of complicated metabolic acidosis/alkalosis **Specific interventions** e.g. single or multiple intervention within or outside of the ICU	nursing staffing levels and resource requirements May allow estimation of overall cost for groups of patients Worse scores correlate with worse outcomes Not standardised

NYHA – New York Heart Association

How can we compare ICUs?

Different units can be compared using structure-based, process-based and outcome-based quality indicators (Table 75.3).

What Is the standardised mortality rate?

The SMR is the ratio of the observed mortality and the expected mortality (estimated using scoring systems) over a specified time period.

$$SMR = \frac{\text{Observed mortality}}{\text{Predicted mortality}}$$

A value of 1 is considered as normal. If the SMR >1, the mortality is worse than predicted. The SMR may be used to compare ICUs as a surrogate for good quality care, however there are limitations to this approach:

1 The case mix is likely to differ between hospitals/units
2 The care received before critical care admission is not standardised between hospitals
3 There may be non-identical application of scoring systems between hospitals

Table 75.2 Examples of disease-specific scoring systems

Disease	Scoring System	Calculation	Notes
Community-acquired pneumonia	CURB-65 Score	**C** – Confusion (AMTS ≤8/10) **U** – Urea >7 mmol/l **R** – RR ≥30 per minute **B** – BP <90/60 mmHg **65** – Age >65 years	Risk of death at 30 days increases as CURB-65 score increases: – 0 – 0.6% – 1 – 2.7% – 2 – 6.8% – 3 –14.0% – 4 – 27.8% – 5 – 27.8% Score ≥4 should prompt ICU referral
Upper GI bleeding	Glasgow-Blatchford Score	Urea Hb **Systolic BP** Others – HR >100 bpm – Melaena at presentation – Syncope at presentation – Liver disease – Cardiac failure	Assesses likelihood for need for endoscopy/treatment and predicts need for hospital admission Each component is scored based on degree of derangement A score ≥6 is associated with ≥50% chance of requiring an intervention
	Rockall Score	**A** – Age **B** – Shock (based on HR and BP) **C** – Comorbidities – Nil – CCF, IHD, other cardiac disease – CKD, cirrhosis, metastatic cancer	Performed after OGD Max score = 11 Score <3 = good prognosis Score >8 = high mortality

		D – Diagnosis
		  – Mallory-Weiss tear
		  – Other
		  – GI malignancy
		E – Evidence of bleeding
		  – None
		  – Adherent clot, spurting vessel, blood visualised	

Acute pancreatitis	**Glasgow Score**	**P** – PaO$_2$ <8 kPa **A** – Age >55 **N** – WCC >15 x 10^9/l (neutrophils) **C** – Calcium <2 mmol/l **R** – Urea >16 mmol/l (renal) **E** – LDH >600 or ALT/AST >200 units/l (enzymes) **A** – Albumin <32 g/l **S** – Glucose >10 mmol/l (sugar)	Each positive finding scores 1 Score ≥3 predicts severe acute pancreatitis (SAP)
	Ranson Score		
	Balthazar CT Grade		Discussed in 'Severe Acute Pancreatitis' (see page 418)
Liver failure	**Model for End-stage Liver Disease (MELD) score**		Discussed in 'Chronic Liver Disease in the ICU' (see page 125–126)
	Childs-Turcotte-Pugh score		
	King's Criteria for referral to transplant centre		Discussed in 'Acute Liver Failure and Paracetamol Overdose' (see page 27)
Pulmonary embolus	**Wells Score**	Clinically suspected DVT ... 3 Other diagnosis unlikely ... 3 HR >100 bpm ... 1.5	Score >6 = high risk for PE Score 2–6 = intermediate risk

Table 75.2 (cont.)

Disease	Scoring System	Calculation		Notes
		Immobilisation or surgery in last 4 weeks	1.5	Score <2 = low risk
		Past history of venous thromboembolism	1.5	Scores used to direct investigation and treatment
		Haemoptysis	1	
		Malignancy	1	
Unstable angina and NSTEMI	GRACE Score	Age		Estimates mortality in ACS:
		HR		i In-hospital
		Systolic BP		ii 6-month
		Creatinine		iii 3-year
		Cardiac arrest at admission		Used to provide a basis for clinical decision-making
		ST changes		
		Abnormal cardiac biomarkers		
		Killip class of cardiac failure		
	Thrombolysis In Myocardial Infarction (TIMI) Score	Age ≥65 years		Estimates the following at 14 days:
		≥3 risk factors for coronary artery disease		i All-cause mortality
		Known CAD with ≥50% stenosis		ii Likelihood of new/recurrent MI
		Aspirin use in last 7 days		iii Likelihood of severe recurrent ischaemia necessitating PCI
		≥2 episodes of severe angina in last 24 hours		Each positive component scores 1
		ST changes ≥0.5 mm		Used to provide a basis for clinical decision-making
		Positive cardiac biomarkers		

Atrial fibrillation	CHA$_2$DS$_2$VASc score	Congestive heart failure	1	Score used to assess likelihood of stroke in patients with AF, to guide anticoagulant therapy
		Hypertension >140/90 mmHg	1	Score 0–1 in women = low risk (no therapy recommended)
		Age >75 years	2	Score 1 in men = moderate risk (consider warfarin or NOAC)
		Diabetes	1	Score ≥2 = high risk (warfarin or NOAC recommended)
		Stroke / clot	2	
		Vascular disease	1	
		Age	1	
		Sex category	1	
Trauma	Injury severity score (ISS)			Discussed in the 'Trauma' topic (page 467)

AMTS – abbreviated mental test score; OGD – oesophagogastroduodenoscopy; CAD – coronary artery disease

Table 75.3 Quality indicators in intensive care medicine

Structure-based	Process-based	Outcome-based
Availability of consultant intensivist	Participation in quality improvement programmes	Number of non-clinical transfers
Two consultant ward rounds per day		
Trainees trained appropriately	Delirium screening	Regular morbidity and mortality meetings
Nurse:patient ratio	Presence of end-of-life pathway	Regular clinical governance meetings
Presence of consultant and nursing lead	Hand hygiene compliance	CRBSI rate
% days at full occupancy	Early EN	Unit-based bacteraemias
MDT ward rounds	Number of readmissions within 48 hours	Unit-acquired MRSA infection
Dedicated physiotherapy and pharmacy teams	Number of overnight discharges (10pm-7am)	Unit-acquired C. difficile infection
Structured handover	Patients being admitted within 4 hours of decision to admit and receiving consultant review within 12 hours	Standardised mortality rate (SMR)
Use of daily plan/goals sheet	Hospital-wide standardised approach to the detection of the deteriorating patient	
Appropriate isolation of infected patients		
Access to an ICU follow-up clinic		

Further Reading

Bouch D C, Thompson J P. Scoring systems in the critically ill. *Contin Educ Anaesth Crit Care Pain* 2008; 8(5): 181–185

The Faculty of Intensive Care Medicine (FICM) and the Intensive Care Society (ICS). 2013. *Core Standards for Intensive Care Units*. London: FICM.

Chapter 76

Sedation

What is remifentanil?

Remifentanil is a synthetic phenylpiperidine derivative of fentanyl. It is a pure μ agonist. It is presented as a white powder consisting of 1, 2 or 5 mg remifentanil hydrochloride with glycine. It is reconstituted most commonly with normal saline and administered as an infusion (0.05–2 mcg/kg/min). It has similar potency to fentanyl and a bolus of up to 1 mcg/kg may be given over 30–60 seconds as co-induction.

Remifentanil is metabolised by non-specific plasma and tissue esterases; its duration of action is determined by elimination rather than distribution, unlike fentanyl. It differs from suxamethonium in that its metabolism is unaffected by cholinesterase deficiency as it is a poor substrate for that enzyme.

Remifentanil may be associated with profound respiratory depression, chest wall rigidity, bradycardia and hypotension. Its effects may be completely reversed with naloxone.

Why might it be used on the ICU?

Remifentanil has a relatively constant context-sensitive half-time (CSHT) of 3–8 minutes, meaning that it has rapid, predictable offset even following prolonged infusions (i.e. is essentially context-insensitive). This pharmacokinetic property lends remifentanil to use in neuro-critical care when frequent partial sedation holds are often required to assess neurology. It may also be useful in patients who are difficult to wean, patients who are expected to be extubated quickly, those with renal or liver impairment, and as analgesia for short procedures.

The analgesic effects wear off rapidly: pain may be a significant problem if inadequate alternative analgesia is not administered before discontinuing the remifentanil infusion. Intra-operative use may be associated with hyperalgesia post-operatively that may necessitate high doses of opioids with their inherent side effects.

What is context-sensitive half-time and why is it relevant?

The CSHT is the time taken for the plasma concentration to halve, after an infusion designed to maintain constant blood levels is stopped. The context is the duration of the infusion. The higher the ratio of *clearance due to redistribution* to *clearance due to elimination*, the greater the possible range of CSHT. It is important because it helps to predict how long a patient will take to wake up from a steady-state infusion of a given sedative drug.

For example, fentanyl redistributes very rapidly and its clearance due to elimination is about 20% of that for distribution. Therefore, the CSHT for fentanyl increases rapidly with increasing duration of infusion. The maximum CSHT for fentanyl is approximately 300 minutes.

In contrast, the clearance due to elimination for propofol is similar to that for redistribution. This rapid elimination means that plasma concentration falls quickly after a propofol infusion is stopped. As a result, the maximum possible CSHT for propofol is approximately 20 minutes.

The distribution clearance of remifentanil is lower than the elimination clearance (i.e. the opposite of fentanyl). Therefore, elimination dictates the clearance of remifentanil from the plasma resulting in very little variation in CSHT.

Tell me about propofol

Propofol is 2,6-di-isopropyl-phenol (Figure 76.1). It is presented as a 1% or 2% lipid-water emulsion containing soya bean oil and purified egg phosphatide. It is highly lipid soluble and poorly water soluble. It is a weak organic acid with a pK_a of 11, and is almost entirely unionised at physiological pH.

Propofol is used for induction (1–2 mg/kg) and maintenance (up to 4 mg/kg/hour, plasma concentration 4–8 mcg/ml) of anaesthesia, and for sedation.

It is 98% protein-bound to albumin with a Vd of 4 l/kg. A bolus dose has a short duration of action due to rapid redistribution. It undergoes mainly hepatic metabolism to inactive compounds that are excreted in the urine (40% glucuronidation, 60% metabolised to a quinol (excreted as a sulphate and a glucuronide)). During prolonged infusion CSHT increases and waking may be protracted due to the slow release of propofol from fat (careful titration may avoid this).

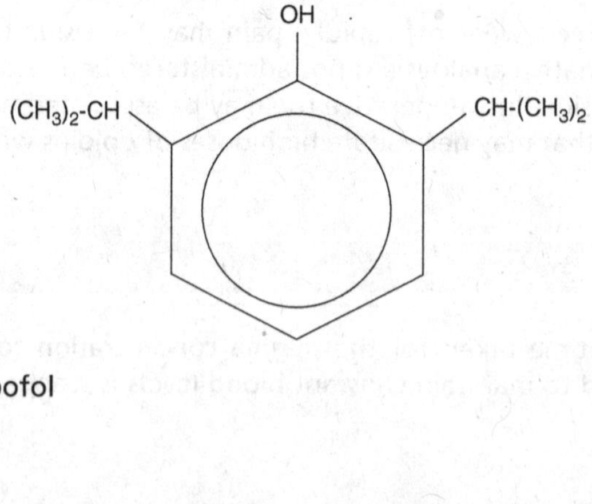

Figure 76.1 Propofol

What are the adverse effects of using propofol as a sedative on the ICU?

Respiratory

- Respiratory depression (can lead to apnoea)

Cardiovascular

- Reduction in SVR leading to hypotension
- Can be associated with a bradycardia (i.e. obtunds baroreceptor reflex)
- Reduced sympathetic activity and myocardial contractility

Metabolic

- Propofol infusion syndrome (PRIS) may follow prolonged infusion in high risk patients

Other

- Green discoloration of urine and hair (no correlation with PRIS)

What is propofol infusion syndrome?

PRIS was first described in the paediatric population, and is characterised by acute refractory bradycardia leading to asystole in the presence of one or more of the following:

1 Unexplained metabolic acidosis (base excess >–10 mmol/l)
2 Rhabdomyolysis (high CK, hyperkalaemia, AKI) or myoglobinuria
3 Lipaemic plasma (hypertriglyceridaemia)
4 Fatty liver or hepatomegaly

What is the pathophysiology?

The mechanism is thought to be related to impaired mitochondrial fatty acid metabolism and direct inhibition of mitochondrial function leading to impaired oxygen utilisation, anaerobic respiration and lactate production. Additionally, propofol is a direct myocardial depressant. There is cardiac and skeletal myocyte ischaemia and necrosis, with accumulation of unutilised fatty acids. This is associated with arrhythmias.

What are the risk factors for PRIS?

1 High dose propofol infusion (>4 mg/kg/hour)
2 Young age
   - Low glycogen stores, high dependence on lipid metabolism
   - The Committee on Safety of Medicines has advised that propofol should be contraindicated for sedation in ICU of children ≤16 years-old
3 Brain injury
4 Low carbohydrate intake, high lipid loads, e.g. PN
   - There is increased lipolysis in periods of starvation precipitated by high energy demands
5 High endogenous or exogenous catecholamine levels
   - Increased propofol clearance, meaning higher infusion rates required
6 High endogenous or exogenous glucocorticoid levels
7 Inborn errors of fatty acid metabolism

How might PRIS present?

PRIS most commonly presents with ECG changes (Figure 76.2):

1 Bradycardia
2 Brugada-like pattern (coved-type ST elevation in V1-V3)
3 Varying degrees of heart block
4 RBBB
5 Unexplained arrhythmias

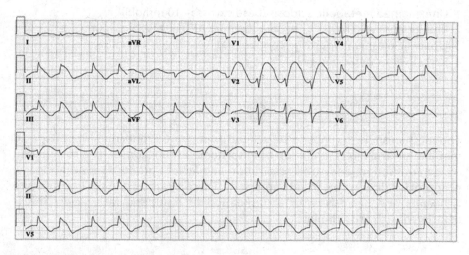

Figure 76.2 Brugada-like coved ST elevation in V1-2 with significant interventricular conduction delay in a patient with PRIS
Reproduced with permission from Mijzen EJ, et al. (*Neurocrit Care* 2012)

There may be unexplained cardiovascular instability and escalating inotrope/vasopressor requirements.

A high index of suspicion should be maintained, particularly in patients on high-dose propofol or with other risk factors. There should be a low threshold for measuring triglyceride levels.

What is the treatment?

The management of PRIS is entirely supportive and should follow an ABCDE approach, treating abnormalities as they are found. Specific management involves:

1 **Stop the propofol infusion** and maintain sedation with an alternative agent, e.g. midazolam
2 Supportive management
   i Titration of vasoactive infusions
   ii Rhabdomyolysis treatment (target urine output 2–3 ml/kg/hour, urinary alkalinisation, diuretics, treatment of hyperkalaemia)
   iii RRT for AKI
   iv Ensure adequate carbohydrate intake (glucose infusion)
2 Consider temporary pacing
3 **VA ECMO** has been used successfully

How is level of sedation assessed on the ICU?

The most commonly used methods are the Richmond Agitation-Sedation Scale (RASS, Table 76.1) and the Ramsay Sedation Scale (below):

Table 76.1 The Richmond Agitation-Sedation Score

Score		Description
+4	Combative	Overtly combative, violent, imminent danger to staff
+3	Very agitated	Pulls or removes tubes or catheters, aggressive
+2	Agitated	Frequent non-purposeful movement, fights ventilator
+1	Restless	Anxious but movements not aggressive or vigorous
0	Alert and calm	
−1	Drowsy	Not fully alert, has sustained awakening with eye contact to voice >10 seconds
−2	Light sedation	Briefly awakens with eye contact to voice <10 seconds
−3	Moderate sedation	Movement or eye opening to voice, no eye contact
−4	Deep sedation	No response to voice, movement or eye opening to physical stimulation
−5	Unrousable	No response to voice or physical stimulation

1 Anxious, agitated or restless
2 Cooperative, oriented and tranquil
3 Responds to commands only
4 Brisk awakening to glabellar tap or loud auditory stimulus
5 Sluggish awakening to glabellar tap or loud auditory stimulus
6 No response to glabellar tap or loud auditory stimulus

What level of sedation should be targeted?

Patients' sedation should be titrated according to clinical need and the sedation score target should be set as part of the daily round. In most situations one should follow the *3 C rule* (aim to have the patient calm, cooperative and comfortable), i.e. a target RASS of 0 to −1 is used. However, there are times when a patient may require deeper sedation, i.e. RASS −3 to −5, such as:

1 Brain injury and raised ICP
2 Use of NMBAs
3 Severe respiratory failure/ARDS
4 Ventilator-patient dysynchrony
5 Strict immobilisation, e.g. unstable spinal fractures
6 Status epilepticus

Further Reading

Loh N H W, Nair P. Propofol infusion syndrome. *Contin Educ Anaesth Crit Care Pain* 2013; **13**(6): 200–202

Peck T, Hill S, Williams M. Applied pharmacokinetic models. In: *Pharmacology for Anaesthesia and Intensive Care* (4th ed). Cambridge University Press, 2014; 71–79

Peck T, Hill S, Williams M. General anaesthetic agents. In: *Pharmacology for Anaesthesia and Intensive Care* (4th ed). Cambridge University Press, 2014; 93–125

Peck T, Hill S, Williams M. Analgesics. In: *Pharmacology for Anaesthesia and Intensive Care* (4th ed). Cambridge University Press, 2014; 126–153

Vincent J L, Shehabi Y, Walsh T S, et al. Comfort and patient-centred care without excessive sedation: The eCASH concept. *Intensive Care Med* 2016; **42**: 962–971

Chapter 77

Sepsis

Define *sepsis*

Sepsis is broadly defined as the presence of pathogenic organisms or their toxins in the blood and tissues.

Until recently, the definition of sepsis focussed on the host response to invasion by microorganisms, i.e. the systemic inflammatory response syndrome (SIRS), as defined by changes in white cell count, respiratory rate, heart rate and temperature. However, there were several problems with the use of SIRS as part of the definition:

1 The criteria for SIRS are not specific to infection – other conditions associated with sterile inflammation can cause a SIRS response, e.g. burns, trauma, pancreatitis
2 Some degree of host response is inherent and appropriate in infection: indeed, its absence may signify immunocompromise
3 Almost every patient with infection (even the common cold) fulfils SIRS criteria, although not all have sepsis or poor outcomes, i.e. poor discriminant validity

In response to this, and in combination with an evolving understanding of the underlying pathophysiology of sepsis, the **SEPSIS-3** definitions were published in 2016 (JAMA, 2016):

Sepsis is life-threatening organ dysfunction caused by a dysregulated host response to infection

– Organ dysfunction can be represented by an increase of ≥2 points in the SOFA score

Septic shock is a subset of sepsis in which particularly profound circulatory, cellular, and metabolic abnormalities are associated with a greater risk of mortality than with sepsis alone

– Patients with septic shock can be clinically identified by:
  i Vasopressor requirement to maintain MAP ≥65 mmHg
  ii Serum lactate level >2 mmol/l in the absence of hypovolemia
– This combination is associated with >40% in-hospital mortality

How should ward staff be trained to recognise high-risk patients with sepsis?

In the ED, general hospital ward and pre-hospital environment, the application of the *quickSOFA* (*qSOFA*) score is useful. If adult patients with suspected infection have ≥2 of the following clinical criteria, they are more likely to have poor outcomes attributable to sepsis:

1 Respiratory rate ≥22/min
2 SBP ≤100 mmHg
3 Altered mentation, i.e. GCS <15

What mechanisms exist to protect the body against microorganisms?

1 **Physical barriers** protect against ~99% of microorganisms
   – Skin
   – Cilia
   – Stomach acidity
   – Flora

2 **Innate immune response** protects against almost 1% of microorganisms (Figure 77.1)
   – Reacts to foreign antigen with *no previous exposure*
   – Rapid, non-specific
   – No memory

Pattern-recognition receptors (PRRs) are present on the surfaces of immune cells such as neutrophils, mast cells, dendritic cells and natural killer cells. These PRRs (e.g. Toll-like receptors [TLR]) respond to *pathogen-associated molecular patterns* (PAMPs), which are unique cellular constituents that are not found in vertebrates and include:

  i Cell surface proteins
 ii Glycoproteins
iii Lipopolysaccharide (LPS) found in Gram-negative bacterial cell walls
 iv Components found in Gram-positive cell walls, e.g. lipotechoic acid (LTA)

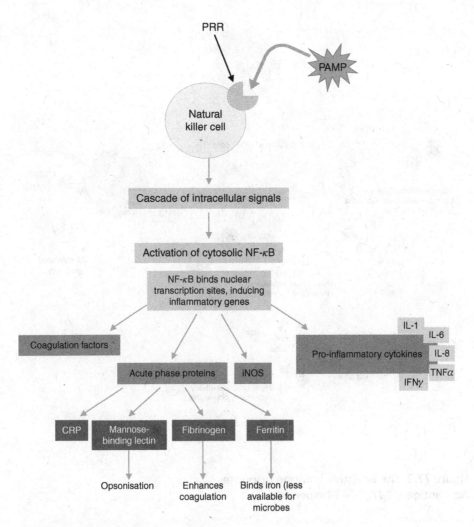

Figure 77.1 The innate immune response
NF-κB – nuclear factor-κB; IL – interleukin; TNFα – tumour necrosis factor-α; IFNγ – interferon-γ; iNOS – inducible nitric oxide synthase
Acute phase proteins are soluble PRRs secreted by the liver, vascular endothelium and innate immune cells, each with a specific function

3 **Adaptive immune response** (Figure 77.2)
  – Retains highly specific memory
  – Subsequent exposure results in a superior response (qualitative and quantitative)

Foreign antigens are presented on an *antigen-presenting cell* (AgPC) by way of major histocompatibility complex (MHC) class II proteins, e.g. dendritic cells, macrophages and monocytes that are within lymphoid tissue.

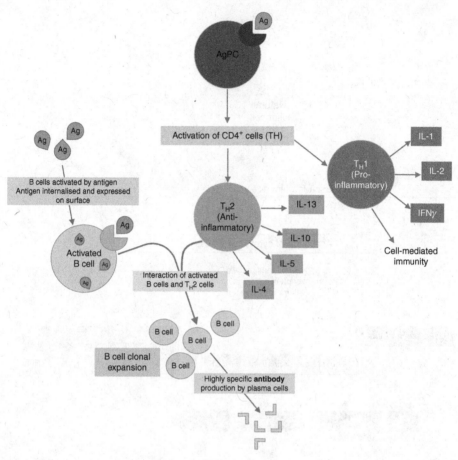

Figure 77.2 The adaptive immune response
Ag – antigen; T$_H$ cells – T-helper cells

What is the pathophysiology of sepsis?

There are several pathophysiological processes that lead to the clinical picture of sepsis and ultimately to tissue hypoxia:

1 *Vasodilatation* (iNOS causes endothelial NO production)
   - Bounding pulses
   - Effective hypovolaemia (distributive shock) leads to hypotension and reflex tachycardia
   - Reduced oxygen delivery as RBCs move more rapidly through capillary beds
2 *Loss of endothelial integrity* due to inflammatory mediator-related disruption of tight junctions
   - Bacterial translocation in the lung, liver and GI tract
   - Interstitial oedema

- Worsens hypovolaemia and hypotension
- Reduces oxygen delivery to tissues, causing lactate production and acidosis
- Causes interstitial pulmonary oedema and can lead to ARDS

3 *Reduced myocardial contractility* (multifactorial)
- Often masked if fluid resuscitation is adequate (i.e. tachycardia with warm extremities and low SVR)

4 *Activation of the coagulation cascade and fibrinolysis* due to IL-1, IL-6 and TNFα release, and reduced protein C levels
- Diffuse endovascular injury
- Microthrombi block capillaries producing shunts

5 *Mitochondrial dysfunction*
- Reduced oxygen utilisation in the face of ample DO_2 leads to increased SvO_2 (Note that an increased oxygen extraction ratio in the absence of mitochondrial dysfunction leads to reduced SvO_2 and implies inadequate resuscitation)
- Effective tissue hypoxia leads to anaerobic metabolism, which produces lactate

The pathophysiology is summarised in Figure 77.3.

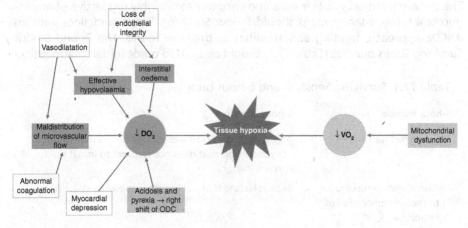

Figure 77.3 The pathophysiology of sepsis
ODC – oxygen dissociation curve; DO_2 – oxygen delivery; VO_2 – oxygen consumption

What are exotoxins/endotoxins?

Exotoxins are polypeptides that are secreted by Gram-positive bacteria, e.g. LTA (Staphylococci, *Str. pyogenes*, Bacillus, Clostridia).

Endotoxins are located within Gram-negative bacterial cell walls, e.g. LPS (*E. coli*, *Salmonella typhi*, Shigella, *Vibrio cholerae*).

A 22-year-old university student is admitted to the ED with a 24-hour history of fevers, rigors, lethargy and increasing confusion. On arrival, she is cool to her knees and elbows with a non-blanching purple discolouration to her toes and shins. She has nuchal rigidity and is photophobic. She opens her eyes and flexes to pain, and is moaning.

Her observations are:

SpO_2 96% on 15 l/min of oxygen via a non-rebreathing mask
RR 28 per minute
HR 126 bpm
BP 89/53 mmHg
Temperature 39.1°C
ABG (taken on 15 l/min oxygen): pH 7.13, $PaCO_2$ 3.2 kPa, PaO_2 47.7 kPa, BE -21.3, HCO_3^- 12.8 mmol/l, lactate 6.9 mmol/l

What is your immediate management?

This patient is critically ill. Her signs and symptoms are highly suggestive of meningococcal sepsis. Management should follow *Surviving Sepsis* guidelines with an ABCDE approach, treating abnormalities as they are found. The 3- and 6-hour *Surviving Sepsis* bundles (Table 77.1) should be used to guide initial treatment.

Table 77.1 Surviving Sepsis 3- and 6-hour bundles

3-hour bundle	6-hour bundle
Measure lactate level	Apply vasopressors to maintain MAP ≥65 mmHg (for hypotension that does not respond to initial fluid resuscitation)
Obtain blood cultures prior to the administration of antibiotics	Repeat lactate if initial lactate was elevated

Administer broad-spectrum antibiotics	If persistent hypotension after initial fluid resuscitation or initial lactate ≥4 mmol/l, reassess volume status and tissue perfusion by either:
	– Repeat focussed exam (vital signs, cardiopulmonary parameters, capillary refill time, pulse, skin findings) *or*
	– Any two of:
	  i Measure CVP
	  ii Measure $ScvO_2$
	  iii Bedside echo
	  iv Dynamic assessment of fluid responsiveness, e.g. straight-leg raise

Table 77.1 (cont.)

3-hour bundle	6-hour bundle
Administer 30 ml/kg crystalloid for hypotension or lactate ≥4 mmol/l	

1 **Airway and breathing**
   - Endotracheal intubation should be considered as she has evidence of neurological obtundation (her GCS is 8 – E2 V2 M4)
   - Significant respiratory failure and ARDS may form part of the initial presentation (particularly in patients with pneumonia), and/or may develop following large-volume fluid resuscitation
2 **Fluid resuscitation** with 30 ml/kg crystalloid
3 **Microbiological samples** taken *before* administering **broad-spectrum IV antibiotics** – this should occur within the first hour of presentation
   - Blood cultures should be taken before administering high-dose IV ceftriaxone in combination with IV aciclovir (but do not delay antibiotic administration)
   - Urine, sputum and stool samples should be sent for MC+S
   - Obtaining CSF samples prior to antibiotic therapy is not practical in this case
4 Blood should also be taken for **serum lactate** level
   - Send FBC, U+Es, CRP, LFTs, clotting screen to detect organ dysfunction simultaneously
5 Consider **vasopressors +/- inotropes** if there is ongoing hypotension despite adequate fluid resuscitation, targeting a MAP ≥65 mmHg
   - Noradrenaline is first-line
   - Add vasopressin to achieve target MAP (or to reduce noradrenaline dose)
   - Consider dobutamine if there is evidence of myocardial dysfunction
6 Other investigations
   - This patient should have a CT brain followed by an LP to aid microbiological diagnosis
7 Lines/catheters
   - Prompt urinary catheterisation to enable accurate urine output measurement and fluid balance
   - Insertion of an arterial line (especially if vasopressors are necessary)
   - Consider the need for CVC insertion (Table 77.1)
8 Other routine interventions in critically ill patients:
   i VAP bundles
   ii Lung-protective ventilatory strategy
   iii Daily sedation holds
   iv Stress ulcer prophylaxis

   v Enteral feeding within 48 hours of diagnosis
  vi Glycaemic control (target glucose 4–10 mmol/l)
 vii Thromboprophylaxis

What is early goal-directed therapy and what is the evidence for/against Its use?

Early goal-directed therapy (EGDT) describes the process of targeting a number of physiological parameters and performing certain procedures during resuscitation in states of sepsis. **Rivers, et al** (NEJM) devised the term in 2001 whilst conducting a single-centre RCT comparing the impact of the introduction of an EGDT care bundle to unprotocolised standard care, on the mortality in patients with severe sepsis and septic shock. The EGDT bundle comprised the following elements:

1 Oxygen +/– intubation and mechanical ventilation
2 CVC and arterial line insertion
3 Continuous $ScvO_2$ measurement
4 500 ml fluid boluses to target CVP 8–12 mmHg
5 Vasopressors or vasodilators to target MAP 65–90 mmHg
6 If $ScvO_2$ <70%, RBC transfusion to target haematocrit ≥0.3
7 If still $ScvO_2$ <70%, add dobutamine 2.5–20 mcg/kg/min until $ScvO_2$ >70%

There was a significant reduction in in-hospital mortality in the EGDT group. Following this trial, there was widespread uptake of the EGDT protocol.

The **ProCESS** trial (NEJM, 2014) was a multi-centre RCT in the US that randomised patients with sepsis to receive strict EGDT protocolised care (based on the Rivers trial) or protocol-based standard therapy for 6 hours. There was no difference detected in 60-day, 90-day or one-year mortality.

The **ARISE** trial (NEJM, 2014) was a primarily Antipodean multi-centre RCT in which patients with septic shock were randomised to receive either protocolised EGDT or usual care (where $ScvO_2$ measurement was not permitted) for 6 hours. There was no difference in 90-day mortality between groups.

The **PROMISE** trial (NEJM, 2015) was an English multi-centre RCT that similarly randomised patients with septic shock to receive protocolised EGDT or usual care (where $ScvO_2$ measurement was not permitted) for 6 hours. Again, they failed to demonstrate a difference in 90-day mortality. There was a reduction in SOFA score and in ICU LOS in the usual care group.

Previous versions of the *Surviving Sepsis* guidelines had recommended a protocolised EGDT approach, using a series of goals including CVP and $ScvO_2$, based on that published by Rivers. This approach has now been challenged following the failure to show a mortality reduction in these three large multi-centre RCTs, and the most recent iteration of the guidelines (2016) reflects this.

Why is a MAP of 65 mmHg targeted in patients with sepsis?

The **SEPSISPAM** trial (NEJM, 2014) was a French multi-centre RCT that looked at the effect of targeting a high (80–85 mmHg) or low (65–70 mmHg) MAP in patients with septic shock. There was no difference in 28- or 90-day mortality. There was a significantly higher incidence of new onset AF in the higher MAP group. Subgroup analysis of patients with chronic hypertension revealed the higher MAP group had a significantly lower incidence of doubling of creatinine (NNT 7.6) and requirement for RRT (NNT 9.5).

The desirable consequences of targeting MAP of 65 mmHg (lower risk of AF, lower doses of vasopressors, and similar mortality) form the basis of the initial MAP target in the *Surviving Sepsis* guidelines. This target can be individualised to the patient if necessary.

Do you know of any evidence surrounding the use of different vasoactive medications in septic shock?

The **VASST** trial (NEJM, 2008) was an international RCT in which patients with noradrenaline-dependent septic shock were randomised to receive either vasopressin (0.01–0.03 units/minute) or noradrenaline infusions. There was no difference in mortality at 28 days. The MAP was similar between the groups. Vasopressin was found to be noradrenaline-sparing. Importantly, this trial did not compare the use of vasopressin with noradrenaline, rather the addition of vasopressin to noradrenaline.

The **VANISH** trial (JAMA, 2016) was a multi-centre RCT that looked at the development of AKI in patients with septic shock. Patients were randomised to receive either noradrenaline or vasopressin, with the addition of hydrocortisone (50 mg qds IV) once maximum dose of the first study drug was reached. There was no difference in numbers of renal failure-free days between any of the resulting study groups. Fewer patients required RRT in the vasopressin group compared with the noradrenaline group.

The **LeoPARDS** trial (NEJM, 2016) was a British multi-centre RCT investigating the effect of levosimendan versus placebo on patients with fluid-resuscitated vasopressor-dependent septic-shock. There was no difference in SOFA scores or mortality between groups. However, there were higher rates of haemodynamic instability, hypotension and vasopressor use in the intervention arm. Furthermore, patients in the levosimendan group were less likely to wean from mechanical ventilation and more likely to develop SVT.

Is there any evidence for steroids in septic shock?

The **CORTICUS** trial (NEJM, 2008) randomised patients with septic shock to receive either hydrocortisone (50 mg qds IV, tapered from day 6) or placebo for 12 days. They demonstrated no improvement in 28-day mortality (even in groups stratified by ACTH response), but there was a reduction in the duration of vasopressor dependence. There was also a non-significant trend towards an increase in the rate of superinfections in the intervention group.

More recently the German multi-centre RCT, **HYPRESS** (NEJM, 2016), investigated the effect of a continuous infusion of hydrocortisone (200 mg/day) compared to placebo on the development of septic shock in patients with sepsis and organ dysfunction. There was no difference between groups.

The international **ADRENAL** trial is currently underway and aims to assess the effect of steroids on 90-day mortality in patients with septic shock.

Should APC be used in sepsis?

The **PROWESS** trial (NEJM, 2001) was an international multi-centre RCT in which patients with severe sepsis or septic shock were randomised to receive either APC (drotrecogin alfa (activated) 24 mcg/kg/hour) or placebo for 96 hours. Mortality at 28 days was lower in the intervention group (NNT 16). Subgroup analysis revealed greater efficacy in patients with an APACHE II score ≥25 (NNT 8).

The subsequent **PROWESS-SHOCK** trial (NEJM, 2012) randomised patients with septic shock and mean APACHE II scores >25 in a similar fashion. There was no evidence of a mortality benefit (28- and 90-day mortality rates were similar) and there was an increase in non-serious bleeding events in the intervention group.

There is controversy regarding whether the original PROWESS trial was flawed, or whether the improvement in the management of sepsis since 2001 has blunted the efficacy of APC seen in the original trial. Nonetheless, drotrecogin alfa was withdrawn from the market in 2011.

Further Reading

Rhodes A, Evans L E, Alhazzani W, et al. Surviving sepsis campaign: International guidelines for management of sepsis and septic shock 2016. *Crit Care Med* 2017; **45**(3): 486–552

Singer M, Deutschman C S, Seymour C W, et al. The third international consensus definitions for sepsis and septic shock (sepsis-3). *J Am Med Assoc* 2016; **315**(8): 801–810

Chapter 78

Severe Acute Pancreatitis

What are the causes of pancreatitis?

Pancreatitis is a multisystem condition that can be caused by a number of different disease processes. Gallstones and alcohol abuse are the most common, causing up to 75–85% of cases of acute pancreatitis. Table 78.1 illustrates the causes of the remaining 15–25%.

Table 78.1 Causes of acute pancreatitis

Obstructive	Systemic/global	Parenchymal
Gallstones	Hypoxaemia/ischaemia	Alcohol
Neoplasm (e.g. head of pancreas)	Drugs (e.g. steroids, furosemide, azathioprine)	Trauma including following ERCP
Cystic fibrosis	Hypothermia	Autoimmune disease (primary sclerosing cholangitis)
Congenital anomalies	Hypercalcaemia, hyperparathyroidism, hypertriglyceridaemia	
	Viruses (e.g. HIV, CMV, mumps, hepatitides)	
	Scorpion bites	

ERCP – endoscopic retrograde cholangiopancreatography

How is the severity and prognosis of acute pancreatitis determined?

Acute pancreatitis can be divided into two types; interstitial oedematous pancreatitis and necrotising pancreatitis. Severe acute pancreatitis (SAP) is characterised by organ dysfunction in the presence of local or systemic complications. There is a protracted clinical course for SAP and a higher mortality rate. Prompt identification of SAP is essential to ensure patients are triaged to the appropriate setting i.e. critical care and ultimately a specialist centre.

A number of scoring systems have been developed to help identify and prognosticate in pancreatitis:

1 *Ranson criteria* (table 78.2)
   - Originally designed for gallstone-induced pancreatitis
   - Uses age, nine laboratory parameters plus fluid requirements to calculate a score over 48 hours
   - A score of >3 at 48 hours indicates the presence of severe pancreatitis, and carries a 15% mortality
2 *Imrie (Glasgow) criteria* (see Table 75.2, p397)
   - Requires 48 hours to complete
   - Uses age and seven laboratory parameters to predict severe pancreatitis
3 APACHE II score
   - A score of >8 at 24 hours defines severe acute pancreatitis

Table 78.2 Ranson's criteria for severe acute pancreatitis

At admission	Non-gallstone pancreatitis	Gallstone pancreatitis
Age (years)	> 55	> 70
WBC (cells/mm³)	> 16000	> 18000
Glucose (mmol/l)	> 11	> 12.2
LDH (U/l)	> 350	> 400
AST (U/l)	> 250	> 250
During initial 48 hours		
Haematocrit decrease (%)	> 10	> 10
Blood urea increase (mmol/l)	> 1.8	> 0.7
Serum calcium (mmol/l)	< 2	< 2
PaO² (kPa)	< 8	< 8
Base deficit (mmol/l)	> 4	> 5
Fluid sequestration (litres)	> 6	> 4

Scoring systems based on CT appearance are also used to grade pancreatitis severity: the CT severity index (CTSI) is the primary example. The Balthazar score is a subscore within the CTSI providing an A–E grade (Table 78.3). In addition to a score for pancreatic necrosis, the Balthazar score provides improved correlation to clinical severity. The maximum score that can be obtained is 10 and predicts a mortality of up to 17%.

Table 78.3 Balthazar CT grading of acute pancreatitis

Grading of pancreatitis (Balthazar score)	Points	Necrosis factor	
		% Necrosis	Points
A: Normal pancreas	0		
B: Enlargement of pancreas	1	0	0
C: Inflammatory of pancreas or peripancreatic fat	2	< 30	2
D: One pancreatic fluid collection	3	30–50	4
E: ≥2 peripancreatic fluid collections	4	>50	6

Points scored (CT grade + necrosis)	% Morbidity	% Mortality
0–3	8	3
4–6	35	6
7–10	92	17

What is the role of imaging in acute pancreatitis?

Imaging is required when the diagnosis is in question or when a certain study might provide specific information. Table 78.4 summarises the different modalities that may be used.

Table 78.4 Imaging in severe acute pancreatitis

Plain AXR	Limited role Will detect free air in the abdomen, ileus, calcified gallstones/pancreas
CXR	May show pleural effusions (usually on the left)
Abdominal ultrasonography	Technique of choice for detecting gallstones
Endoscopic ultrasonography	Used mainly for detection of microlithiasis and periampullary lesions not easily revealed by other methods
Abdominal CT (+/- contrast)	Always indicated in SAP Used to detect necrosis, fluid collections, haemorrhage, pseudoaneurysm etc. Can guide interventional procedures
ERCP	Patients with signs/symptoms of cholangitis should have early ERCP to relieve biliary obstruction
MRI / Magnetic resonance cholangiopancreatography (MRCP)	MRCP not as sensitive as ERCP but safer and non-invasive MRI may be indicated in patients unable to receive CT contrast Can delineate necrotic areas

When should a patient with acute pancreatitis be managed within critical care?

Strong indicators for admission to critical care in patients meeting the criteria for SAP include:

1 Age >70 years
2 Obesity (BMI >30 kg/m^2)
3 Patients requiring ongoing volume resuscitation
4 Presence of indicators of more severe disease:
   i Substantial pancreatic necrosis (>30%)
   ii ≥3 Ranson criteria present
   iii Pleural effusions
   iv CRP >150 mg/dl at 48 hours

What general principles govern the management of acute pancreatitis?

Severe acute pancreatitis is an archetypal example of a sterile inflammatory process with a clinical picture often indistinguishable from severe sepsis. It should be managed with an ABCDE approach, treating abnormalities as they are found. Specific management of acute pancreatitis depends largely on severity and follows these general principles:

1 Initial resuscitation and supportive care
   i Fluid resuscitation
      – Maintain a urine output ≥0.5 ml/kg/hour
      – Inadequate volume repletion is associated with higher rates of pancreatic necrosis
   ii Correction of electrolyte abnormalities
   iii Close monitoring
2 Control of symptoms
   – Pain may be severe and a PCA is often required
3 Organ support
4 Nutritional support
5 Prevention and treatment of infection
6 Treatment of associated or causative conditions
7 General supportive care
   i Thromboprophylaxis
   ii VAP bundles (head up, supraglottic suction ETT, daily sedation holds, PPI and thromboprophylaxis, oral chlorhexidine)
   iii Physiotherapy

What local complications are associated with severe acute pancreatitis?

The main local complications of SAP are:

1. *Pseudocyst formation*
   - Complicates approximately 5% of cases of acute pancreatitis
   - Results from pancreatic duct leakage
   - Consists of a collection of pancreatic secretions encased in granulation tissue
   - May be asymptomatic, present with pain alone or present with complications including bleeding, infection or rupture
   - Rarely, pseudocysts can cause gastric outlet and/or biliary obstruction and thrombosis of splenic or portal veins
2. *Pancreatic necrosis*
   - Infected necrosis is associated with significant morbidity and mortality
   - Image-guided needle aspiration of pancreatic tissue is required to confirm the diagnosis
   - Proven infection necessitates drainage/debridement

What is the role of surgery in SAP?

Open or minimally invasive surgery is indicated in selected cases:

1 *Pseudocysts*
   - No intervention necessary in most cases
   - Percutaneous aspiration, or endoscopic or surgical techniques for large or symptomatic pseudocysts
2 *Pancreatic duct disruption*
   - Image-guided percutaneous placement of a drainage tube into the fluid collection
   - Distal pancreatectomy or Whipple's procedure in refractory cases
3 *Pancreatic abscess*
   - Percutaneous catheter drainage and antibiotics
   - Surgical drainage if no response
4 *Infected pancreatic necrosis*
   - Image-guided aspiration, or a necrosectomy
   - It is important to distinguish sterile from infected pancreatic necrosis
     - Around half of patients with pancreatic necrosis will develop infection in the necrotic tissue by weeks 3–4
     - Debridement and/or drainage is *not* recommended in sterile necrosis
   - The timing of surgery is important: early surgery (within the first 2 weeks) is associated with very high mortality
   - Necrosectomy to remove infected tissue should be delayed until clear demarcation of infected tissue can be demonstrated – this also minimises the number of surgical procedures required

– Clinical picture (severity and evolution) should be the primary determinant of timing of intervention

How should patients with pancreatitis be fed?

Enteral feeding is advocated for patients with pancreatitis in order to help maintain the intestinal mucosal barrier and hence prevent translocation (a major source of infection). Post-pyloric (NJ) feeding may be required as gastric emptying is frequently impaired; however, NG feeding is equivalent if gastric emptying is adequate.

Parenteral nutrition is used when patients are unable to tolerate oral feeding (ileus, pain, nausea etc.).

What is recommended regarding antimicrobial prophylaxis?

International consensus guidelines from 2004 recommend against the use of systemic prophylactic antimicrobials in patients with necrotising pancreatitis, given a consistent lack of evidence of benefit and a real risk of harm.

Further Reading
Balthazar E J. Acute pancreatitis: assessment of severity with clinical and CT evaluation. *Radiology* 2002; **223**: 603–613

Nathens A B, Curtis J R, Beale R J. Management of the critically ill patient with severe acute pancreatitis. *Crit Care Med* 2004; **32**(12): 2524–2536

Ranson J H. Etiological and prognostic factors in human acute pancreatitis: a review. *Am J Gastroenterol* 1982; **77**: 633–638

Young S P, Thompson J P. Severe acute pancreatitis. *Contin Educ Anaesth Crit Care Pain*. 2008; **8**(4): 125–128

Chapter 79

Spinal Cord Injury

How is spinal cord injury classified?

Spinal cord injury is classified according to the ASIA (American Spinal Injury Association) impairment scale (A-E), which is scored as soon as possible after the injury:

A *Complete*
  No sensory or motor function is preserved in the sacral segments S4-S5
B *Incomplete*
  Preservation of sensory but not motor function below the neurological level and includes the sacral segments S4-S5
C *Incomplete*
  Preservation of motor function below the neurological level
  More than half of key muscles below the neurological level have a power grade <3
D *Incomplete*
  Preservation of motor function below the neurological level
  More than half of key muscles below the neurological level have a power grade ≥3
E *Normal*
  Sensory and motor function is normal

What is *neurogenic shock?*

Neurogenic shock is a distributive shock resulting from interruption of autonomic pathways that leads to hypotension, bradycardia and hypothermia. It is common in injuries involving the cardiac sympathetic nerves (T2-5) resulting in a decrease in systemic vascular resistance and inotropy, with an increase in vagal tone.

What is *spinal shock?*

Spinal shock is the loss of reflexes below the level of spinal cord injury resulting in flaccid areflexia. It is often combined with hypotension and neurogenic shock. Reflex activity returns when the reflex arcs below the level of the lesion redevelop (3–6 weeks post-injury). Spasticity and autonomic dysreflexia are common: up to 50–80% of patients with lesions above T7 develop autonomic dysreflexia.

What is autonomic dysreflexia?

Stimulation below the level of the lesion causes a mass spinal sympathetic reflex that would normally be inhibited from above. Patients suddenly develop marked hypertension with a compensatory bradycardia, and cutaneous flushing and sweating above the lesion (due to compensatory vasodilatation). In extreme circumstances, seizures, stroke or cardiac arrest may result.

Common precipitants include:

1 Bladder and bowel distension
2 Pressure sores
3 Medical intervention

Management is largely preventative, and careful preparation of drugs including magnesium and vasodilators should precede any medical intervention (whether under general anaesthesia or not).

What are the main clinical syndromes associated with spinal cord injury?

There are a number of clinical syndromes associated with spinal cord injury (Table 79.1).

What are the principles of initial management after acute spinal cord injury and what are the specific considerations for airway, breathing and circulation?

The immediate management of a patient who has suffered a spinal cord injury should follow an ABCDE approach, treating abnormalities as they are found. Consider the presence of other associated major injuries. It is essential to preserve spinal alignment at all times and prevent secondary spinal cord injury by avoiding hypoxia, hypotension and hypercapnia.

1 **Airway**
   - Low threshold for intubation (particularly with high cervical injuries)
   - Rapid sequence induction (RSI) maintaining manual in-line stabilisation (MILS)
   - Higher incidence of difficult intubation given the possibility of associated maxillofacial trauma, blood or vomit in the upper airway, airway oedema and the necessity for cervical immobilisation
   - Increased risk of regurgitation and aspiration (paralytic ileus, loss of gastro-oesophageal sphincter tone)
   - From 72 hours post-injury, suxamethonium must be avoided given the risk of life-threatening hyperkalaemia

Table 79.1 Clinical syndromes associated with spinal cord injury

Syndrome	Cause	Clinical effects
Anterior spinal artery syndrome	Interruption of the anterior spinal artery which supplies the anterior 2/3 of the cord Usually caused by a hyperflexion injury	Paralysis and loss of pain and temperature sensation below the level of the lesion Sparing of the dorsal columns Preservation of proprioception, fine touch and vibration
Brown Séquard syndrome	Lateral cord damage, i.e hemisection of the cord	Ipsilateral loss of motor function, fine touch, proprioception and vibration sense below the level of the lesion Contralateral loss of pain and temperature below the lesion
Cauda equina syndrome	Injury to the lumbosacral nerve roots (not spinal cord itself)	Bladder and bowel dysfunction, upper motor neurone symptoms and signs in the legs Unilateral and asymmetric sensory deficit Asymmetric motor deficit Knee and ankle reflexes may be absent
Conus medullaris syndrome	Injury to sacral cord and lumbar nerve roots Injury at T12-L2 is most likely to result in conus medullaris syndrome	Areflexic bladder, faecal incontinence Absent ankle reflex, knee reflexes preserved Signs similar to cauda equina; more likely to be bilateral
Central cord syndrome	Bleeding, infarction or oedema involving the central grey matter of the spinal cord (most common in the cervical region)	Upper motor neurone signs in the legs and mixed upper and lower motor signs in the arms Loss of pain and temperature sensation in the arms Motor impairment > sensory impairment Upper limbs affected > lower limbs Relative proximal sparing
Posterior cord syndrome	Damage to the posterior spinal artery (very rare)	Loss of vibration and proprioception below the level of the lesion

2 Breathing

The impact on breathing is dependent on the site of injury (Table 79.2). In the acute phase, patients with high cervical spine injures will have better respiratory function when supine because the diaphragm has greater excursion in inspiration as it is pushed into the chest by abdominal contents, acting as a fulcrum.

Table 79.2 Level of injury and impact on respiratory function

Level of injury	Effect	Vital capacity	Need for ventilation
Above C3	Diaphragmatic paralysis as a result of loss of phrenic nerves	< 10%	Immediate and long-term
C3-C5	Partial phrenic nerve denervation leads to diaphragmatic weakness/paralysis	10–30%	80% will require ventilation within 48 hours
Above T8	Loss of intercostal and abdominal muscles	30–80%	Impaired sputum clearance may necessitate short-term ventilation
Below T8	Loss of abdominal muscles	80–100%	Short-term ventilation occasionally required secondary to weak cough/impaired sputum clearance

3 Cardiovascular system

A hyper-adrenergic state is initially present following acute spinal cord injury, resulting in dramatic hypertension and tachycardia. Following this phase, loss of sympathetic tone leads to hypotension. Unopposed vagal tone can lead to profound bradycardia and atropine may be required, especially before vagally stimulating procedures such as tracheal suctioning.

Other important considerations in the ICU:

1 Thromboprophylaxis (high incidence of DVT in these immobilised patients)
2 Gut protection (unopposed vagal activity increases gastric acid production)
3 Nutrition (unopposed vagal activity may lead to gastroparesis; hence nausea and vomiting may occur)
4 Pressure areas (pressure sores can lead to sepsis and prolonged immobility)

What are the prognostic factors after spinal cord injury?

1 Level of injury
2 Age of patient (higher mortality is seen in patients >60 years of age)
3 Injury severity

Further Reading

Bonner S, Smith C. Initial management of acute spinal cord injury. *Contin Educ Anaesth Crit Care Pain* 2013; **13**(6): 224–231

Consortium for Spinal Cord Medicine. Early acute management in adults with spinal cord injury. Clinical practice guidelines. *J Spinal Cord Med* 2008; **31**: 403–479

Ditunno J F Jr, Young W, Donovan W H, Creasey G. The international standards booklet for neurological and functional classification of spinal cord injury. American spinal injury association. *Paraplegia* 1994; **32**(2): 70–80

Chapter 80

Subarachnoid Haemorrhage

Why is subarachnoid haemorrhage important?

Subarachnoid haemorrhage (SAH) accounts for 5% of all strokes and is associated with high mortality (~50%) and significant disability: approximately one third of survivors are dependent on carers and almost half have life-changing cognitive deficits.

What are the causes of SAH? Can you outline the pathophysiology?

Subarachnoid haemorrhage may result from:

1 Intracranial aneurysms (85%)
   - Most occur close to bifurcations on the Circle of Willis
     i Anterior cerebral artery/anterior communicating artery bifurcation (40%)*
     ii MCA bifurcation (34%)
     iii Posterior communicating artery/internal carotid artery take-off (20%)*
     iv Basilar artery bifurcation (4%)
   * – most common sites for rupture
2 Arterio-venous malformations
3 Trauma
4 Rare conditions, e.g. Moyamoya disease (intimal proliferation of the cerebral arteries, which leads to stenosis and the development of a collateral circulation, whose vessels are weak and prone to rupture)

Risk factors include:

1 Age (peak incidence between 40–60 years-old)
2 Male gender (1.5 times more common in men)
3 Hypertension
4 Atherosclerosis
5 Cocaine use
6 Alcohol abuse
7 Smoking
8 Inherited conditions:
   i Autosomal dominant polycystic kidney disease
   ii Collagen vascular disease, e.g. Ehlers Danlos type 4
   iii Familial intracerebral aneurysms

Pathophysiologically, haemodynamic stress causes a sudden increase in pressure within the cerebral vasculature with subsequent rupture of the vessel. This results in bleeding into the subarachnoid space.

How does SAH present?

The classical presentation is a *thunderclap* headache. Associated features include nausea and vomiting, altered mental state or coma, neck stiffness, photophobia, focal neurological signs, seizures or cardiorespiratory arrest. Patients occasionally have a preceding history of more minor headaches that may represent a sentinel bleed.

How is SAH diagnosed?

1 Unenhanced CT head is first-line
   - Highly sensitive (95–100%) for the presence of subarachnoid blood on day one
   - Can visualise intracranial complications, e.g. obstructive hydrocephalus
   - MRI is an alternative
2 Lumbar puncture ≥12 hours after symptom onset if CT is non-diagnostic and there is a high index of suspicion
   - CSF sent for xanthochromia
3 CT angiography is used to differentiate the underlying cause
4 Cerebral angiography remains the gold standard

Do you know of any grading systems used for SAH?

Subarachnoid haemorrhage may be graded clinically or radiologically (Table 80.1).

What is your immediate management of a patient with SAH?

The management of a patient with SAH should follow an ABCDE approach, treating abnormalities as they are found. Specific points include:

1 Airway control and ventilatory support
   - Indications for intubation include:
     i GCS <8
     ii Drop in GCS ≥2 points
     iii Optimisation of ventilation
     iv Seizures
     v To facilitate transfer to neurosurgical centre
     vi Uncontrolled hypertension in the presence of an unsecured aneurysm

Table 80.1 Grading of SAH

Grade	World Federation of Neurosurgeons	Hunt and Hess	Fischer (CT appearances)
1	GCS 15 No motor deficit	Asymptomatic Minimal headache, slight nuchal rigidity	No blood seen
2	GCS 13–14 No motor deficit	Moderate-severe nuchal rigidity Cranial nerve palsy only, no other deficits	Diffuse deposition or thin layer of subarachnoid blood All vertical layers of blood <1 mm thick
3	GCS 13–14 With motor deficit	Drowsiness, confusion Mild neurological deficit	Localised clots Vertical layers of blood ≥1 mm thick
4	GCS 7–12 +/– motor deficit	Stupor Moderate-severe hemiparesis Early decerebrate rigidity Vegetative disturbance	Diffuse or non-subarachnoid blood Intracerebral clots Intraventricular involvement
5	GCS ≤6 +/– motor deficit	Deep coma Decerebrate rigidity Moribund	

Adapted with permission from Luoma A., Reddy U. (*Contin Educ Anaesth Crit Care Pain* 2013)

- Ensure the ETT is taped rather than tied
- Mechanical ventilation should be targeted to PaO_2 >10 kPa and $PaCO_2$ 4.5–5.0 kPa to minimise secondary brain injury
- $EtCO_2$ and ABG monitoring should be instituted rapidly to ensure ventilatory targets are met
2 Optimisation of cardiovascular physiology
   - A SBP <160 mmHg or MAP <110 mmHg should be targeted using IV antihypertensive therapy e.g. labetalol, nitrates, hydralazine or SNP
   - A SBP <100 mmHg should be supported with appropriate fluid resuscitation and vasopressors or inotropes
3 Monitor pupils closely following sedation and ventilation
4 Prompt CT imaging
5 Neuroprotective measures should be instituted (normothermia, normoglycaemia, adequate cerebral venous drainage – see page 480)
6 Liaison with neurosurgical team and transfer for definitive treatment

What are the definitive management options for securing an aneurysm? Is there any evidence that one method is superior?

Treatment of aneurysmal SAH is threefold:

1 Securing the ruptured aneurysm by *surgical clipping* or *endovascular coiling*
2 Minimising secondary brain injury and delayed neurological deficit (DND)
3 Preventing and treating non-neurological complications

The **ISAT** trial (Lancet, 2002) randomised patients with ruptured intracranial aneurysms to receive either endovascular coiling or neurosurgical clipping. The primary outcome (risk of death or dependence at 1 year) was significantly less common in the coiling group (absolute risk reduction (ARR) 6–9%). However, long-term follow-up of these patients (Lancet Neurology, 2009) has revealed that patients who were treated with coiling have a higher risk of re-bleeding and require significantly more delayed retreatment. Despite this, clipping is now reserved for aneurysms that are unsuitable for coiling, which includes those with a wide neck or those in locations such as the middle cerebral artery.

What is vasospasm and delayed cerebral ischaemia? How is it diagnosed?

Vasospasm and delayed cerebral ischaemia (DCI) occurs in ≥60% of patients with SAH.

The Neurocritical Care Society defines DCI as *neurological deterioration related to ischaemia (unrelated to treatment of the aneurysm) that persists for one hour and has no other cause*.

Vasospasm can be diagnosed when a patient exhibits symptoms and signs of DND following SAH secondary to arterial narrowing that is demonstrable angiographically or with TCD. Incidence peaks at 4–10 days post-SAH, persists for several days and is associated with a worse outcome. It is more common in smokers and patients with high grade SAH or large clot size.

Transcranial Doppler is non-invasive and images flow velocity in the basal cerebral arteries. It is highly specific and moderately sensitive. Vasospasm is diagnosed if:

1 Flow velocities are >120 cm/s
2 Velocities increase >50 cm/s/day from baseline
3 Lindegaard ratio >3 (ratio of flow velocity in ipsilateral MCA and internal carotid artery)

CT angiography is highly specific but may overestimate the degree of vasospasm. Digital subtraction angiography is the gold standard but is rarely used.

How is vasospasm prevented or treated?

Prevention and treatment of vasospasm includes:

1 *Nimodipine*
   L-type CCBs relax arterial smooth muscle, and nimodipine appears to have a particularly cerebro-selective effect. Nimodipine is administered routinely (60 mg PO 4 hourly) for 21 days following SAH.
   In 2006, the Cochrane collaboration performed a meta-analysis collecting data from 12 randomised trials of the use of calcium antagonists including nimodipine in patients following acute SAH. Administration of CCBs reduced the risk of death or severe dependency (ARR 5.1%, NNT 20).

2 *Triple H therapy*
   Triple therapy has been advocated traditionally and consists of:
   i Hypertension – with vasopressor support if required to maintain cerebral perfusion pressure
   ii Haemodilution – to a haemoatocrit of 30–35%
   iii Hypervolaemia – using crystalloid infusion targeting a CVP of 12 mmHg
   The use of triple H therapy is controversial, with some small trials supporting benefit with hypertension alone. However, it is important to avoid hypovolaemia and hypotension.

3 *Magnesium sulphate*
   The **MASH-2** trial (Lancet, 2012) showed no improvement in outcome with IV magnesium after aneurysmal SAH. Its routine use is not recommended (see page 283).

4 *Statins*
   Statins are HMG-CoA (3-hydroxy-3-methyl-glutaryl-CoA) reductase inhibitors and have been shown to have anti-inflammatory effects. However, the **STASH** trial (Lancet, 2014) did not detect any difference in long-term or short-term outcome when compared with placebo. Patients with SAH should not be treated routinely with simvastatin during the acute stages.

5 *Antiplatelet therapy*
   Due to an increased risk of haemorrhagic complications, antiplatelets are only recommended in situations in which stenting has been performed.

6 *Endovascular intervention*
   Aggressive endovascular treatment (angioplasty and/or intra-arterial vasodilator therapy) may improve neurological outcome. Suggested criteria for the use of endovascular treatment include a new neurological deficit without other cause, absence of cerebral infarction on CT, failure of medical therapy, and vasospasm on angiography. There is no substantial evidence for optimal timing or technique at present, although prophylactic use is thought to involve greater risk than benefit and is not recommended.

What other neurological complications can arise following SAH and how are they managed?

1 *Obstructive hydrocephalus* (20–30%)
   - More common in those with high clinical grade or large amounts of sub-arachnoid and/or intraventricular blood
   - Should be suspected in patients with a neurological deterioration within the first three days (although 25% will present later)
   - CT is diagnostic
   - Treatment is with placement of an external ventricular drain (EVD)
2 *Re-bleeding* (5–10% in first 72 hours)
   - Highest risk immediately following primary bleed, and in patients with high clinical grade or larger aneurysms
   - May occur following rapid reduction in ICP, e.g. following EVD insertion in a patient with an unsecured aneurysm
3 *Seizures* (up to 7%)
   - May indicate a re-bleed and should be treated aggressively
   - Routine seizure prophylaxis (particularly with phenytoin) is associated with a worse outcome and is not recommended
   - Perform an EEG in patients with neurological deterioration or those who fail to recover to exclude non-convulsive status epilepticus (NCSE)

What non-neurological complications may result from SAH?

Non-neurological complications occur in ~40% of patients with SAH and are responsible for 25% of the mortality.

Respiratory

 i Aspiration pneumonitis
 ii Neurogenic pulmonary oedema (massive catecholamine surge following SAH causes pulmonary arterial hypertension and injury to the capillary-alveolar membrane with increased transudation)
 iii ARDS

Cardiovascular

 i Neurogenic stunned myocardium syndrome (NSMS) occurs in ~15%
   - This is due to noradrenaline release from sympathetic nerve terminals, resulting in intracellular calcium depletion and myocyte death
   - Causes reversible ECG changes, arrhythmias, transient LV dysfunction (usually of little clinical consequence), and a troponin rise (lower than in primary myocardial event)
   - Associated with regional wall motion abnormalities (RWMAs) in 15% of cases
 ii Takotsubo's cardiomyopathy occurs more rarely

Metabolic

i Fever
  - Associated with worse outcomes
  - Full septic screen is mandatory and infection should be treated aggressively
  - Patients should be cooled to normothermia and antipyretics used
ii Hyperglycaemia
  - Marker of severity in SAH
  - Associated with worse outcomes
  - Hypoglycaemia worsens outcome and should be avoided
  - Optimal blood glucose targets are 4–10 mmol/l
iii Disorders of sodium balance

Venous thromboembolism

  - Mechanical thromboprophylaxis is mandatory
  - LMWH is usually held until the aneurysm is secured

Which disorders of sodium balance may be associated with SAH?

1 Syndrome of inappropriate ADH (see page 240)
2 Cerebral salt-wasting syndrome (CSWS)
3 Cranial DI (see page 124)

What is cerebral salt-wasting syndrome? Describe the pathophysiology

Cerebral salt-wasting syndrome may occur following brain injury (typically SAH or TBI) and is characterised by renal loss of sodium. There is polyuria, hyponatraemia and hypovolaemia. The precise pathogenesis is unknown but is likely to be mediated by increased levels of ANP and BNP in combination with increased sympathetic tone, contributing to increased renal perfusion pressure and subsequent natriuresis.

How is CSWS diagnosed and what is the management?

The biochemical criteria for a diagnosis of CSWS are:

1 Low or normal serum Na^+
2 High or normal serum osmolality
3 High or normal urine osmolality
4 Urinary sodium >40 mEq/l
5 Biochemical evidence of hypovolaemia (increased haematocrit, urea, bicarbonate and albumin)

Importantly, the daily sodium excretion exceeds intake resulting in low total body sodium, and the patient will exhibit symptoms and signs of hypovolaemia.

In addition to treatment of the underlying cause, specific management of CSWS involves correction of fluid and sodium depletion (see page 239 for detailed management of hyponatraemia).

1 Fluid resuscitation with 0.9% saline is the mainstay
2 In acute symptomatic hyponatraemia, hypertonic (1.8% or 3%) saline is recommended
   - Furosemide may be used to minimise the risk of fluid overload
3 Once the patient is normovolaemic and normonatraemic, ongoing losses should be matched with IV crystalloid and sodium tablets until CSWS resolves (usually 2–4 weeks)
4 Refractory CSWS may necessitate fludrocortisone therapy (0.1–0.4 mg/day)
   - Limits natriuresis by increasing sodium reabsorption from the renal tubule (aldosterone agonist)
   - Monitor for hyperkalaemia

What are the differences between SIADH and CSWS?

The principal differences are outlined in Table 80.2.

It is extremely important to distinguish between the two conditions, as the treatment of SIADH (water restriction) will worsen the symptoms of CSWS.

Table 80.2 Comparison of SIADH and CSWS

		Syndrome of inappropriate ADH	Cerebral salt wasting syndrome
Serum	Na$^+$	↓	↓
	Osmolality	↓	↑
	Plasma volume	↑	↓
Urine	Na$^+$	↑	↑
	Osmolality	↑	↑ or→
	Volume	Low, concentrated	High
Na$^+$ balance		Even	Negative
Urea and creatinine		↓ or→	↑
Haematocrit		↓ or→	↑
Volaemic status		Euvolaemic or hypervolaemic	**Hypovolaemic**
CVP		→ or↑	↓

Further Reading

Bradshaw K, Smith M. Disorders of sodium balance after brain injury. *Contin Educ Anaesth Crit Care Pain* 2008; **8**(4): 129–133

Diringer M N, Bleck T P, Hemphill J C, et al. Critical care management of patients following aneurysmal subarachnoid hemorrhage: Recommendations from the neurocritical care society's multidisciplinary consensus conference. *Neurocrit Care* 2011; **15**: 211–240

Dorhout Mees S M, Rinkel G J, Feigin V L et al. Calcium antagonists for aneurysmal subarachnoid haemorrhage. *Cochrane Database Syst Rev* 2007; CD000277

Luoma A, Reddy U. Management of aneurysmal subarachnoid haemorrhage. *Contin Educ Anaesth Crit Care Pain* 2013; **13**(2): 52–58

Chapter 81

Tetanus

What causes tetanus?

Clostridium tetani is a Gram-positive spore-forming rod-shaped anaerobic bacterium which is ubiquitous in the environment in soil, saliva, dust and faeces.

The clinical syndrome of tetanus results from the production of neurotoxin within a host infected with the bacteria.

Who is at risk of developing tetanus?

Tetanus is an entirely preventable disease. Widespread immunisation programmes have resulted in this being a rare disease in the developed world. However, tetanus remains endemic in the developing world.

At risk groups include:

1 Those who have not completed the tetanus vaccination schedule, e.g. certain immigrant groups
2 Elderly
3 Intravenous drug users

In developing countries, the mortality from tetanus exceeds 50%. Modern intensive care has achieved a dramatic drop in mortality. In one series, all-age mortality from tetanus fell from 44% to 15% after the introduction of an ICU.

Summarise the pathophysiology of tetanus

The tetanus toxin, *tetanospasmin*, is a 150 kDa polypeptide that is released into the systemic circulation following germination of the spores under anaerobic conditions. It binds irreversibly to neuronal membrane proteins and travels in a retrograde fashion to the spinal cord. Once in the spinal cord it prevents synaptic transmission of neurotransmitters from the presynaptic GABAergic inhibitory interneurons. This leads to uncontrolled motor neuron activity and produces the increased muscle tone and spasms characteristic of the disease. Disinhibited autonomic nervous system activity is also observed, with subsequent cardiovascular instability.

What are the clinical features of tetanus?

Tetanus is characterised by a triad of:

1 Rigidity
2 Muscle spasms
3 Autonomic instability

The incubation period averages 7–10 days, whilst the clinical onset time varies between 1–7 days. Muscle spasms and rigidity predominate during the first week, with autonomic disturbance developing several days after the spasms. Early symptoms include neck stiffness, sore throat and dysphagia.

Clinical features of concern:

1 Trismus
2 *Risus sardonicus* (the pathognomic sardonic grin that results from severe facial muscle spasm)
3 Muscle spasms or abdominal rigidity
4 Laryngeal spasm causing airway compromise – common and rapidly fatal if unrecognised
5 Autonomic instability reflected in heart rate, blood pressure and temperature

There are four recognised forms of tetanus. The most common form is *generalised tetanus* (80%), which affects muscles throughout the body. *Localised tetanus* is seen with lower toxin loads or peripheral injuries. Mortality is lower in this group unless the cranial nerves are involved *(cephalic tetanus). Neonatal tetanus* has a particularly high mortality and is seen in the developing world. Infected neonates present within a week of birth with fever, vomiting and convulsions.

Recovery from tetanus only occurs once the terminal axons have regrown.

How is tetanus diagnosed?

There is no diagnostic test to confirm tetanus and as such the diagnosis is based on history, clinical findings and rate of disease progression.

C. tetani may be cultured from the primary wound, although this is rare. In addition to routine blood tests, ABG and CXR are helpful to assess the severity of the disease (aspiration is common).

The Ablett Tetanus Severity Score can be used to determine the severity of infection (Table 81.1).

What are the differential diagnoses of tetanus?

Differential diagnoses to consider are:

1 Dystonic reactions to antidopaminergic drugs
2 NMS

Table 81.1 Ablett classification of tetanus severity

Grade	Clinical features
I (mild)	Mild trismus, general spasticity, no respiratory compromise, no spasms, no dysphagia
II (moderate)	Moderate trismus, rigidity, short spasms, mild dysphagia, moderate respiratory involvement, ventilatory frequency >30
III (severe)	Severe trismus, generalised rigidity, prolonged spasms, severe dysphagia, apnoeic spells, pulse >120, ventilatory frequency >40
IV (very severe)	Grade 3 with severe autonomic instability

3 Hypocalcaemic tetany
4 Strychnine poisoning
5 Epilepsy
6 Stiff person syndrome
7 Meningoencephalitis
8 SAH
9 Rabies

How is tetanus treated?

The patient with suspected tetanus should be managed on the ICU with an ABCDE approach, treating abnormalities as they are found. Airway management is paramount. Particular care must be taken to avoid provoking laryngeal spasm during laryngoscopy (primary tracheostomy is recommended) and precipitating spasms (nurse in a quiet, darkened room).

Four principles apply to the management of tetanus:

1 **Prevention of further toxin release**
   - Adequate wound toilet including surgical debridement of wounds
   - Administration of IV antibiotics: metronidazole 500 mg tds is the first line choice. Erythromycin, tetracycline, chloramphenicol and clindamycin are also effective agents. Penicillin has been used historically but has been associated with an increase in mortality.
2 **Neutralise toxin present in the body**
   - Unbound toxin can be neutralised by administering human tetanus immunoglobulin (HTIG)
   - HTIG does not affect toxin that is already fixed to nerve terminals
   - There is some evidence that intrathecal administration may result in a shorter duration of mechanical ventilation
   - Recovery from tetanus does not result in immunity, and vaccination with tetanus toxoid is indicated during the convalescent stage of the disease

3 **Minimise the effects of the toxin already in the CNS**
   - Muscle spasms can be effectively controlled using a combination of sedative agents including benzodiazepines (GABA agonists), propofol and opioids such as morphine and remifentanil
   - Other agents that can be used for spasm control include baclofen, dantrolene and barbiturates
   - Heavy sedation may be required and subsequently necessitate airway protection and mechanical ventilation
   - Muscle relaxation is indicated when sedation alone is inadequate: atracurium or vecuronium are the agents of choice
   - Autonomic instability can be managed with a number of agents including magnesium sulphate, clonidine and esmolol (beta-blockers such as propranolol have been used in the past, but can cause hypotension and sudden death)
4 **Supportive ICU treatment**
   - A multidisciplinary approach is essential as most cases require 4–6 weeks of supportive treatment
   - Establish enteral nutrition early
   - Meticulous mouth care, tracheal suction and chest physiotherapy to prevent respiratory complications
   - Thromboprophylaxis
   - Rhabdomyolysis is a common finding after prolonged tetanic spasm and AKI may result
   - Psychological support is often essential during and following the slow recovery

How is tetanus prevented?

Routine vaccination began in the UK in 1961. It is given as a combined vaccine along with diphtheria and pertussis (DPT). Immunity to tetanus may not be lifelong and booster injections may be required after an individual sustains a tetanus-prone wound.

What are the complications of tetanus?

The main complications of tetanus are:

1 Severe painful muscular spasms
2 Airway compromise
3 Respiratory failure
4 Autonomic instability

There are also the inherent risks related to prolonged intensive care admission such as protracted requirement for invasive ventilation, tracheostomy insertion, skin complications etc.

Further Reading

Taylor A M. Tetanus. *Contin Educ Anaesth Crit Care Pain* 2006; **6**(3): 101–104

Trujillo M H, Castillo A, Espana J, Manzo A, Zerpa R. Impact of intensive care management on the prognosis of tetanus. Analysis of 641 cases. *Chest* 1987; **92**: 63–65

Chapter 82

Thyroid Emergencies

Thyroid Storm

What is a thyroid storm?

A thyroid storm is a rare life-threatening disorder occurring in approximately 1% of patients with hyperthyroidism.

Describe the pathophysiology of a thyroid crisis

The most common underlying mechanism is primary overproduction of thyroid hormone. Additional causes include damage to the gland precipitating release of thyroid hormone and excessive iodine intake which may cause thyrotoxicosis.

There are causes and precipitants of a thyroid storm. Please can you give examples of each?

Causes

1 Grave's disease (most common) – due to autoimmune process involving thyroid-stimulating antibodies
2 Toxic multinodular goitre
3 Thyroid adenoma
4 Trauma
5 Excessive exogenous thyroid hormone

Precipitants

1 Sepsis
2 Trauma
3 Surgery
4 MI
5 Administration of iodinated contrast load in previous 6 weeks
6 Poorly-controlled DM
7 The puerperium
8 Drugs (anticholinergic, adrenergic, NSAIDs)

How does it present?

Patients typically present with features reflecting a hypermetabolic state. It may be difficult to differentiate from other conditions such as NMS, MH and sepsis.

Cardiovascular

- Tachycardia, tachyarrhythmias (especially AF)
- Flushing, sweating
- High output cardiac failure

Neuropsychiatric

- Agitation, confusion, psychosis and coma

Metabolic

- Hyperpyrexia
- Rhabdomyolysis
- Dehydration
- Electrolyte disturbance (hypernatraemia and hypokalaemia)

Gastrointestinal

- Abdominal pain, nausea and vomiting

Signs of underlying hyperthyroidism

- Eye signs: lid retraction, proptosis, exophthalmos
- Hot, moist skin
- Hair loss

What investigations would you request if you suspected a thyroid storm?

1 Blood tests
   - FBC, CRP and cultures looking for infection
   - U+Es (prerenal AKI, hypokalaemia)
   - LFTs
   - Clotting screen
   - TFTs ($\uparrow T_3$, $\uparrow T_4$, $\downarrow$thyroid stimulating hormone (TSH))
   - CK
   - Cortisol, ACTH
   - Glucose (usually high due to sympathetic activity)
   - ABG (metabolic or mixed acidosis)
2 Urinalysis
   - MC+S
   - Myoglobin
   - Catecholamines (phaeochromocytoma is a differential)
3 CXR looking for pulmonary oedema; lower respiratory tract infection (LRTI) is a potential precipitant
4 ECG looking for arrhythmias and evidence of myocardial ischaemia (may be causative or secondary to hyperthyroid state)
5 Echo to assess LV function and look for RWMAs (MI is a potential precipitant)

How would you manage a patient with a thyroid storm?

A patient presenting with a thyroid crisis should be managed with an ABCDE approach, and abnormalities treated as they are found. Treatment is both supportive and directed at correcting the underlying endocrine abnormality, precipitant or cause.

1 **Supportive management**
   i Supplemental oxygen should be given as the underlying metabolic rate is high
   ii Sedation and mechanical ventilation may be required to reduce metabolic rate – be aware of difficulty in intubation in patients with goitre (usually causes either difficult direct laryngoscopy or difficulty passing the ETT due to external compression causing subglottic narrowing)
   iii Fluid resuscitation
   iv Treat life-threatening arrhythmias
   v Provide cardiovascular support
   vi Electrolyte replacement
   vii Cool patient
      – Passive: remove clothing, cool cloths
      – Active: cold IV infusions, bladder irrigation, intravascular devices, extracorporeal circuits
      – Antipyretics (aspirin is best avoided as it competes with thyroxine for thyroid-binding globulin (TBG))
2 **Treat precipitating cause**
3 **Treat endocrine abnormality**
   i Betablockade – **propranolol** IV
      – Sympatholysis for symptomatic control
      – Reduced peripheral conversion of T4 to T3
   ii Thionamides (anti-thyroid medication)
      – **Propylthiouracil** enterally
         – Blocks iodination of tyrosine and peripheral conversion of T4 to T3
      – **Carbimazole** (slower onset but longer acting than propylthiouracil) enterally
         – Blocks thyroid hormone production
         – Often associated with short-lived leucopenia
   iii **Steroids** (reduce peripheral conversion of T4 to T3)
      – This is a glucocorticoid-deficient state and correction of thyrotoxicosis may precipitate an Addisonian crisis
      – Dexamethasone or hydrocortisone can be given
4 Additional measures
   i **Digoxin** and **amiodarone** (after giving propylthiouracil, as may exacerbate crisis) can be used
   ii **Vitamin B complex**
      – Vitamin B1 (thiamine) requirements are increased in thyrotoxicosis
      – There is a risk of precipitating Wernicke's when thyrotoxicosis is treated if vitamin B complex is not given
   iii **Dantrolene** has been used in case reports of significant muscle hyperactivity
   iv **Plasma exchange** may be needed in rare cases
      – May be particularly useful in Grave's disease to clear the antibodies

What Is the prognosis of a thyroid storm?

Mortality approaches 30%.

Myxoedema Coma

What is myxoedema coma?

Myxoedema coma is a rare, potentially fatal clinical syndrome caused by deficiency of thyroid hormone.

What are the causes of a hypothyroid crisis?

Myxoedema coma most commonly occurs in patients with undiagnosed or undertreated hypothyroidism. The causes of hypothyroidism are:

1 Iodine deficiency (most common cause worldwide)
2 Hashimoto's thyroiditis (autoimmune condition caused by anti-thyroid antibodies)
3 Previous treatment with radioactive iodine or thyroid surgery
4 Thyroid or pituitary injury
5 Medications including amiodarone

The common precipitants include:

1 Sepsis
2 Trauma
3 Surgery
4 Drugs, including sedatives
5 Hypothermia
6 (Over)treatment of hyperthyroidism

How does myxoedema coma present?

Respiratory

– Hypoventilation, hypoxaemia

Cardiovascular

– Bradycardia, long QTc, T wave flattening / inversion
– Pericardial effusion

Neuropsychiatric

– Seizures
– Stupor, obtunded, coma

Metabolic

- Hypothermia
- Electrolyte disturbance (hyponatraemia, hyperphosphataemia)
- Hypoglycaemia

Signs of underlying hypothyroidism

- Coarse, dry skin
- Peripheral and periorbital oedema, macroglossia
- Slow-relaxing reflexes

How is myxoedema coma managed?

A patient presenting with a hypothyroid crisis should be managed with an ABCDE approach, and abnormalities treated as they are found. Treatment is both supportive and directed at correcting any underlying endocrine abnormality, precipitant or cause.

1 **Supportive management**
   i Airway control may be necessary due to reduced GCS
   ii Fluid resuscitation using normal saline (these patients have a dilutional hyponatraemia with high total body water but intravascular hypovolaemia)
   iii Provide cardiovascular support with inotropes
   iv Correction of hypoglycaemia and electrolyte abnormalities
   v Warming (avoid rewarming too rapidly as vasodilatation in an under-resuscitated circulation will produce cardiovascular collapse)
2 **Treat the precipitating cause**
3 **Treat endocrine abnormality** using small incremental doses of thyroxine (there is no evidence of any prognostic benefit of using parenteral over enteral thyroid hormone). Use cautiously in the elderly or those with IHD to avoid precipitating myocardial ischaemia.
   i **Liothyronine** IV (quicker onset)
   ii **Levothyroxine** enterally or IV (gastric absorption may be impaired)
      - Blocks iodination of tyrosine and peripheral conversion of T4 to T3
   iii **Corticosteroids**
      - Adrenal function is impaired in hypothyroidism
      - Give steroid *before* thyroxine to avoid precipitating an Addisonian crisis

What is the prognosis of myxoedema coma?

The mortality is between 30–50%.

Further Reading

Eledrisi M S, 2016. Myxedema coma or crisis [online]. Qatar: Medscape. Available at: http://emedicine.medscape.com/article/123577 (Accessed 18 December 2016)

Schraga E D, 2016. Hyperthyroidism, thyroid storm, and Grave's disease treatment & management [online]. California: Medscape. Available at: http://emedicine.medscape.com/article/767130 (Accessed: 18 December 2016)

Chapter 83

Toxicology and Overdose

There are a multitude of drugs and poisons that, when ingested, can result in a patient becoming critically ill. Table 83.1 provides a summary of the presentation and specific management of the drugs most commonly taken in overdose. Please see also the 'Acute Liver Failure and Paracetamol Overdose' and 'Hyperthermia' topics.

Table 83.1 Summary of presentation and specific management of common toxins

Drug	Presentation	Specific Management
Amphetamines, MDMA	Sympathomimetic toxidrome May result in ICH, hyponatraemia, rhabdomyolysis and acute renal and hepatic failure	**Benzodiazepines** for agitation **Beta-blockers** for arrhythmias/ cardiovascular toxicity
Anticholinergic agents	Anticholinergic toxidrome	Supportive care **Physostigmine** (an anticholinesterase) may be useful
Aspirin	Biphasic toxicity: i Hyperventilation (central respiratory stimulant, causes respiratory alkalosis), tinnitus, vasodilatation ii Metabolic acidosis (direct effect of acid), non-cardiogenic pulmonary oedema, ↓GCS	**AC** may be used up to 4 hours post-ingestion **Bicarbonate** (urinary alkalinisation to enhance renal excretion) **Haemodialysis** if salicylate level >700 mg/l
Benzodiazepines	Sedative toxidrome	Supportive care is usually sufficient **Flumazenil** (specific antagonist at benzodiazepine receptor) is used with caution as it has inverse agonist effects and may precipitate seizures
Beta-blockers	Bradyarrhythmias, high grade AV block, hypotension, ↓GCS,	**Atropine/isoprenaline** for bradycardia

Table 83.1 (cont.)

Drug	Presentation	Specific Management
	delirium, seizures, hypoglycaemia Sotolol prolongs the QTc and may cause VT	**Pacing** may be necessary **Glucagon 50–150 mcg/kg IV** +/- infusion works as an inotrope and chronotrope (mechanism is independent of β-receptors)
Calcium channel-blockers (see below)	Bradyarrhythmias, high grade AV block, hypotension, cardiac arrest, ↓GCS, seizures, GI effects, hyperglycaemia	**Atropine/isoprenaline** for bradycardia **Pacing** may be necessary **Calcium** replacement **Inotropes/vasopressors** **High-dose euglycaemic insulin therapy** **Intralipid** (especially with verapamil overdose)
Digoxin	Nausea, vomiting, yellow vision, any type of arrhythmia/conduction abnormality	Correct hypokalaemia and hypomagnesamia (worsen toxicity) Ventricular arrhythmias may respond to **phenytoin, lignocaine** or **amiodarone** **Digoxin-specific antibody fragments (Digibind)** indicated for haemodynamic compromise due to arrhythmias
Ethanol	Alcohol poisoning results in coma and hypoventilation due to cortical and brainstem depression, high anion gap metabolic acidosis, hypoglycaemia (reduced gluconeogenesis)	Supportive care Correction of fluid and metabolic imbalance
Ethylene glycol (antifreeze)	Hyperthermia, hypoglycaemia, hypocalcaemia Similar clinical picture to ethanol poisoning, high osmolar gap Toxicity due to hepatic metabolites	Supportive care **Ethanol** (competes for metabolic pathway) infusion **Haemodialysis** may be helpful if severe
Lithium	Polyuria, polydipsia (nephrogenic DI may occur) vomiting, diarrhoea, tremor, ↓GCS and seizures Very narrow therapeutic window (serum [Li$^+$] >1.5 mmol/l is toxic)	Supportive care Correct fluid and electrolyte imbalance **Haemodialysis** if serum [Li$^+$] ≥2 mmol/l

Table 83.1 (cont.)

Drug	Presentation	Specific Management
Methanol	Nausea, vomiting, abdominal pain, GI bleeding, visual disturbance, high anion gap metabolic acidosis with high osmolar gap Toxicity due to hepatic metabolites	Supportive care **Ethanol** (competes for metabolic pathway) infusion Consider **haemodialysis** if: – Peak serum [methanol] >15 mmol/l – AKI – Visual impairment – Cognitive disturbance – Acidosis resistant to bicarbonate
Opioids	Narcotic toxidrome Aspiration is a risk Seizures are usually due to cerebral hypoxia	Supportive care **Naloxone** titrated to effect (caution in habitual users as may precipitate acute withdrawal and seizures)
Organophosphates	Cholinergic toxidrome Rapid onset	**Strict isolation** (very lipid soluble, skin to skin contact should be avoided) **Atropine** should be given as soon as possible to treat bradycardia and bronchorrhoea **Pralidoxime** (specific reactivator of cholinesterase) effective only if given <24 hours post-exposure Many agents are irreversible and recovery necessitates generation of new plasma cholinesterase
Selective serotonin reuptake inhibitors	Tachycardia, ↓GCS, tremor Serotonin syndrome may develop if taken in conjunction with another serotoninergic drug	If asymptomatic 3 hours post-overdose, discharge Organ support and active cooling, sedation and paralysis may be needed Serotonin receptor antagonists may be used, e.g. **cyproheptadine**
Tricyclic antidepressants	Myocardial depression, arrhythmias, ↓GCS, seizures, anticholinergic effects QRS duration is useful to predict toxicity: – 0.1–0.15 s associated with	AC can be used up to 24 hours post-ingestion **Bicarbonate** alkalinises blood, increases protein binding and prevents renal reabsorption – Also treats ventricular

Table 83.1 (cont.)

Drug	Presentation	Specific Management
	greater risk of seizures – >0.16 s associated with increased risk of seizures and arrhythmias	arrhythmias **Lignocaine, phenytoin** and **magnesium** may be of help in arrhythmias. Procainamide is contraindicated (worsens cardiovascular toxicity)

What is meant by the term *toxidrome*?

A toxidrome is a pattern of symptoms and signs observed when the patient has taken a certain class of drug.

What different toxidromes Are you aware of?

There are six commonly described toxidromes (Table 83.2).

Table 83.2 Toxidromes

Toxidrome	Examples	Presentation	
Anticholinergic	Antihistamines Antidepressants, especially TCAs Antipsychotics Antispasmodics Anti-Parkinsonian drugs	CVS CNS Neuropsychiatric GU GI Metabolic	Tachycardia, arrhythmias Myoclonus, seizures, mydriasis Delirium Retention Reduced bowel sounds Hyperthermia, flushed/dry skin
Cholinergic S – salivation, sweating L – lacrimation U – urination D – diarrhoea G – GI pain E – emesis	Organophosphates Nerve agents Cholinesterase inhibitors, e.g. in patients with MG	RS CVS CNS GU GI Metabolic	Bronchorrhoea, bronchospasm, progressive paralysis leading to respiratory failure/arrest, asphyxiation Tachy-/bradycardia Lacrimation, miosis, weakness, paralysis, seizures Urinary incontinence Salivation, cramping, nausea and vomiting, diarrhoea Diaphoresis

Table 83.2 (cont.)

Toxidrome	Examples	Presentation	
Narcotic	Opioids	RS	Respiratory depression
		CVS	Bradycardia, hypotension
		CNS	↓GCS, hyporeflexia, miosis
		Metabolic	Hypothermia, rhabdomyolysis
Sedative	Benzodiazepines Alcohol Barbiturates	RS	Respiratory depression
		CVS	Bradycardia, hypotension
		CNS	↓GCS, hyporeflexia
		Metabolic	Hypothermia
Serotoninergic (see also 'Serotonin Syndrome', page 234)	TCAs, SSRIs, MAOIs Cocaine Amphetamines Tramadol, pethidine	CVS	Tachycardia, hypo-/hypertension
		CNS	Tremor, fasciculations, extrapyramidal side effects, hyperreflexia, seizures
		Neuropsychiatric	Confusion, agitation
		Metabolic	Hyperthermia, rhabdomyolysis
Sympathomimetic	Cocaine Amphetamines Decongestants Caffeine Theophyllines	CVS	Tachycardia, hypo-/hypertension, arrhythmias
		CNS	Hyperreflexia, myoclonus, seizures, mydriasis
		Neuropsychiatric	Agitation, delusions, paranoia
		Metabolic	Hyperthermia, diaphoresis, rhabdomyolysis

GU – genitourinary

What methods of gastrointestinal decontamination are you aware of and what are the potential complications of these?

The main methods of GI decontamination are detailed in Table 83.3.

Table 83.3 Methods of GI tract decontamination

Method	Use	Disadvantages
Gastric lavage	Of no proven benefit even if performed within one hour of ingestion	Aspiration Electrolyte disturbance Oropharyngeal/oesophageal/gastric injury
Activated charcoal (AC)	Multiple-dose AC used in: Salicylate Digoxin Carbemazepine Barbiturates Theophylline Quinine	Some drugs are poorly adsorbed to charcoal: Acids Alcohols Ethylene glycol Alkali Heavy metals Inorganic salts Iron Lithium Pesticides Potassium
	May be used in sustained-release preparations	Aspiration risk mitigated by intubation
Whole bowel irrigation	Administration of large volumes of polyethylene glycol solution flushes drug through the gastrointestinal tract Mixed data on efficacy – insufficient to recommend routine use Possible option in body-packers and in ingestion of toxic heavy metals and sustained release preparations	May result in considerable discomfort to the patient

Which drugs are cleared by renal replacement therapy?

Drugs which are dialysable are those which have a small volume of distribution, are hydrophilic and are poorly protein-bound. They are listed in Table 83.4.

Table 83.4 Drugs cleared by RRT

V	Valproate
A	Aspirin
L	Lithium
A	Aminoglycosides (+ other antibiotics except quinolones and macrolides)
C	Carbemazepine
T	Theophyllines
E	Ethylene glycol
M	Methanol
M	Metformin
M	Methotrexate

What are the clinical features of calcium channel blocker overdose?

The presentation of CCB overdose is similar to beta-blocker overdose.

Symptoms:

1 Chest pain
2 Palpitations
3 Weakness
4 Dizziness, syncope, confusion, seizures
5 Diaphoresis, flushing
6 Headache
7 Nausea and vomiting

Signs:

1 Bradycardia (reflex tachycardia *may* result with peripheral vasodilatation and hypotension)
2 Arrhythmias
3 Heart block, bundle branch block
4 Hypotension
5 Low GCS
6 Weakness
7 Signs of GI dysmotility; may progress to bowel ischaemia +/- perforation if severe

What tests would you perform in a patient with suspected CCB overdose?

1 Blood tests:
   FBC, U+Es, LFTs, calcium level (used as a baseline to guide therapy), magnesium and phosphate levels, glucose, clotting screen, ABG, paracetamol and salicylate levels, TFTs (hypothyroidism is a differential), troponin
   Common biochemical abnormalities include:
     i Hyperglycaemia (impaired insulin release) – beta-blockers often cause *hypo*glycaemia
     ii Hypokalaemia
     iii Lactic acidosis (hypoperfusion)
2 Urine toxicology screen
3 CXR – looking for signs of pulmonary oedema
4 ECG – arrhythmias (and MI is a differential)
5 CT brain – differential diagnosis of low GCS and weakness
6 Echo – assessment of LV function, presence of RWMAs etc.

What is the mechanism of toxicity?

L-type calcium channel blockers decrease calcium influx in the cardiac conduction pathway. This leads to an inhibition of the rapid depolarisation in cardiac pacemaker cells and slows the plateau phase in cardiac myocytes and vascular smooth muscle cells. Myosin and actin binding is diminished and muscle contraction reduced, causing decreased myocardial contractility and peripheral arterial vasodilation.

Cardiovascular effects

1 Peripheral and coronary vasodilatation
2 Negative chronotropy via SA node blockade, causing bradycardia
3 Negative dromotropy via AV blockade, producing conduction abnormalities
4 Negative inotropy, causing myocardial depression

Other effects

1 Suppression of pancreatic insulin release, resulting in hyperglycaemia
2 Decreased utilisation of free fatty acids by myocardium, causing myocardial depression

What is the management of a patient with CCB OD?

The management of CCB overdose should follow an ABCDE approach, treating abnormalities as they are found. Specific management is as follows:

1 100% oxygen
2 **Activated charcoal** may be of use up to 4 hours after ingestion of sustained-release preparations
3 **Cardiovascular support**
   - Fluid boluses as required
   - Inotropes/vasopressors as required
   - Treatment of arrhythmias
   - Atropine (often ineffective) +/– isoprenaline +/– pacing may be necessary
   - VA ECMO may be considered in refractory cases
4 **Calcium** therapy
   - Calcium chloride is preferred, given slowly via CVC if possible
   - Serum calcium levels of 1.5–2 times normal have shown to have beneficial effect on myocardial contractility
5 **Glucagon** therapy
   - Glucagon promotes calcium entry into cells via a mechanism separate to adrenergic receptors
   - Note its action opposes insulin but both can be used in the treatment of CCB OD
6 **High-dose insulin euglycaemic therapy** (HIET) – associated with improved survival in animal models
   - Positively inotropic, increases intracellular calcium transport and improves CCB-associated vasodilatation
   - High doses combined with 50% glucose infusion
   - 1–10 units/kg may be required
   - Caution: hypokalaemia, hypoglycaemia – careful monitoring of bloods and GCS
   - Targets of HIET:
     i Improvement in myocardial ejection fraction (LVEF >50%)
     ii Adequate heart rate (>60 bpm)
     iii Restoration of acid-base balance, normoglycaemia and adequate urine output (1–2 ml/kg/hour)
     iv Reversal of cardiac conduction abnormalities (QRS <120 ms)
     v Improved GCS
7 **Intralipid** (1.5 ml/kg bolus followed by infusion 0.25 ml/kg/hour) – acts as a lipid sink for lipophilic molecules (e.g. verapamil)
   - Used anecdotally with good effect

Further Reading

Dignam G, Bigham C. Novel psychoactive substances: a practical approach to dealing with toxicity from legal highs. *BJA Educ* 2017; **17**(5): 172–177

Ward C, Sair M. Oral poisoning: an update. *Contin Educ Anaesth Crit Care Pain* 2010; **10**(1): 6–11

Chapter 84

Transfusion

What do you understand by the term *patient blood management* and why is it important?

Peri-operative anaemia is an independent risk factor for increased ICU and hospital LOS, post-operative complications, and increased mortality. It is found in approximately one third of patients at pre-assessment and is associated with increased likelihood of peri-operative transfusion.

Patient blood management (PBM) is a concept directed at preventing unnecessary transfusion and improving patient safety. The three cornerstones of PBM are:

1 *Detection and management of pre-operative anaemia (Hb <130 g/l in men, <120 g/l in women)*
   - Attend pre-assessment 4–6 weeks before operation date (not always practicable, e.g. cancer 2-week wait)
   - Treat absolute or functional iron deficiency with iron (oral or IV)
   - Consider erythropoietin (EPO) following discussion with haematology (has been associated with thrombotic complications)
   - Consider referral to other specialities, e.g. gastroenterology
2 *Minimising perioperative blood loss*
   - Review bleeding risk including family and personal history
   - Review antiplatelet or anticoagulant medications, involving relevant specialities if necessary
   - Meticulous surgical haemostasis
   - Physiological optimisation of coagulation at all stages peri-operatively
   - Additional techniques, e.g. patient positioning, central neuraxial blockade, use of point of care testing
   - Intra-operative cell salvage
3 *Management of postoperative anaemia*
   - Optimise cardiopulmonary reserve at all stages peri-operatively
   - Optimise cardiac output and oxygen delivery peri- and post-operatively
   - Continue iron/EPO post-operatively
   - Avoid secondary bleeding
   - Treat infection promptly
   - Use evidence-based transfusion thresholds

What is cross-matching?

Cross-matching is the process of mixing donor cells with recipient serum and observing for signs of agglutination.

A *group and save* involves determining the patient's ABO and rhesus blood group and storing the sample for cross-matching at a later date if necessary.

A few important points:

– O^- is the universal donor
– AB^+ is the universal recipient
– O^+ is the most common blood group in the UK, followed by A^+
– AB^- is the rarest group in the UK
– 85% of people in the UK are Rh^+

What is donor blood tested for?

WHO has issued guidelines stating that donated blood should routinely be tested for:

1 HIV antibodies
2 HCV antibodies
3 Hepatitis B surface antigen
4 Syphilis serology

This is highly sensitive, but lacks specificity (high false positive rate).

How is blood stored?

Packed red blood cells (PRBCs) are stored with the following preservatives (CPDA), ensuring a shelf-life of 35 days:

1 Citrate – binds calcium (acts as anticoagulant)
2 Phosphate – substrate for ATP
3 Dextrose – energy substrate for glycolysis
4 Adenine – increases RBC ATP levels

In the US, SAG-M (saline, adenine, glucose, mannitol) is used, which extends shelf-life to 42 days.

Table 84.1 outlines how the various blood components are prepared and stored.

Table 84.1 Preparation and storage of blood products

Product	Contents	Preparation	Notes
PRBCs	Haematocrit 0.6–0.7	Whole blood is centrifuged and leucodepleted	Shelf-life 35 days
FFP	Clotting factors Albumin	Supernatent that remains following centrifuging whole blood Frozen within 8 hours to maintain factor V and VIII activity Stored at –30°C	Lasts ≥1 year at –30°C Use within 24 hours of thawing
Octaplas	Solvent-detergent-treated FFP More standardised clotting factor concentration	Pooled from 1500 donors	Solvent-detergent process inactivates encapsulated viruses thereby reducing infection risk Used in neonates as standard
Platelets	55×10^9 platelets in 50 ml plasma	Pooled from 4–6 FFP donations Stored at 20–24°C (increased risk of infection) Agitated during storage to prevent clumping	Shelf-life 3–5 days Not usually cross-matched Will increase platelet count by $10–20 \times 10^9/m^2$ BSA One third sequestered in spleen following transfusion
Cryoprecipitate	One unit contains: – 150–300 mg fibrinogen – 70 IU factor VIII – vWF	FFP thawed to 1-6°C and liquid collected Stored at -24°C Ten units combined to form one pack (~200 ml)	

What is the *storage lesion*?

Storage lesion refers to the haematological and biochemical changes that occur in stored blood:

1 Hyperkalaemia (a unit of PRBCs stored for 4–5 weeks may contain between 5–30 mmol/l K^+)
2 Acidosis – pH ~6.8
3 Reduced 2,3-DPG – oxygen dissociation curve shifted to the left (normalises within a few hours of transfusion)
4 Platelet count tends towards 0 after ~48 hours
5 Factor V and VIII activity falls to 50% after 24 hours

What adverse effects may result from transfusion of blood products?

Transfusion is independently associated with increased risk of death and organ dysfunction. It is unclear whether the association of anaemia with disease severity contributes to this.

It was previously thought that transfusion of older PRBCs was associated with worse outcomes, but the recent **ABLE** study (NEJM, 2015) showed no difference in 90-day mortality between critically ill patients who were transfused with fresh (stored <8 days) or older (stored up to 42 days) blood.

Other complications are outlined in Table 84.2, including prevention and management strategies.

Define *massive transfusion*

There are several definitions of *massive transfusion*:

1 Transfusion of whole circulating volume (~70 ml/kg in adults) in 24 hours
2 Transfusion of ≥50% circulating volume <3 hours
3 Transfusion of ten units of blood

Table 84.2 Complications of transfusion

Complication		Prevention	Management
Immediate haemolytic reaction	Recipient antibodies attack donor cells causing haemolysis	Blood transfusion training	Crystalloid fluid resuscitation +/– vasoactive infusions
	↑LDH, ↓Hb, +ve direct Coombs' test, haemoglobinuria	Policies and protocols to reduce transfusion of ABO incompatible blood	Administer oxygen, consider ventilatory support as needed
	Fever, chills, flushing, urticarial, angioedema, tachycardia, hypotension, bronchospasm		Aim urine output >2 ml/kg, consider furosemide once volume replete
			Send blood for FBC, clotting, direct Coombs' test and repeat cross-match
Delayed haemolytic reaction (after 3–10 days)	Previous alloimmunisation to minor antibodies, e.g. Rh/Kidd		
	Anaemia, fever		
	Haemoglobinuria or AKI rare		
Non-haemolytic reactions	Febrile – very common, temperature increases by 2°C	Universal leucodepletion has reduced the incidence of febrile reactions	Transfusion can be continued if symptoms are mild
	Donor leucocyte antigens react with recipient white cell antibodies		Oral paracetamol
			Other treatment usually not required
			Severe reactions may necessitate discontinuation of transfusion, e.g. rigors, myalgia, nausea, hypotension
	Allergic – probably reaction to donor antigens in previously sensitised recipient	Plasma reduction or use of solvent detergent treated FFP may reduce the incidence of allergic reactions	Discontinue transfusion and return to blood bank
	Anaphylaxis 1:20 000 – 1: 50 000		See 'Anaphylaxis' topic (page 50)

Metabolic	**Hyperkalaemia** **Hypocalcaemia** **Metabolic alkalosis** due to metabolism of citrate to bicarbonate (Rarely a problem in clinical practice)		Prompt active management of electrolyte and acid-base disturbance as they emerge
	Iron overload with *chronic transfusion*, e.g. in SCD, exceeds transferrin binding capacity and is deposited in organs including the heart and the liver – causes free-radical formation resulting in progressive tissue injury, cirrhosis and cardiomyopathy	Iron chelation therapy, e.g. desferrioxamine Recurrent venesection	Iron chelation therapy Management of organ-specific symptoms and signs
Transfusion-transmitted infection	**Bacterial** – contamination PRBCs 1:500 000 Platelets (stored at 20–24°C) 1:2000	Disinfection of donor site Discarding initial bloodflow	Discontinue transfusion and return unit to blood bank Crystalloid fluid resuscitation +/– vasoactive infusions Administer oxygen, consider ventilatory support as needed Send blood for FBC, clotting, MC+S and repeat cross-match Start broad-spectrum antibiotics
	HIV 1: 5 000 000 Hepatitis B 1:450 000 Hepatitis C 1:32 000 000 CMV New-variant CJD	Careful donor screening and exclusion of high-risk groups Leucodepletion reduces risk of viral infection Products screened for CMV in	

Table 84.2 (cont.)

Complication		Prevention	Management
		high-risk recipients, e.g. pregnant women, neonates	Leucodepletion Patients born after 1996 are transfused with FFP from the USA (where BSE and nvCJD are uncommon)
Transfusion-associated circulatory overload (TACO)	Acute LVF or CCF occurring within 6–24 hours of transfusion Presents with respiratory distress, tachycardia, hypertension, raised CVP, positive fluid balance and pulmonary oedema	Pre-transfusion assessment for cardiac failure, renal impairment, hypoalbuminaemia or pre-existing fluid overload Close monitoring during transfusion	Sit patient upright Administer oxygen, consider ventilatory support as needed Inotropic support if indicated Furosemide +/– GTN infusion
Transfusion-related acute lung injury (TRALI)	The onset of ARDS within 6 hours of transfusion Immune-mediated – donor antibodies attack recipient white cells Non-immune-mediated – due to underlying condition, e.g. trauma, sepsis; worsened by second insult from biological mediators in stored blood Mortality ~10% (compared to 40–50% with ARDS due to other causes) Risk is increased with FFP and platelets from female donors	Universal leucodepletion Pooled plasma donations to dilute any antibodies present Exclusive use of male donors for all FFP and plasma for platelet pools Additional screening and exclusion of donors at high risk of having anti-leucocyte antigen antibodies	Administer oxygen, consider ventilatory support as needed (see 'ARDS' topic, page 33) Negative fluid balance (although furosemide not necessary if TACO not suspected)

What are the complications specific to massive transfusion?

1 Coagulopathy (both dilutional and consumptive)
2 Hypothermia
3 Acidosis (usually due to impaired oxygen delivery rather than a direct result of the low pH of stored blood)
4 Electrolyte disturbance
   i Hyperkalaemia (due to high potassium level in stored blood and acidosis)
   ii Hypocalcaemia (due to calcium in stored blood being bound to citrate (less important if liver function is normal) and consumption of calcium in clotting cascade)
   iii Hypomagnesaemia (due to binding to circulating citrate)

What transfusion trigger do you use in critically ill patients? What is the evidence base for your practice?

A transfusion threshold of 70 g/l with a target Hb of 70–90 g/l is accepted in the general critical care population. Transfusion thresholds should not exceed 90 g/l in most patient groups.

The **TRICC** study (NEJM, 1999) randomised patients with an Hb <90 g/l to either a liberal (trigger 100 g/l, target 100–120 g/l) or restrictive (trigger 70 g/l, target 70–90 g/l) transfusion strategy. There was a trend towards lower mortality with the restrictive approach; this reached significance in patients with a lower APACHE II score (<20) and in those aged >55 years. There were also lower rates of new organ failure in the restrictive group and a trend towards higher rates of ARDS in the liberal group.

Following this, the **TRACS** study (JAMA, 2010) found no difference in a composite endpoint of 30-day mortality and severe comorbidity in cardiac patients randomised prospectively to a liberal or restrictive transfusion approach. The **FOCUS** trial (NEJM, 2011) randomised high-risk (but not critically ill) elderly patients with cardiovascular disease to a restrictive or liberal transfusion strategy following hip surgery. There was no difference in mortality or morbidity between the study groups.

Most recently, the **TRISS** study (NEJM, 2014) found no difference in mortality or ischaemic events in patients with septic shock and Hb ≤90 g/l, who were managed either with a restrictive or liberal approach. Patients with IHD were excluded from this study.

The **TITRe2** study (NEJM, 2015) again found no difference in a composite endpoint of infective and ischaemic complications in patients following cardiac surgery randomised to a restrictive (Hb 75 g/l) or liberal (Hb 90 g/l) transfusion strategy. However, there was a statistically significant increase in mortality in the restrictive group, suggesting that transfusion thresholds should be tailored on an individual basis.

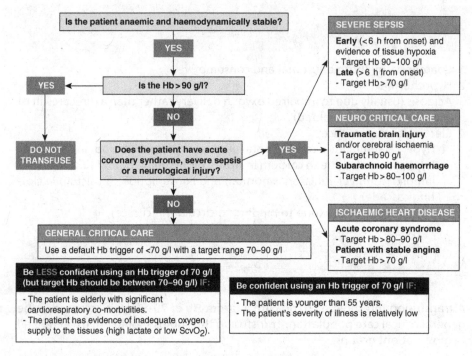

Figure 84.1 A suggested approach to transfusion in critical care
Reproduced with permission from Retter, et al. (*Br J Haematol* 2013)

Figure 84.1 shows a suggested approach to transfusion in critical care.

Further Reading

Clevenger B, Kelleher A. Hazards of blood transfusion in children and adults. *Contin Educ Anaesth Crit Care Pain* 2014; **14**(3): 112–118

Retter A, Wyncoll D, Pearse R, et al. Guidelines on the management of anaemia and red cell transfusion in adult critically ill patients. *Br J Haematol* 2013; **160**: 445–464

Thakrar S V, Clevenger B, Mallett S. Patient blood management and perioperative anaemia. *BJA Educ* 2017; **17**(1): 28–34

Chapter 85

Trauma

You are called as part of the advanced trauma team to the ED resuscitation room to review a 43-year-old pedestrian who was hit by a lorry 45 minutes ago. On arrival, he has three-point immobilisation and a pelvic binder in situ. He is moaning, and opens his eyes and localises to pain. He has a large scalp wound that is bleeding profusely and bruising with paradoxical movement of the right chest wall. There is an open fracture of his right tibia and fibula with associated crush injury to the foot.

His observations are:

SpO$_2$ 96% on 15 l/min of oxygen via a non-rebreathing mask
RR 31 per minute
HR 126 bpm
BP 89/53 mmHg

What is your immediate management?

This patient is severely injured and should be managed in a Major Trauma Centre. Management should involve a multidisciplinary trauma team and follow an ATLS approach, treating life-threatening injuries as they are identified. Given the mechanism and pattern of injury, there should be a high index of suspicion for significant head, thoracic, abdominal and pelvic injuries. The priorities are a **rapid primary survey** with treatment of life-threatening injuries, and stabilisation to facilitate CT imaging from head to pelvis with CT angiography of the lower limbs. Plain chest and pelvic X-rays may be used and FAST (focussed assessment with sonography for trauma) scanning can identify pneumothoraces or evidence of free fluid in the abdomen.

1 **Catastrophic external haemorrhage control**
   - This involves direct pressure, elevation, and application of haemostatic dressings or tourniquets to active external haemorrhage

2 **Airway** with C-spine control
   - High concentration oxygen should be administered via a facemask with a reservoir bag
   - Endotracheal intubation is indicated if the airway is at risk, e.g. airway swelling, significant neck or facial injuries or burns, ongoing haemorrhage or cardiovascular instability, or low GCS

- Intubation may also be required in the presence of hypoxia secondary to chest trauma, e.g. pulmonary contusions
- A RSI should be performed, using agents that avoid excessive changes in blood pressure
- MILS is mandatory, and a bougie should be used as a matter of course

3 **Breathing** – life-threatening chest injuries (TOM-FC) require urgent treatment at this stage:
   i Tension pneumothorax
      - Needle decompression in the 2nd–4th intercostal space, mid-clavicular line to relieve the tension followed rapidly by intercostal drain placement
   ii Open pneumothorax
      - Three-sided dressing (to create one-way valve) and intercostal drain insertion
   iii Massive haemothorax (>1500 ml)
      - Intercostal drain insertion +/– thoracotomy if ongoing blood loss >200 ml/hour
   iv Flail chest (likely in this patient)
      - Usually associated with significant underlying pulmonary contusion and severe hypoxia, which may require intubation and ventilation
      - Necessitates excellent analgesia (e.g. morphine or ketamine in the resuscitation room, followed by consideration of a thoracic epidural or para-vertebral block)
   v Cardiac tamponade (identified on FAST scan)
      - *Beck's triad* (distended neck veins, hypotension and muffled heart sounds) is rarely seen in trauma
      - High index of suspicion in penetrating chest or upper abdominal trauma
      - Resuscitative thoracotomy and pericardotomy may be carried out in the resuscitation room if necessary

4 **Circulation**
   - Assume all hypotension is due to haemorrhage until proven otherwise
     - Other causes include tension pneumothorax, tamponade, myocardial contusions, neurogenic shock
   - Haemorrhage may be concealed in the chest, abdomen, retroperitoneum and pelvis
   - The **massive transfusion protocol** should be activated (rapid delivery of pre-packed blood products to the resuscitation room) as this patient fulfils criteria for class 3 haemorrhagic shock
   - A pelvic binder should be applied in suspected pelvic injury
     - Pelvic bleeding is most frequently due to injury to pelvic veins
     - If due to arterial injury, it may be amenable to radiological embolisation
     - *Resuscitative endovascular balloon occlusion of the aorta* (REBOA) is becoming increasingly popular in the management of exsanguinating pelvic injuries in both the pre-hospital environment and within the emergency department: REBOA achieves endoluminal vascular control and increases myocardial and cerebral perfusion pressure
   - IV access should be obtained quickly

- A trauma line (7–8 French short rapid infusion cannula) may be inserted into a subclavian vein (the internal jugular and femoral veins are usually inaccessible in trauma patients)
    - Short large-bore peripheral cannulae or intraosseous access are alternatives
    - A level one rapid infusor should be available
    - All IV fluid should be warmed
- Resuscitation with clear fluids is potentially detrimental: blood products are preferable
- This patient should undergo a trial of filling guided by haemodynamics and ABG
    - If he remains unstable, or destabilises following initial response to resuscitation, he should be transferred directly to theatre for exploratory/damage-control surgery *without* CT imaging
- A resuscitative endpoint of SBP 80–90 mmHg is targeted (100 mmHg if concurrent TBI)
- Lactate and base deficit should be monitored closely
- Give tranexamic acid 1 g IV stat and start an infusion of 1 g over 8 hours

5 **Disability** – see 'Traumatic Brain Injury' topic (page 476)
- This man has a GCS of 9 (E2 V2 M5) with an obvious head injury and is likely to be actively bleeding – he requires intubation
- Titration of IV analgesia in an unanaesthetised trauma patient is paramount, e.g. ketamine, morphine

6 **Exposure**
- Remove the patient's clothes and examine from top to toe (including log-roll) to ensure no immediately life-threatening injuries have been missed
- Cover the patient with a blanket +/– forced-air warmer
- Increase the ambient temperature in the ED and operating theatre

How do you classify haemorrhagic shock?

The ATLS classification of haemorrhagic shock is outlined in Table 85.1.

What is the injury severity score?

The ISS involves the use of the abbreviated injury scale (AIS, Table 85.2) to score six body regions:

1 Face
2 Head and neck
3 Chest (including diaphragm and thoracic spine)
4 Abdominal and pelvic contents (including lumbar spine)
5 Extremities and pelvic girdle
6 External

Table 85.1 The ATLS classification of haemorrhagic shock

	Class 1	Class 2	Class 3	Class 4
% Circulating volume lost	≤15%	15–30%	30–40%	≥40%
Blood loss (ml) in 70 kg patient	750	750–1500	1500–2000	>2000
SBP (mmHg)	→	→	↓	↓↓
DBP (mmHg)	→	↑ (↓ pulse pressure)	↓	↓↓
HR (bpm)	<100	100–120	120–140	>140
RR (breaths per minute)	14–20	20–30	30–40	30–40
Urine output (ml/hour)	>30	20–30	10–20	0
Mental state	Alert	Anxious / aggressive	Confused	Drowsy / unconscious

Table 85.2 The abbreviated injury scale

1	Minor
2	Moderate
3	Serious
4	Severe
5	Critical
6	Maximal (untreatable)

Each body region is given a score using the AIS. The ISS is calculated by taking the AIS from the three most injured regions, squaring them and then adding the three squared numbers together. The maximum score is 75. An AIS score of 6 in any region automatically equates to an ISS of 75 as it is deemed unsurvivable.

$$ISS = A^2 + B^2 + C^2$$

Where A, B and C are the AIS scores from the three most injured ISS body regions

Severe trauma is defined as an ISS ≥16.

What is *damage control resuscitation*?

Damage control resuscitation (DCR, also known as haemostatic resuscitation) describes the process of restoring and sustaining normal tissue perfusion to the patient presenting in uncontrolled haemorrhagic shock (i.e. until definitive anatomical control of the haemorrhage has occurred), with an emphasis on preservation of effective clotting. It is associated with increased survival in victims of major trauma who are bleeding.

In contrast to traditional *goal-directed therapy* (which is the approach once haemorrhage control has been achieved), DCR focuses on providing the lowest cardiac output necessary to sustain vital organ function. This requires experienced clinical judgement because thresholds for ischaemic injury to specific organs differ between patients.

There are four pillars of DCR:

1 *Early administration of blood products in a balanced ratio*
   - Give PRBCs, FFP and platelets in a ratio that most closely resembles reconstituted whole blood
   - This is facilitated by the implementation of a *massive transfusion protocol* that allows for automatic dispatch of blood products from the blood bank
   - Minimise the use of non-blood resuscitation fluid as it reduces blood viscosity and dilutes the concentration of red cells, clotting factors and platelets
   - Crystalloid fluid is also associated with endothelial injury, which contributes to extravasation
2 *Permissive hypotension*
3 *Prevention and immediate correction of coagulopathy*
   - Hypothermia worsens coagulopathy and all exogenous fluids should be warmed
4 *Expedited damage control surgery*
   - Aimed at minimising operative time to reduce the secondary insult in a critically injured unstable patient
     i Resuscitative thoracotomy and aortic control to optimise cerebral and myocardial perfusion
     ii Exploratory laparotomy with wide exposure, rapid ligation of bleeding vessels, excision of badly injured organs, control of contamination (without anastomosis) and packing
     iii External fixation of long bone or pelvic fractures
   - May occur in conjunction with DCR – DCR should continue intra-operatively until the patient is well enough for transfer to the ICU
   - The patient then returns to theatre for definitive/anatomical corrective surgery at a later date

What ratio of blood products should be used in DCR?

The early use of balanced ratios of blood products became the standard of care in battlefield trauma surgery over ten years ago. Observational data have subsequently documented increased survival with early use of FFP and platelets in physiological ratios. This has since been supported by two large multi-centre RCTs.

The **PROMMTT** study (JAMA Surgery, 2013) showed that in trauma patients who had received at least one unit of PRBCs within 6 hours of admission, earlier use of higher amounts of plasma and platelets (albeit without consistent ratios) was associated with improved 6-hour survival.

The **PROPPR** trial (JAMA, 2015) compared the use of FFP, platelets and red cells in a 1:1:1 ratio to a 1:1:2 ratio in patients with severe trauma and major bleeding. There was no difference in all-cause 24-hour or 90-day mortality, but more patients in the 1:1:1 group achieved haemostasis and fewer died as a result of exsanguination in the first 24 hours.

What is *permissive hypotension* and is there any evidence for its use?

Intravascular volume repletion augments CO, which contributes to increased arterial pressure and reflex vasodilatation. This can promote extravasation and mechanical disruption of early extravascular clots. *Permissive hypotension* is the term employed to describe the technique of targeting volume resuscitation to a lower than normal blood pressure. Small volume (~250 ml) boluses, preferably of blood or plasma, are used to target a SBP 80–90 mmHg or MAP 50–65 mmHg until haemorrhage control is achieved. Prolonged permissive hypotension (>1 hour) is likely to be associated with poor outcome.

Bickell, et al (NEJM, 1994) randomised hypotensive victims of penetrating thoraco-abdominal trauma at the scene of injury to receive conventional fluid therapy or minimal fluid therapy during the pre-hospital and ED phases of care. They demonstrated significant survival advantage in the cohort given minimal fluid.

Dutton, et al (Journal of Trauma, 2002) randomised hypotensive trauma patients to resuscitation targeted to a MAP of 60 or 80 mmHg until definitive haemorrhage control had been achieved. There was no difference in survival between the groups.

Preliminary results from an RCT by **Morrison, et al** (Journal of Trauma, 2011) suggest that hypotensive resuscitation (targeting a MAP of 50 mmHg) is associated with a significant reduction in postoperative coagulopathy and lower risk of early postoperative death compared to targeting a minimum MAP of 65 mmHg.

What is coagulopathy of trauma and how is it prevented/treated?

Acute traumatic coagulopathy (ATC) is one of the three components of the *Triad of Death*: coagulopathy, hypothermia and acidosis. Patients presenting with coagulopathy have a four-fold increase in mortality, and are more likely to require transfusion and to develop multi-organ failure. The underlying mechanism appears to include a systemic activation of the protein C pathway and generation of APC (which inhibits factors V and VIII and decreases fibrino-gen utilisation) leading to a reduction in thrombin generation and increased fibrinolysis.

There are four main factors that worsen ATC (collectively termed trauma-induced coagulopathy (TIC)):

1 *DIC*
   - Results from activation of clotting pathways by thromboplastin exposed following the traumatic insult
   - This is accompanied by a physiological increase in fibrinolysis leading to consumptive coagulopathy
   - The incidence of DIC is positively correlated with increasing ISS and decreasing GCS
2 *Dilutional coagulopathy*
   - Stored blood undergoes progressive loss of clotting factors and functional platelets
   - Non-blood resuscitation fluid contributes to this
3 *Hypothermia*
   - Impairs platelet and coagulation factor function, even in undiluted blood
   - Body temperature <35°C is associated with significantly increased blood loss
   - In severely injured patients (ISS >25) mortality rates rise precipitously with each degree drop in core temperature <34°C
   - Use of heat and moisture exchanger (HME) filters, fluid warmers and forced air warming devices during resuscitation is advocated
4 *Acidosis*
   - Associated with reduced factor VII activity, reduced activation of factor X and prothrombin, and reduced platelet function
   - Correction of acidosis rests on improvement in tissue perfusion and avoidance of iatrogenic acidosis (i.e. hypercapnia, hyperchloraemia)

What is the role of tranexamic acid in major trauma?

The use of TXA in trauma patients who are actively bleeding or at risk of haemorrhage has been advocated since the **CRASH-2** trial (Lancet, 2010), which randomised such patients to receive either TXA or placebo as a loading dose followed by infusion. They demonstrated a significant reduction in mortality (but no reduction in the volume of blood products transfused) with no associated increase in adverse vascular occlusive events. The first dose of TXA should be given within three hours of injury.

How would you guide blood product replacement in major trauma?

In addition to haemodynamic parameters, point-of-care tests including ABG and FBC are used to guide resuscitation and PRBC transfusion. Viscoelastic haemostatic assays, i.e. Thromboelastography (TEG®) or Rotational Thromboelastometry (ROTEM®), may be used to assess ATC/TIC and guide FFP, platelet and cryoprecipitate/fibrinogen concentrate therapy.

TEG®

- Blood placed into a cup, which rotates
- A pin is inserted into the cup, which remains stationary
- An electrical transducer measures torsion
- Kaolin may be added to activate coagulation
- Heparinase removes the effect of heparin
- Tissue factor and glycoprotein IIb/IIIa inhibitors may be added to produce a trace that represents the contribution of fibrinogen to the clot firmness

ROTEM®

- Blood is placed into a cup, which remains stationary A pin is inserted into the cup, which rotates
- An optical system detects torsion
- EXTEM uses tissue factor (extrinsic pathway)
- INTEM uses contact activator (intrinsic pathway)
- Heparinase option as with TEG®
- FIBTEM uses platelet inhibitor, producing a trace that represents the contribution of fibrinogen to the clot firmness
- APTEM uses aprotinin and calcium, and rapidly detects fibrinolysis

Figure 85.1 illustrates a typical TEG® and ROTEM® trace, and the components of each are broken down in Table 85.3. Figure 85.2 demonstrates how the trace

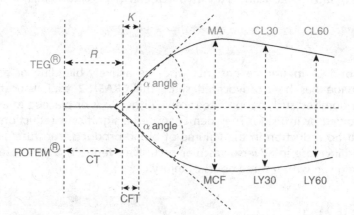

Figure 85.1 Typical TEG® and ROTEM® tracings
Reproduced with permission from Srivastava A., Kelleher A. (*Contin Educ Anaesth Crit Care Pain* 2013)

Table 85.3 Interpretation of TEG® and ROTEM® parameters

TEG®	ROTEM®	Definition	Significance	Intervention
R (reaction) time 4–8 minutes	CT (clotting time) INTEM 137–246 seconds EXTEM 42–74 seconds	Time till initiation of fibrin formation (until amplitude reaches 2 mm)	Concentration of stable clotting factors	FFP
K time 1–4 minutes	CFT (clot formation time) INTEM 40–100 seconds EXTEM 46–148 seconds	Time for amplitude to increase from 2 to 20 mm	Measurement of clot kinetics	FFP Platelets
α angle 47–74°	α angle INTEM 71–80° EXTEM 63–80°	Angle between tangent to tracing at 2 mm amplitude	Rapidity of fibrinogen build-up and cross-linking	Fibrinogen (cryoprecipitate or fibrinogen concentrate)
MA (maximum amplitude) 55–73 mm	MCF (maximum clot firmness) INTEM 52–72 mm EXTEM 49–71 mm	Greatest vertical width	Number and function of platelets and fibrinogen concentration	Platelets Fibrinogen
CL30/60 (clot lysis at 30/60 min) <7.5%	Ly30/60 (lysis at 30/60 min) <7.5%	% reduction in amplitude after 30/60 minutes following MA/MCF	Fibrinolysis	TXA

Adapted with permission from Srivastava A, Kelleher A. (*Contin Educ Anaesth Crit Care Pain* 2013)

looks in various coagulopathy states, and Figure 85.3 is an example algorithm for use in trauma patients.

A Cochrane review in 2015 demonstrated that there is currently a paucity of evidence supporting the use of viscoelastic testing in trauma. The **iTACTIC** study is currently recruiting and aims to address this question. Trauma patients who are actively bleeding will be randomised to blood product transfusion guided by VHA versus local empiric massive transfusion protocol.

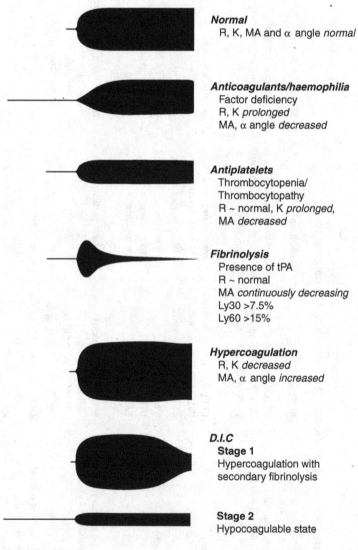

Normal
R, K, MA and α angle *normal*

Anticoagulants/haemophilia
Factor deficiency
R, K *prolonged*
MA, α angle *decreased*

Antiplatelets
Thrombocytopenia/
Thrombocytopathy
R ~ normal, K *prolonged*,
MA *decreased*

Fibrinolysis
Presence of tPA
R ~ normal
MA *continuously decreasing*
Ly30 >7.5%
Ly60 >15%

Hypercoagulation
R, K *decreased*
MA, α angle *increased*

D.I.C
Stage 1
Hypercoagulation with
secondary fibrinolysis

Stage 2
Hypocoagulable state

Figure 85.2 Abnormal VHA traces

CODE RED TRAUMA
Management of Trauma Induced Coagulopathy

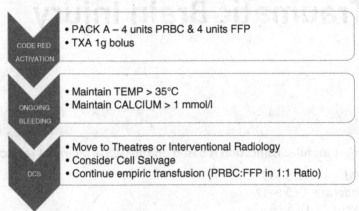

CODE RED
ACTIVATION
- PACK A – 4 units PRBC & 4 units FFP
- TXA 1g bolus

ONGOING
BLEEDING
- Maintain TEMP > 35°C
- Maintain CALCIUM > 1 mmol/l

DCS
- Move to Theatres or Interventional Radiology
- Consider Cell Salvage
- Continue empiric transfusion (PRBC:FFP in 1:1 Ratio)

ROTEM Algorithm

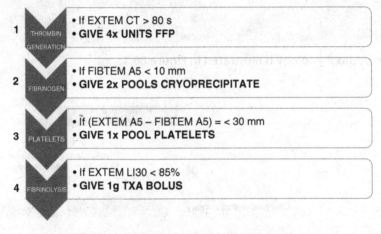

1 THROMBIN GENERATION
- If EXTEM CT > 80 s
- **GIVE 4x UNITS FFP**

2 FIBRINOGEN
- If FIBTEM A5 < 10 mm
- **GIVE 2x POOLS CRYOPRECIPITATE**

3 PLATELETS
- If (EXTEM A5 – FIBTEM A5) = < 30 mm
- **GIVE 1x POOL PLATELETS**

4 FIBRINOLYSIS
- If EXTEM LI30 < 85%
- **GIVE 1g TXA BOLUS**

*ROTEM repeatable 15 min after blood products to assess
treatment response and to further guide therapy*

Figure 85.3 Example algorithm for ROTEM® use in major trauma
Reproduced with kind permission from the Trauma Anaesthesia Group, Royal
London Hospital

Further Reading

Alam H B, Velmahos G C. New trends in resuscitation. *Curr Probl Surg* 2011; **48**(8): 531–564

Brohi K. Diagnosis and management of coagulopathy after major trauma. *Br J Surg* 2009; **96**: 963–964

Dutton R P. Haemostatic resuscitation. *Br J Anaesth* 2012; **109** (suppl 1): i39–i46

Srivastava A, Kelleher A. Point of care coagulation testing. *Contin Educ Anaesth Crit Care Pain* 2013; **13**(1): 12–16

Chapter 86

Traumatic Brain Injury

How can traumatic brain injury be classified?

The most useful classification is based on the GCS *after* initial resuscitation:

Mild   GCS ≥13
Moderate GCS 9–12
Severe   GCS ≤8

What is the pathophysiology of primary traumatic brain injury?

The pathophysiology is illustrated in Figure 86.1.

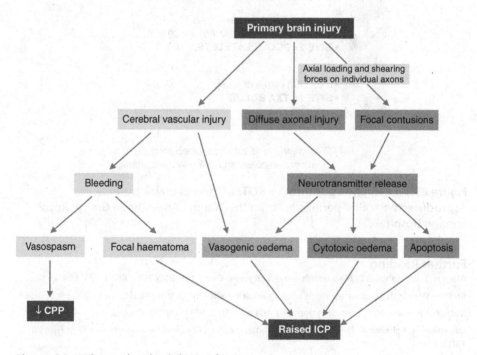

Figure 86.1 The pathophysiology of primary brain injury

What is the pathophysiology of secondary brain injury?

There are a number of mechanisms by which the injured brain may suffer a secondary insult. These are divided into three categories:

1 *Reduced cerebral oxygen delivery*
   i Anaemia, e.g. due to bleeding from associated injuries
   ii Hypoxaemia, e.g. hypoventilation, V/Q mismatch due to aspiration, pulmonary contusions, haemo/pneumothorax
   iii Hypotension, e.g. hypovolaemia, neurogenic shock, myocardial contusions
   iv Increased ICP, e.g. DAI, intracranial bleeding, obstructive hydrocephalus
2 *Increased cerebral oxygen requirement* ($CMRO_2$)
   i Seizures
   ii Pyrexia
3 *Cellular mechanisms*
   i Excitotoxicity due to neurotransmitter release
   ii Inflammation
   iii Hyperglycaemia
   iv Free radical damage

Hypotension (SBP <90 mmHg) and hypoxaemia (SpO_2 <90%) are independent risk factors for mortality following severe head injury and should be treated aggressively.

How is diffuse axonal injury graded?

Diffuse axonal injury results from accelerating, decelerating or rotational forces applied to the brain. This type of trauma causes traumatic shearing of axons, which results in widespread cell damage and death. It is associated with a significant level of morbidity and mortality including coma, persistent vegetative state and ultimately death. Classical CT findings are diffuse brain swelling and loss of grey-white differentiation. The *Marshall system* is used to grade DAI using CT findings (Table 86.1).

Table 86.1 Marshall grading system for diffuse axonal injury

Grade	CT Findings	Mortality
I	No visible intracranial injury	10%
II	Cisterns present Midline shift <5 mm Small, high- or mixed-density lesions <25 cc	14%
III	Cisterns compressed or absent	34%
IV	Midline shift >5 mm	56%

What forms of monitoring are useful in severely brain injured patients?

All patients should have invasive arterial monitoring in addition to ECG, pulse oximetry and end-tidal CO_2 monitoring. In addition, the Brain Trauma Foundation (BTF) recommends:

1 *ICP monitoring*
   The gold standard monitoring device is a surgically-placed intraventricular catheter (which also permits removal of CSF). A CPP of 50–70 mmHg should be targeted.

$$CPP = MAP - ICP$$

The BTF recommends ICP monitoring in:

   i All salvageable patients with severe TBI and an abnormal CT brain
   ii Patients with severe TBI and a *normal* CT if the following risk factors are present (50–60% increased risk of intracranial hypertension in these patients):
      – Age >40
      – Motor posturing
      – SBP <90 mmHg
2 *Jugular bulb oxygen saturation (SjvO$_2$)*
   A fibreoptic catheter inserted into the IJV and directed cranially to lie at the level of the C1 vertebral body allows measurement of global cerebral VO_2 and is useful in guiding therapy such as controlled hyperventilation and osmotherapy. The normal range for SjvO$_2$ is 50–75% and a value <50% necessitates intervention.

Other forms of monitoring include:

1 *Transcranial Doppler*
   This visualises the blood flow within the Circle of Willis and allows a pulsatility index to be calculated:

$$\text{Pulsatility index} = \frac{\text{systolic velocity} - \text{diastolic velocity}}{\text{mean velocity}}$$

2 *EEG*
   Often used to detect sub-clinical seizures or to titrate sedation

Why may intubation and ventilation be required in the head injured patient?

The reasons to intubate and ventilate in head injury are:

1 Airway protection
   i GCS ≤8, or decrease in motor score by ≥2 points
   ii Associated airway trauma, e.g. bleeding, bilateral fractured mandible

2 To facilitate maintenance of ventilatory targets
   i Spontaneous hyperventilation leads to hypocapnia, which causes cerebral vasoconstriction and worsens perfusion to injured and normal brain tissue
   ii Hypoventilation (due to reduced central drive following the brain injury or secondary to drugs administered pre-hospital) results in hypercapnia, which causes cerebral vasodilatation and increases ICP, which in turn compromises global cerebral perfusion
3 To protect/prevent worsening of the TBI and/or coexisting injuries
   i Associated high cervical spine injury (and resulting apnoea)
   ii Seizures
   iii Haemodynamic instability (caused either by the head injury itself or by associated extracranial injuries)
4 To facilitate safe neuroimaging or transfer to a neurosurgical/major trauma centre

What is the immediate management of TBI?

The patient with TBI should be managed according to ATLS principles, with particular focus on preventing secondary brain injury. Specific management involves:

1 **Primary survey** to detect any associated life-threatening injury with concomitant resuscitation as required
   - A rapid neurological assessment, with documentation of GCS and limb movement on scene and on arrival to hospital

2 **Secure the airway and control ventilation** if needed
   - Assume coexisting cervical spine injury: use MILS
   - Assume a full stomach: use cricoid pressure and insert an orogastric tube post-intubation
   - Avoid significant BP fluctuations during laryngoscopy/intubation:
     - Haemodynamically stable induction, e.g. ketamine 1–2 mg/kg and fentanyl 1–3 mcg/kg (ketamine has traditionally not been used in head injured patients due to concerns that it may increase ICP; however, this notion has now been challenged, with evidence to suggest that ketamine may even have a protective effect)
     - Muscle relaxation with rocuronium 1 mg/kg or suxamethonium (has been reported to increase ICP but the effect is clinically insignificant)
     - Ensure a vasopressor is immediately available
   - Have a low threshold to use a bougie, and consider other advanced airway techniques including videolaryngoscopy or Airtraq®
   - Tape ETT in place rather than tie
   - End-tidal CO_2 and ABG monitoring should be instituted rapidly to ensure ventilatory targets are met

3 **Cardiovascular support**
   - Damage control resuscitation principles are employed, using a target SBP of 100 mmHg in major trauma patients with associated head injury

- Avoid large-volume crystalloid resuscitation as it worsens cerebral oedema in the context of a disrupted blood-brain barrier (BBB) in animal models: small volume boluses are preferred, preferably of blood and plasma in the multiply injured patient
- Colloids are avoided as post-hoc analysis of data from the **SAFE** trial revealed a higher mortality in TBI patients resuscitated with albumin vs saline (see page 139)
- Once hypovolaemia is excluded, vasopressor therapy can be used to maintain BP

4 **Monitor pupils closely** following sedation and ventilation

5 Prompt **imaging**
- Major trauma patients should receive a full body CT with contrast

Importantly, concurrent resuscitative and/or cranial surgery may be required in the polytrauma patient.

How should we care for brain injured patients on the ICU?

Such patients should continue to be treated using *neuroprotection* strategies to prevent further secondary brain injury. Specific treatment aims are as follows:

1 **Normoxia** (PaO$_2$ >10 kPa)
2 **Normocapnia** (PaCO$_2$ 4.5–5.0 kPa)
3 **Normotension** (MAP ≥80 mmHg after haemorrhage control)
- This assumes normal cerebral autoregulation with an ICP of ~20 mmHg, to achieve CPP ≥60 mmHg
4 **Normoglycaemia** (blood glucose 6–10 mmol/l)
5 **Normothermia** (avoid hyperthermia)
6 **30° head-up position** (tilt the whole bed if patient under spinal precautions) and avoidance of positioning, cervical collars, ties etc. that would interrupt venous drainage

Additionally, routine ICU measures are important in this group:

1 VAP care bundles
2 Thromboprophylaxis (pharmacological prophylaxis is usually guided by neurosurgeons)
3 Early enteral feeding (within 5 days) is associated with improved outcomes
4 Stress ulcer prophylaxis
5 Physiotherapy

The **CRASH** trial (Lancet, 2004) showed a significantly increased mortality in head injured patients treated with corticosteroids compared to placebo, hence there is no place for steroids in the management of TBI.

The **CRASH-3** trial is currently recruiting and aims to assess the effect of tranexamic acid on the risk of death or disability in patients with TBI.

How is raised ICP managed?

The BTF recommend treating a sustained ICP ≥22 mmHg, as values above this are associated with increased mortality. A cause should be sought: repeat CT scanning should be considered and neurosurgical input is essential.

1 Optimise **sedation** and commence **neuromuscular blockade** to reduce $CMRO_2$

2 **Treat seizures** aggressively
   - Benzodiazepines are first-line
   - Load with phenytoin 18 mg/kg
   - There is little evidence for prophylactic anticonvulsant therapy to prevent late post-traumatic seizures in TBI; early post-traumatic seizures are not associated with adverse outcomes

3 **Osmotherapy**
   - Causes early volume expansion and reduced viscosity, which improves microvascular blood flow and increases circulating volume and cardiac output
   - This is thought to improve regional blood flow, and result in vasoconstriction in areas of intact autoregulation, thus reducing ICP and vasogenic oedema formation
   - There is a secondary osmotic effect, which moves fluid from the intracellular to intravascular and interstitial spaces, increasing CBF and reducing cytotoxic oedema
   - Agents used:
     i *Hypertonic saline* (1–2 ml/kg of 5% solution)
        - Acts predominantly via osmotic shift of fluid
        - May also improve CBF and have an immunomodulatory function
        - Can be repeated every 4–6 hours provided serum osmolality <320 mOsm/kg and Na+ <155 mmol/l
     ii *Mannitol* (0.25–1 g/kg of 20% solution)
        - In addition to the beneficial effects on blood rheology and oedema formation, there is an osmotic diuresis (reduces extravascular fluid volume)
        - Potential side effects include hypovolaemia, hypotension, hyperkalaemia and rebound intracranial hypertension
        - Can be repeated as needed provided serum osmolality <320 mOsm/kg and patient is normovolaemic

4 **Moderate hyperventilation** to $PaCO_2$ 4.0–4.5 kPa to reduce cerebral blood volume and ICP
   - This is reserved for intractable intracranial hypertension as a temporising measure, e.g. before transfer to theatre for surgical intervention
   - Ideally should be guided by $SjvO_2$ monitoring to ensure adequate cerebral VO_2

5 **Barbiturate coma**
   - Thiopentone-induced burst suppression is used to reduce $CMRO_2$ in refractory cases
   - EEG or bispectral index monitoring is recommended to guide treatment

6 **Therapeutic hypothermia**
   – Not used following the **Eurotherm3235** trial (NEJM, 2015), which showed worse neurological outcome and increased mortality in the intervention group (see page 249)
   – Hyperthermia should be avoided as it is associated with increased $CMRO_2$

7 **Decompressive craniectomy** is considered in intractable intracranial hypertension

The **DECRA** trial (NEJM, 2011) randomised patients with severe non-penetrating TBI to receive DC or standard care. There was a reduction in ICP, duration of mechanical ventilation and LOS on the ICU in the intervention group. However, the chance of unfavourable neurological outcome (as measured by the GOSE – see Table 86.2) was increased. Mortality was similar in both groups.

The **RESCUEicp** trial (NEJM, 2016) was an international RCT in which TBI patients with abnormal CT brain and ICP >25 mmHg for 1–12 hours were randomised to receive usual therapy with either decompressive craniectomy or barbiturate coma. Mortality was significantly lower in the intervention group; however, DC was associated with significantly increased rates of poor neurological outcomes (severe disability or vegetative state on the EGOS) in survivors. Importantly, 37% of patients in the control group underwent rescue DC, so the observed treatment effect may have been attenuated.

It is important to rapidly identify patients who have a surgically correctable cause for their raised ICP. Indications for emergency neurosurgery include:

1 Craniotomy and evacuation of intracranial haematoma
2 Insertion of an EVD for obstructive hydrocephalus
3 Elevation of depressed skull fracture
4 Evacuation of traumatic ICH

The **STITCH (trauma)** trial (Journal of Neurotrauma, 2015) was an international RCT that looked at patients with traumatic intraparenchymal haemorrhage. Patients were randomised to early surgical intervention or medical therapy with delayed (>12 hours after randomisation) surgery if indicated. There was a non-significant trend towards increased favourable outcomes and a significant reduction in mortality at 6 months in the intervention group. A larger trial is needed to explore the potential improvement in functional outcome.

Table 86.2 The extended Glasgow Outcome Score

	Score	Outcome
Favourable	5	Good recovery
	4	Moderate disability
Unfavourable	3	Severe disability
	2	Vegetative state
	1	Dead

What is the *Lund concept*?

The *Lund concept* is a volume-targeted (as opposed to ICP-targeted) protocol notionally based on cerebral oedema formation as a result of alterations in Starling's forces across an injured BBB. A CPP of 60–70 mmHg is considered optimal. The principles are:

1 **Reduction of stress response and cerebral energy metabolism**
   - Stress response is reduced by liberal use of sedative agents and analgesia
   - This is achieved using low-dose thiopentone
2 **Reduction of capillary hydrostatic pressure**
   - Administer metoprolol and clonidine to target physiological BP (based on the age of the patient)
   - Pre-capillary vasoconstriction with low-dose thiopentone or dihydroergotamine
3 **Maintenance of colloid osmotic pressure**
   - Transfusion of packed red cells and HAS are used to preserve normal oncotic pressure and favour transcapillary absorption
   - Aim serum albumin >40 g/l, Hb 125–140 g/l
4 **Reduction of cerebral blood volume**
   - Pre-capillary vasoconstriction with thiopentone and dihydroergotamine
   - Post-capillary vasoconstriction with dihydroergotamine
   - Avoid hypervolaemia
   - Avoid dobutamine use (causes cerebral vasodilatation)

There is a single small trial that supports the use of the Lund concept in TBI. However, there have been a number of large trials that provide evidence *against* components of the protocol. The concept is not, therefore, in widespread use.

What are the indicators of poor prognosis in TBI?

1 Extremes of age
2 Reduced GCS motor score
3 Bilateral unreactive pupils
4 Absent oculocephalic reflex
5 Low GCS eye and verbal score
6 Untreatable raised ICP with DAI (vs surgically amenable discrete intracranial lesion)
7 Presence of extracranial complications

Further Reading

Brain Trauma Foundation. 2016. *Guidelines for the Management of Severe TBI*, 4th ed [online]. Campbell, CA: Brain Trauma Foundation. Available at: https://braintrauma.org/guidelines/guidelines-for-the-management-of-severe-tbi-4th-ed#/ (Accessed: 4 March 2017)

Dinsmore J. Traumatic brain injury: an evidence-based review of management. *Contin Educ Anaesth Crit Care Pain* 2013; **13**(6): 189–195

Gründe P O. The Lund concept for the treatment of severe head trauma – physiological principles and clinical application. *Intensive Care Med* 2006; **32**: 1475–1484

Chapter 87

Tuberculosis

What is the causative organism of tuberculosis?

Mycobacterium tuberculosis is the causative bacteria for tuberculosis. Mycobacteria are aerobic bacilli and classically *acid-fast* (resist decolourisation by acids used during laboratory staining procedures).

Other *atypical* or *non-tuberculous* mycobacterium exist, such as *M. kansasii*, that can result in a similar clinical picture to that of TB. These will not be discussed here.

What are the risk factors for tuberculosis?

WHO have identified the following risk factors for TB:

1 Immunosuppression
  i HIV
  ii Diabetes
  iii Malnutrition
  iv Smoking and substance abuse
  v Alcohol excess
  vi Organ transplant recipients or other conditions requiring immunosuppressant regimens
2 General exposure factors
  i Close contact with infectious TB disease
  ii Immigration from areas of the world with high rates of TB
  iii Groups with high rates of TB transmission, e.g. homeless persons

How is tuberculosis diagnosed?

The presentation of TB can be indistinguishable from other more common conditions. Tuberculosis should therefore form part of the differential diagnosis in all patients who exhibit the non-specific signs and symptoms alongside an abnormal CXR and positive risk factors.

1 Clinical symptoms and signs
  i Fever
  ii Weight loss
  iii Night sweats

    iv Persistent cough

    v Haemoptysis

    vi Chest pain

2 Imaging

    i CXR

      – Cavitating lesions, bilateral infiltrates, calcification, patchy/nodular sha-
dowing in upper zones

      – May be normal in extrapulmonary disease

    ii CT chest

      – Allows identification of active TB

      – Can differentiate from old fibrotic lesions – centrilobular nodules and
tree in bud pattern often seen in active disease

      – Mediastinal lymphadenopathy, cavitation and miliary shadowing may be
present on CT even with a normal CXR

      – May help in gathering diagnostic information in an intubated patient
where TB is suspected

      – Can help target bronchoscopy

3 Microbiology

Microbiological cultures should be obtained to confirm diagnosis and
facilitate drug sensitivity testing

    i Two sputum samples should be obtained where possible

    ii BAL samples may be obtained for microbiology in the intubated patient

      – Transbronchial biopsy may increase the diagnostic yield

    iii Induced sputum may have a role

    iv Transtracheal aspirates have shown a high sensitivity in smear-negative
patients

    v Auramine or Ziehl-Neelsen stain help to confirm TB (new liquid culture
techniques also exist for diagnosis)

If there are signs, symptoms and imaging results consistent with TB,
treatment should be started without waiting for culture results

4 Non-pulmonary samples

Extrapulmonary TB is common in ICU patients with pulmonary TB. Whilst
positive cultures are central to confirmation of the mycobacterium, PCR for
TB may have a role in establishing a diagnosis.

The following samples may therefore be useful:

    i Pleural biopsies

    ii Lymph node aspiration

    iii Pleural fluid tap – TB may be associated with a lymphocytic effusion

    iv Urine culture for TB in miliary disease

In what situations might a patient with tuberculosis require critical care?

1 Acute respiratory failure

2 Massive haemoptysis

3 DIC as a consequence of miliary TB

4 Cardiogenic shock secondary to pericardial effusion
5 Complications of anti-tuberculous drugs, particularly renal/liver failure
6 Tuberculous meningitis
7 Stroke/pituitary apoplexy secondary to cerebral tuberculoma

What is the medical management of tuberculosis?

The standard first-line treatment of non-drug resistant TB should be guided by an infectious disease specialist and involves the drugs outlined in Table 87.1. Combination therapy is essential and regimens commonly have an intensive phase of two months, followed by a continuation phase of either four or seven months (to total six or nine months' treatment).

Table 87.1 Standard drugs used in the treatment of non-drug resistant TB

Drug	Side effects	Comments
Rifampicin	Hepatotoxicity Autoimmune reactions	Parenteral preparations available Interaction with oral contraceptives, anticoagulants, hypoglycaemics, anticonvulsants, antifungals, corticosteroids, antiretrovirals
Isoniazid	Hepatotoxicity Peripheral neuropathy Drug-induced lupus	Parenteral preparations available Peripheral neuropathy is preventable with vitamin B6 (pyridoxine)
Ethambutol	Optic nerve toxicity Colour blindness	Visual field assessment (if possible) prior to initiation Dose adjustment is required for eGFR <30 ml/min/1.73 m^2
Pyrazinamide	Hepatotoxicity Hyperuricaemia	Dose adjustment is required for eGFR <30 ml/min/1.73 m^2

Other drug treatments include:

1 Fluroquinolones (i.e. moxifloxacin)
2 Aminoglycosides (i.e. streptomycin)

The management of HIV co-infection is complicated and necessitates an awareness of the potential for the development of IRIS (see page 224). It is recommended that HAART be initiated as soon as is practicable in the very immunosuppressed (CD4 <100 cells/mm^3).

Figure 87.1 illustrates a proposed algorithm for the treatment of pulmonary TB on the ICU.

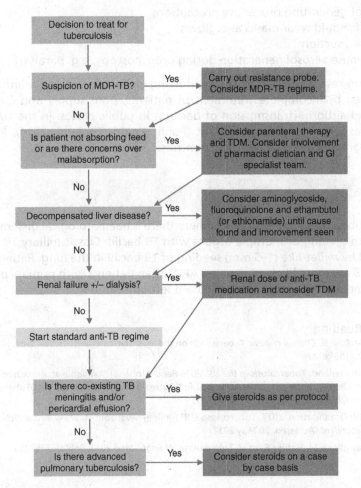

Figure 87.1 Proposed algorithm for the treatment of suspected or actual pulmonary TB on the ICU
Adapted with kind permission from Hagan G, Nathani N. (*Critical Care* 2013)
TDM – therapeutic drug monitoring

Infection control measures should be instigated, which include:

1 Isolation room
   – Negative pressure room
   – Warning signs on room
   – Door kept closed
   – Minimise healthcare worker contact where possible
2 Surgical masks should be worn by patients who are transported outside an isolation room

3 Aerosol-generating procedure precautions
   - Staff should wear masks and gloves
   - Closed suction
   - Minimise aerosol generation during bronchoscopy, e.g. paralysis

Multi-drug-resistant TB (MDR-TB) is a growing global concern. It is multifactorial and driven by incomplete treatment of patients, poor supply and quality of drugs and airborne transmission of bacteria in public places. In the UK, 1.6% of isolates were multi-drug-resistant (Public Health England, 2014). Rates of MDR-TB are much higher in other countries.

What is miliary tuberculosis?

Miliary tuberculosis is a form of TB where there is haematological dissemination leading to seeding of multiple organs with TB bacilli. Classic miliary TB is characterised by *millet-like* (1–5 mm) seeding of TB bacilli in the lung. Patients with miliary TB are more likely to develop ARDS than patients with primary pulmonary TB, and mortality approaches 100% if left untreated.

Further Reading

Hagan G, Nathani N. Clinical review: Tuberculosis on the intensive care unit. *Critical Care* 2013; **17**(5): 240 DOI: 10.1186/cc12760

Public Health England. *Tuberculosis in the UK: 2014 Report* [online]. Available at: www.lstmed.ac.uk/sites/default/files/content/news_articles/files/Public%20Health%20England%20-%20Tuberculosis%20in%20the%20UK.pdf (Accessed: 30 May 2017)

World Health Organisation. 2017. Tuberculosis (TB) [online]. Available at: www.who.int/tb/areas-of-work/laboratory/en/ (Accessed: 30 May 2017)

Zumla A, Raviglione M, Hafner R, et al. Tuberculosis. *N Engl J Med* 2013: **368**(8): 745–755

Chapter 88

Venous Thromboembolism and Heparin-Induced Thrombocytopenia

Why does venous thromboembolic disease matter?

Venous thromboembolism is an important complication of hospital admission and of critical illness, and as such is a major cause of *potentially preventable* morbidity and mortality. An estimated 25% of patients who have one or more risk factors will develop a DVT. Pulmonary embolism complicates approximately one third of cases of DVT, and may be life-threatening. Critically ill patients are at particular risk of thrombosis due to their acute and chronic illness, immobility, interventions including organ support and central venous access, sedation and paralysis.

Tell me about the pathophysiology of VTE

Virchow's triad describes three factors that are necessary to be present in order for a thrombus form:

1 Perturbation in blood flow, e.g. stasis or turbulence
2 Injury to the vascular endothelium
3 Alterations in blood coagulability

Typically, venous thrombosis occurs following vascular trauma, in response to an indwelling venous device, or in regions of poor flow. Platelets and fibrin are deposited, and the clot grows rapidly (in the direction of flow). It may occlude the vein distally, causing the acute presentation of venous congestion (most commonly of the limbs in a DVT) or pulmonary infarction, or even obstructive shock with RVF in massive PE. Endogenous fibrinolysis then breaks down the clot over a period of time, but this may be incomplete and result in chronic venous insufficiency.

What are the risk factors for VTE?

The risk factors for venous thrombosis are summarised in Table 88.1.

Table 88.1 Risk factors for venous thrombosis

Venous stasis	Immobility, including anaesthesia >30 mins
	Long travel
	Varicose veins
Endothelial injury	Indwelling devices
	Surgery
	Trauma
	Burns
Hypercoagulabilty	Malignancy
	Pregnancy and puerperium
	Obesity
	Medical conditions (stroke, IBD, nephrotic syndrome (loss of ATIII), history of VTE, HIT)
	Drugs (combined oral contraceptive, hormone replacement therapy, chemotherapy)
	Smoking
	Ageing
	Thrombophilia (factor V Leidin, activated protein C resistance, antiphospholipid syndrome, antithrombin and protein C and S deficiencies)

How would you classify pulmonary embolism?

Pulmonary embolism can be classified on the basis of haemodynamic stability:

Massive PE

Acute PE with one or more of the following:

  i Sustained hypotension
    SBP <90 mmHg for at least 15 min or requiring inotropic support
    Not due to a cause other than PE, e.g. arrhythmia, hypovolemia, sepsis, or LVF
 ii Pulselessness
iii Persistent profound bradycardia (heart rate <40 bpm with signs or symptoms of shock)

Submassive PE

Acute PE without systemic hypotension (i.e. SBP ≥90 mmHg) but with either RV dysfunction or myocardial necrosis

PE may also be classified according to clinical severity, and is based on the estimated in-hospital or 30-day mortality:

High-risk – suspected or confirmed PE in the presence of shock or sustained hypotension

Not high-risk – suspected or confirmed PE in the absence of shock or sustained hypotension

What are the echocardiographic findings in acute pulmonary embolus?

Acute PE may lead to RV pressure overload and dysfunction, which can be detected by echocardiography. Right ventricular dilatation is found in 25% of cases of PE and is used to risk stratify the disease.

McConnell's sign (reduced RV free wall contractility with sparing of the apex) has a high positive predictive value for PE even in the presence of respiratory disease.

In suspected cases of high-risk PE, the absence of echocardiographic signs of RV overload or dysfunction can help to exclude PE as the cause of the haemodynamic instability.

Do you know of any guidelines for the treatment of high-risk PE?

A taskforce for the European Society of Cardiology (ESC) released guidelines on the diagnosis and management of acute PE in 2014 (Figure 88.1).

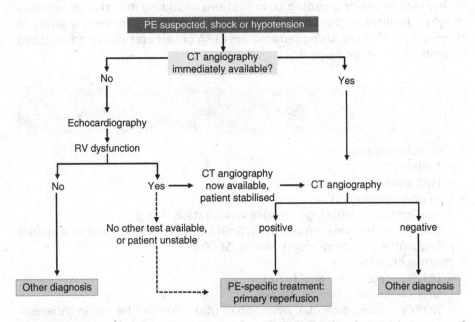

Figure 88.1 European Society of Cardiology algorithm for the management of patients with suspected high-risk PE
Reproduced with permission from the European Society of Cardiology (*Eur Heart J* 2014)

The ESC recommend that treatment of pulmonary embolus is coordinated with MDT input including that of an interventional cardiologist with the following approach:

1 Haemodynamic and respiratory support
2 Anticoagulation
   – IV UFH is the preferred mode of initial anticoagulation
3 Primary reperfusion therapy
   i **Thrombolysis** is first line
   ii **Surgical embolectomy** in patients with contraindications to systemic thrombolysis or in whom initial thrombolysis has failed to improve the haemodynamic status
   iii **Percutaneous catheter-directed treatment** if available

Is there any evidence for thrombolysis in submassive PE?

The **PEITHO** trial (NEJM, 2014) was a multi-centre, randomised, double-blind comparison of thrombolysis with a single bolus of IV tenecteplase plus heparin compared to placebo plus heparin. Patients with acute PE were eligible for the study if they had objective (biochemical or radiographic) evidence of RV dysfunction. There was a significant reduction in the composite endpoint of cardiovascular decompensation plus all-cause mortality within seven days of randomisation. However, there was a significantly higher rate of major bleeding complications including intracranial haemorrhage in the intervention arm, highlighting the need to improve the safety of thrombolytic therapy. Using reduced dose tPA or catheter-delivered localised thrombolysis may be helpful.

What methods are available to help prevent venous thromboembolic disease?

1 General measures
   – Mobilisation
   – Hydration
2 Non-pharmacological
   – Anti-embolism stockings – reduce venous stasis in legs
     Caution with arterial insufficiency, limb fractures, cellulitis and neuropathy
   – Sequential calf compression devices (SCCDs)
3 Pharmacological
   – LMWH – caution in renal failure
   – UFH – bd dosing, similar efficacy
   – NOACs – dabigatran (IIa), rivaroxaban (Xa) – licensed for use in thromboprophylaxis following TKR/THR
   – Regional anaesthesia peri-operatively

Tell me about heparin

Heparin is a large polysaccharide (5–40 kDa) and is a naturally occurring anticoagulant that exerts its action by binding to endogenous antithrombin III. This complex then inhibits factor Xa and IIa (thrombin). Unfractionated heparin has a predictable effect on the activated partial thromboplastin time (APTT) when administered intravenously (which is used to monitor therapeutic anticoagulation with heparin), although less so when given subcutaneously. UFH is cleared rapidly by the reticuloendothelial system.

Low molecular weight heparins are short chain polysaccharides (<8 kDa) and work in a similar manner to UFH, although exhibit limited antithrombin activity. There is a lower risk of bleeding and complications including HIT and osteoporosis when compared with UFH. LMWHs are renally excreted and their dose should be adjusted in renal impairment. LMWHs require no monitoring (anti-Xa assay may be performed if overdose/accumulation are suspected) and are given on a once daily basis for prophylaxis against VTE.

Protamine may be given to reverse the action of UFH (1 mg will neutralise 100 units of UFH). It must be given slowly to avoid pulmonary vasoconstriction and hypotension. Protamine may partially reverse the effects of LMWH, but the effects are inconsistent.

What are the causes of an isolated APTT rise, and what would you do in this situation?

The causes of an isolated rise in APTT are:

1 Haemophilia A (factor VIII deficiency)
2 Haemophilia B (factor IX deficiency)
3 Factor XI deficiency
4 Factor XII deficiency
5 Heparin therapy
6 Antiphospholipid syndrome (the antibodies can have a variable effect on the clotting screen)
7 Artifact

Appropriate action:

1 Review the patient – history, examination, review the notes and drug chart
2 Repeat the APTT and perform a full coagulation screen
   – It is important to realise that the results from a clotting screen can be greatly affected simply by alterations in the volume of blood placed in the bottle (due to the dilutional effect on the anticoagulant)
3 Request a heparinase test
4 Perform a clotting factor assay
5 Request an antiphospholipid screen (anticardiolipin antibodies and lupus anticoagulant)

What are the contraindications to the use of heparin?

1 Documented allergy to heparin
2 Previous history of HIT (caution)
3 Active major bleeding or risk of serious re-bleeding including intracranial haemorrhage or recent ischaemic stroke
4 Platelets <50 x 10^9/l, coagulopathy
5 Recent neuraxial block/catheter removal
   - Heparin may be given >4 hours after uncomplicated neuraxial blockade or epidural catheter removal
   - Neuraxial anaesthesia should be avoided for 12 hours after prophylactic LMWH has been given

How might your approach to VTE prophylaxis differ in a multiply injured trauma patient who is at high risk of bleeding and of developing VTE?

The patient should be managed using an ABCDE approach, treating abnormalities as they are found and ensuring all steps are taken to stop the bleeding. Other measures include:

1 Involve haematology early
2 SCCDs +/– anti-embolism stockings if appropriate
3 Consider IVC filter or Angel® Catheter

The Angel® Catheter is a retrievable IVC filter that can be placed via the femoral vein on the ICU in a manner similar to CVC insertion. It is intended for use in patients in whom anticoagulation is contraindicated or in whom the risk of VTE is very high, e.g. pelvic trauma

Importantly, the emphasis in these patients may change quickly from the management of life-threatening haemorrhage, to prevention and management of life-threatening thromboembolism. Any decision with regards to whether to anticoagulate or not should be carefully documented in the notes and communicated to the patient and their relatives.

What is HIT?

Heparin-induced thrombocytopenia is a life-threatening prothrombotic complication of heparin therapy. There are two types:

1 Type I
   - Non-immune mediated
   - More common (10–20% of patients on heparin)
   - Occurs early in treatment – within three days
   - Platelet count 100–150 x 10^9/l

- No bleeding/thrombotic complications
- Resolves spontaneously
2 Type II
    - Immune mediated – IgG to heparin/platelet factor 4 complex causes platelet activation and results in arterial and venous thrombosis
    - ~0.6% of patients treated with heparin – >10 times more common with UFH than LMWH
    - Occurs 5–10 days after starting treatment
    - Platelets fall to ~50 x 10^9/l or by >50%
    - Thrombosis occurs in 20–50%
    - Skin necrosis occurs in up to 20%

How do we diagnose HIT?

The pre-test probability of HIT is calculated (the 4 Ts, see Table 88.2), and on this basis a HIT screen may be carried out after consulting a haematologist. The HIT screen may be functional (measure heparin-dependent platelet activation by the heparin/PF4 antibody) or use immunoassays (measure antibody level in the blood; however, only 5–30% of patients with heparin/PF4 antibodies will have clinically relevant HIT).

Table 88.2 The pre-test probability of HIT: The 4 Ts

	2 points	1 point	0 points
Thrombocytopenia	>50% fall Nadir ≥ 20	30–50% fall Nadir 10–19	<30% fall Nadir < 10
Timing	Days 5–10	> 10 days	< 4 days
Thrombosis	Confirmed Skin lesions Acute SIRS after heparin	Worsening/recurrent/silent +/– skin lesions	None
oTher causes	None	Possible	Definite
Points	0–3 4–5 6–8	Low probability (<5%) Moderate probability (10–30%) High probability (20–80%)	

How is HIT managed?

1 HIT is a prothrombotic state and although **heparin should be immediately withdrawn**, an alternative anticoagulant should be introduced:
    - Argatroban (direct thrombin inhibitor) – first line, IV, half-life ~20 minutes, only licensed for use in HIT
    - Dabigatran (direct thrombin inhibitor)

- Danaparoid (indirect Xa inhibitor) – LMW heparinoid + dermatan sulphate + chondroitin sulphate
- Fondaparinux (indirect Xa inhibitor) – synthetic heparin pentasaccharide
- Lepiridun and bivalirudin are no longer used in the UK

2 Avoid giving platelets as this will worsen the condition (cf. TTP)

3 Warfarin will worsen the skin necrosis – only consider once plts >150

4 Avoid reintroduction of heparin for 100 days to minimise the risk of thrombosis
  - Does not contraindicate the use of UFH/LMWH but caution is advised – no IgM antibodies are produced, so the body does not retain immunological memory
  - In extreme circumstances it is possible to measure the antibody titre to assess response and timing of reintroduction of heparin

In exceptional circumstances, e.g. the patient post-cardiothoracic surgery who needs to return to theatre, it is possible to use heparin but the patient should be anticoagulated using an alternative agent immediately post-operatively.

Further Reading

Barker R C, Marval P. Venous thromboembolism: Risks and prevention. *Contin Educ Anaesth Crit Care Pain* 2011; **11**(1): 18–23

Meyer G, Vicaut E, Danays T, et al. Fibrinolysis for patients with intermediate-risk pulmonary embolism. *N Engl J Med* 2014; **370**(15): 1402–1411

The Task Force for the Diagnosis and Management of Acute Pulmonary Embolism of the European Society of Cardiology. Guidelines on the diagnosis and management of acute pulmonary embolism. *Eur Heart J* 2014; **35**: 3033–3073

Chapter 89

Viral Infection and Antiviral Therapy

Tell me about hepatitis B. How does it present? What is the specific treatment?

Hepatitis B is a DNA virus transmitted through contact with infected bodily fluids. Acute infection is normally asymptomatic. Fulminant hepatic failure occurs in 1% of patients and approximately 5% will develop chronic infection. Patients can be asymptomatic carriers: these patients have persistent HBV in the liver but no significant inflammation, and may still be infectious. Chronic HBV infection is treated with lamivudine.

Table 89.1 summarises the five main viral hepatitides.

You perform a hepatitis screen on a patient who presents with decompensated undifferentiated chronic liver failure. He is positive for anti-HAV IgG, HBsAb and HBcAb. What does this mean?

This patient has evidence of previous hepatitis A infection and chronic hepatitis B infection. The serological findings in viral hepatitis are summarised in Table 89.2.

What is *Herpes simplex* virus?

Herpes simplex is a double-stranded DNA virus from the Herpes family. HSV-1 is usually associated with orofacial disease (i.e. coldsores) and HSV-2 usually causes genital herpes. HSV shows neurovirulence and exhibits latency in nerve ganglia, with the potential for recurrent reactivation. HSV is the commonest cause of viral encephalitis, producing fronto-temporal changes that are visible on neuroimaging. It is diagnosed using HSV PCR and treated with aciclovir.

What is cytomegalovirus? How might it present?

Cytomegalovirus is a double-stranded DNA virus belonging to the Herpes family (human herpes virus 5). CMV has an affinity for lymphocytes and monocytes, and causes them to become enlarged (hence the name). Infection is manifested in four different ways:

Table 89.1 Viral hepatitis

Virus	Virology	Transmission	Presentation	Clinical Course	Treatment
Hepatitis A (HAV)	RNA virus	Faeco-oral Incubation 2–6 weeks	Fever, fatigue, malaise, jaundice, abdominal pain Transaminitis	Usually self-limiting FHF <1%	Supportive Vaccine available
Hepatitis B (HBV)	DNA virus	Blood-borne / bodily fluid	Acute infection usually asymptomatic Fatigue, malaise, nausea, vomiting, headache, arthralgia and low-grade fever Obstructive jaundice may be apparent	FHF ~1% Chronic hepatitis B ~5% Asymptomatic carrier state	Lamivudine Vaccine available
Hepatitis C (HCV)	RNA virus	Blood-borne (1:30 chance of transmission)	Acute infection usually asymptomatic 20–30% may have self-limiting illness similar to above	70–85% develop chronic hepatitis C infection	Ribavirin Pegylated interferon-α
Hepatitis D (HDV)	RNA virus	Blood-borne / bodily fluid	Only causes infection in presence of HBV May occur as simultaneous co-infection or as super-infection when HDV infection occurs in a patient with chronic HBV	Higher likelihood of FHF More rapid progression to cirrhosis Increased chance of HCC	
Hepatitis E (HEV)	RNA virus	Faeco-oral		Similar to HAV but increased risk of FHF	

FHF – fulminant hepatic failure; HCC – hepatocellular carcinoma

Table 89.2 Serology in viral hepatitides

Virus	Serology	Interpretation
Hepatitis A	Anti-HAV IgM	Active infection (persists for 3–6 months)
	Anti-HAV IgG	Past infection
Hepatitis B	HBsAg	HBV surface antigen (used in vaccine)
		Active infection (persists for 6–12 weeks)
	HBsAb	HBV surface antibody
		Previous HBV infection/immunity (develops 6 weeks after exposure)
	HBcAb	HBV core antibody
		IgM – early or chronic HBV infection
		IgG – past or chronic infection
	HBeAg	HBV e antigen (released during viral replication)
		Indicates infectious state and higher risk of progression to cirrhosis
	HBV DNA	Chronic HBV infection
Hepatitis C	HCV Ab	Antibody develops 4–10 weeks following infection
		Remains positive for life (even in absence of chronic HCV infection)
	HCV RNA PCR	Indicates active infection
		Genotyping may be used to determine likely response to treatment

1 *Asymptomatic*
   - Infection is usually asymptomatic in immunocompetent individuals
   - Seropositivity is highly prevalent in the general population (60–80% in adults), increasing with age
2 *Infectious mononucleosis-like illness* (fever, pharyngitis, headache, malaise, and lethargy, often with lymphadenopathy and splenomegaly)
3 *Placental transfer*
   - Occurs in 40% of patients after primary CMV infection during pregnancy
   - Congenital CMV infection is an important cause of sensorineural hearing loss and learning disability
   - Neonatal CMV is associated with significant morbidity and mortality
4 *Immunocompromised patients* (particularly those following organ transplantation)
   - May cause retinitis, colitis or pneumonitis

How is CMV infection diagnosed and treated?

Infection with CMV is diagnosed using PCR, which can be performed on various bodily fluids or tissues. CMV IgM appears in the serum within a week of infection and will decrease over the following few months. IgG levels become detectable a few days after the appearance of IgM, and remain positive lifelong (indicating previous infection). The treatment is with ganciclovir, or foscarnet in ganciclovir-resistant CMV.

What is Ebola virus? How does it present?

Ebola virus is an RNA virus of the Filoviridae family that is responsible for causing viral haemorrhagic fever (VHF). It is transmitted via direct mucous membrane or percutaneous exposure to infected body fluids. The most recent outbreak in West Africa was caused by the Zaire strain of the virus. Mammalian reservoirs include primates and fruit bats. Incubation varies between 2 and 21 days.

The typical clinical course is:

1 *Non-specific febrile illness*
   - Associated with fatigue, malaise, anorexia, arthralgia, myalgia and conjunctival injection
2 *Gastrointestinal phase* characterised by uncontrollable high volume diarrhoea and vomiting resulting in:
   - Electrolyte disturbance
   - Hypovolaemia
   - Shock, multi-organ failure and death
3. *Haemorrhagic phase*
   - Often manifest as GI bleeding
   - Does not occur universally, but is frequently fatal

Reported mortality in the developing world ranges from 38–70%.

How is VHF diagnosed?

1 Blood tests including cultures and Ebola serology (IgM, IgG, viral PCR)
2 Urine MC+S and viral PCR
3 Throat swabs for PCR
4 CXR looking for pneumonitis and ARDS

In addition to organ support and routine critical care, what specific obstacles are present when managing a patient with confirmed VHF?

1 Patient will require isolation in a *High-Level Isolation Unit (HLIU)* at the Royal Free Hospital in London
   i *Trexler negative pressure isolator system*
      - Large plastic tent with five half-suits built into the walls to allow patient access
      - Also contains components to permit passage of wires and tubing safely

- Utilises negative pressure filtered air flow
- Interventions are more complicated and necessitate unique and unfamiliar equipment and techniques

ii PPE (gloves, hand hygiene, gowns, N95 masks)
- Alternative to Trexler system
- Can be used in the management of high numbers of patients with VHF
- Used for transfer of patient to HLIU
- Moderate likelihood of VHF transmission to healthcare workers, highly likely to contaminate environment
- Potentially complicated and protracted training required

2 Access to investigations
- Point of care laboratory available in HLIU, facilitating a wide range of blood tests including cultures and cross-matching

3 Endotracheal intubation
- Potentially very challenging
- Should be regularly rehearsed in simulation scenarios
- Drugs and equipment have to be moved into the isolator before any intervention, which requires planning and is time consuming

4 Ventilation
- A small portable ventilator should be placed entirely within the Trexler tent so expired gases are vented via the filtered airflow system
- HME filters are changed every 24 hours

5 Central venous access
- Should be performed early in the patient's admission
- Internal jugular is the preferred site (high risk of infection with femoral access due to diarrhoea)
- Minimises venepuncture episodes (and hence risk to healthcare workers)

6 Administration of drugs
- All pumps and bags of fluid, including transducer sets, should be placed within the isolator in case of accidental disconnection
- Avoid IM injections in the haemorrhagic phase of VHF

7 Renal replacement therapy
- Any extracorporeal circuit represents a risk to the healthcare workers; the filtrate fluid may also contain live virus
- HLIU use a standalone isolator containing a haemofilter and its circuit
- Low volume CVVHF (15–20 ml/kg/hour) minimises effluent production
- Anticoagulation may be used to prolong circuit life in the absence of haemorrhagic symptoms

8 Ebola is a notifiable disease

Tell me about aciclovir

Table 89.3 summarises the commonly used antiviral agents. Most have action on viral DNA polymerase during the replication phase.

Table 89.3 Antiviral agents

Agent	Mechanism of Action	Uses	Side Effects
Aciclovir	Nucleoside analogue Phosphorylated in virus to produce active compound	HSV	Nephrotoxicity Neurotoxicity
Ganciclovir	Nucleoside derivative Phosphorylated in virus to produce active compound Resistance due to mutations in phosphorylation enzyme	CMV	Myelosuppression Neurotoxicity Liver impairment
Foscarnet	Reversible non-competitive inhibitor of DNA polymerase	Resistant CMV or HSV	Nephrotoxicity
Cidofovir	Nucleoside diphosphate analogue Phosphorylated in virus to produce active compound	CMV retinitis Resistant HSV	Nephrotoxicity Neutropenia
Oseltamivir	Neuraminidase inhibitor Early treatment can reduce functional time to recovery by 1–3 days and reduce risk of lower respiratory tract complications	Influenza A and B	Rash Hepatitis Thrombocytopenia

Further Reading

Johnstone C, Hall A, Hart I J. Common viral illnesses in intensive care: presentation, diagnosis, and management. *Contin Educ Anaesth Crit Care Pain* 2014; **14**(5): 213–219

Martin D, Howard J, Agarwal B et al. Ebola virus disease: the UK critical care perspective. *Br J Anaesth* 2016; **116**(5): 590–596

Chapter 90

Weaning from Mechanical Ventilation

What is weaning from mechanical ventilation?

Weaning is the process of liberating the patient from mechanical ventilation and achieving extubation.

What common conditions or situations may impact on the ability to wean a patient from mechanical ventilation?

Respiratory load

i *Increased work of breathing:* inappropriate ventilator settings (inadequate inspiratory flow rate or flow trigger)
ii *Increased resistance:* bronchospasm, thick secretions
iii *Reduced compliance:* pneumonia, pulmonary oedema, pneumothorax, diaphragmatic splinting, pleural effusions
iv *Increased ventilatory requirement:* metabolic acidosis, shock, pulmonary embolism

Cardiac load

i Ischaemic heart disease
ii Valvular heart disease
iii Systolic or diastolic dysfunction

Neuromuscular factors

i *Depressed central drive:* sedative/hypnotic medication, metabolic alkalosis, brainstem haemorrhage/ischaemia, loss of hypoxic drive
ii *Neuromuscular pathology:*
   - Primary neurological disorders, e.g. GBS, myasthenia, botulism
   - Critical illness polyneuropathy
   - Critical care myopathy/malnutrition
   - Electrolyte abnormalities (hypokalaemia, hypophosphataemia, hypocalcaemia, hypomagnesaemia)
   - Hypothyroidism
iii *Neuropsychological factors:* delirium, anxiety, depression

Nutrition

i Anaemia
ii Malnutrition
iii Obesity: reduced FRC, reduced compliance

What is the usual process of initiating weaning from the ventilator?

1 Assess readiness to wean
  i Clinical assessment
    – The causes of acute respiratory failure (or reasons for requiring intubation) have resolved or are resolving
    – Absence of excessive tracheobronchial secretions
    – Adequate cough
    – Cooperative patient
  ii Objective measurements
    – Haemodynamically stable; no or minimal vasopressors
    – PaO_2/FiO_2 >200, FiO_2 <0.5, pH>7.25, PEEP <10 cmH_2O
2 Predicting successful weaning
  i RR <35
  ii Vt >5 ml/kg
  iii Rapid shallow breathing index (RSBI = RR/Vt):
    <65   likely to be successful
    65–105 may be successful
    >105   likely to fail
  iv Airway occlusion pressure at 0.1 second >5 cmH_2O
  v Maximal inspiratory pressure <20 cmH_2O
3 Conduct *SBT*
    – The original description involved disconnecting the patient from the ventilator and connecting a T-piece
    – Other variations involve CPAP and low-level pressure support ventilation as tube compensation
    – Duration: studies have shown that SBTs for 30 or 120 minutes are equivalent
    – Patients who fail SBTs may require a slower period of weaning involving SBTs of a gradually increasing duration
4 Extubation:
    – Extubate if SBT passed, neurological status adequate, no excessive secretions and no airway obstruction

How is failure of SBT defined?

Objective indices of failure:

1 Respiratory rate >35 bpm
2 SpO_2 <90%

3 Heart rate >140 bpm or a change of >20%
4 Systolic blood pressure >180 or <90 mmHg

Subjective indices:

1 Agitation
2 Sweating
3 Anxiety or signs of increased work of breathing

What is the role of tracheostomy in weaning?

Tracheostomy is often performed in patients who require a prolonged respiratory wean. The benefits are:

1 Reduced sedation and hence incidence of delirium (and potentially reduced CINM)
2 Reduction of dead space and improved work of breathing
3 Tracheal toilet
4 Communication (cuff down and speaking valve)

Is there anything you can do to try to minimise the need for re-intubation in patients at high risk of failed extubation?

Extubation on to NIV (even in those who fail SBT) has been associated with reduced ventilator days, reduced LOS on ICU, reduced VAP and reduced 60-day mortality rate. It is particularly useful in patients with acute exacerbation of COPD.

Further Reading

Lermitte J, Garfield M J. Weaning from mechanical ventilation. *Contin Educ Anaesth Crit Care Pain* 2005: **5**(4); 113–117

McConville J F, Kress J P. Weaning Patients from the Ventilator. *N Engl J Med* 2012; **367**: 2233–2239

Chapter 91

Withdrawal of Treatment and End-of-Life Care on the ICU

When should treatment be withdrawn?

In general, treatment is withdrawn when death is felt to be inevitable despite continued treatment, e.g. when a patient has dysfunction in three or more organ systems that persists or worsens despite active treatment.

Establishing the wishes and values of patients is of utmost importance. However, this is not always possible, particularly in a critical care setting. An advanced refusal of treatment (advance directive) is legally binding providing certain conditions are met.

What are the ethical principles governing the decision to withdraw care of a patient?

As per 2010 GMC guidance, the following principles should be adhered to:

1 Equalities and human rights
    - Ensure patients at the end of life receive the same quality of care as all other patients
2 Presumption in favour of prolonging life
    - This presumption will normally require you to take all reasonable steps to prolong a patient's life; however, there is no absolute obligation to prolong life
3 Presumption of capacity
    - Work on the premise that every adult patient has the capacity to make decisions about their care and treatment
4 Maximising capacity to make decisions
    - If the patient's capacity to make a decision may be impaired, you must provide the patient with all the appropriate help and support to understand, weigh-up and retain the information needed to make that decision
5 Overall benefit
    - If the patient lacks capacity, the decisions made must be based on whether treatment would be of overall benefit to the patient

What other factors are necessary regarding the decision to withdraw care?

1 Prognostic information
   - Valid prognostic information is a fundamental component of end-of-life discussions
2 Input from specialists/parent clinical team
   - The shared decision-making model is the archetypal decision-making tool in which physicians and patients (or their surrogates) share information and participate equally in the decision
3 Involve relatives, partners and others close to the patient
   - They may have been granted legal power by the patient/court to make decisions
   - Relatives that have not been given legal authority to make decisions must not be given the impression they are being asked to make the decision
   - Their role is to *advise the healthcare team about the patient's wishes, views or beliefs*
4 Seek a second opinion if you are in doubt about the benefits/burdens and risks about a particular option for a patient

What problems can arise from decisions to withdraw treatment and how can these be resolved?

1 Discord between intensive care and the parent team, e.g. the referring team request continued therapy when the intensive care team feel treatment is futile
   - A second opinion should be sought from another intensive care consultant
2 Discord between intensive care team and the patient's family, e.g. the patient's family requests continued therapy or discontinuation of therapy in opposition to the thoughts of the intensive care team
   - Conflict can be resolved by explaining the rationale again and offering a second opinion from within or outside of the intensive care team
   - Communication is key here: ongoing and honest discussion between the clinician and the family is an important aspect of conflict resolution. Use of the *VALUE* mnemonic (University of Washington End-of-Life Care Research Program) is advocated:
   V Value statements made by family
   A Acknowledge emotions
   L Listen to family members
   U Understand who the patient is as a person
   E Elicit questions from family members
   - Ultimately the duty of care is to the patient not the family
3 Discord between intensive care team and the patient, e.g. the patient requests discontinuation of therapy

- – Again, good communication is key to ensure the patient understands that in the opinion of the intensive care team, a chance of recovery exists
- – Ultimately, the competent patient has the right to refuse treatment
4 Expected outcome changes, e.g. the patient doesn't pass away
  - – This scenario will generate mixed emotions in the family who have previously been prepared for a different outcome
  - – A particularly important issue that will arise is where will the continued care of the patient be based, and whether transferring them out to a ward is appropriate
  - – Offer appropriate support to the family and ensure they are updated regularly

What patient-centred goals/processes should be considered prior to withdrawal of life-supporting therapy?

The following practical points should be considered prior to withdrawal of life support:

1 Emphasise to patients and their surrogates that care focused on symptomatic management and palliative care will continue
2 Prepare the patient's room/environment and family
  - – Optimise lighting, temperature for comfort and consider the presence of patient's possessions
  - – Nurse the patient in a side room if possible; ensure noise outside the room is kept to a minimum
  - – Remove visiting restrictions where possible/practical allowing families to spend time with their loved one
  - – Remove unnecessary equipment but consider bringing extra chairs into the room
  - – Consult the family with regard to spiritual, religious and cultural rituals, and honour these
  - – Ensure family have access to a quiet space away from the patient's bed
  - – Offer families the opportunity to meet with ancillary staff for emotional or psychological support (e.g. clergy)
3 Prepare the patient
  - – Stop unnecessary procedures that do not provide comfort (e.g. blood taking, dialysis, enteral feeding)
  - – Review drug chart – start comfort medications and stop all other unnecessary medications (e.g. vasopressors, antibiotics)
  - – Consider stopping routine monitoring, or dim lighting on screens to make it less distracting
  - – Ensure patient is positioned comfortably and is distress-free prior to withdrawing life support

What cautions/considerations must be taken into account when preparing the withdrawal of individual organ support?

1 *RRT*
   - Low level of physical distress
   - Death may be prolonged if this is the only form of organ support
2 Discontinuation of *mechanical ventilation*
   - Risk of dyspnoea
   - Death may occur quickly if the patient requires high FiO_2 or ventilatory pressures, however it may be prolonged if the patient requires minimal support
   - Preemptive sedation is frequently necessitated to blunt air hunger (doctrine of double effect)
3 Discontinuation of *inotropes or vasopressors*
   - No risk of distress
   - Death may not occur quickly if the patient requires low doses
4 *Extubation*
   - Avoids discomfort of an ETT
   - Facilitates verbal communication and conveys a natural appearance
   - Glycopyrrolate may be necessary to reduce secretions causing noisy breathing
   - Airway obstruction/snoring may occur
   - Communication with the family regarding what to expect following extubation is essential

What is the *doctrine of double effect*?

The *doctrine, or principle, of double effect* distinguishes consequences that are intended from those that are foreseeable though unintended. For example, the management of a terminally ill patient's pain with an opiate (an otherwise legitimate act) may also cause an effect that physicians would normally be obliged to avoid (sedation and a slightly shortened life). Given these side effects were not the intention, the action of providing pain relief is ethically justified.

What medications are available for symptom management in end of life care?

The goal of drug therapy at the end of life is the alleviation or prevention of pain, dyspnoea and other distressing symptoms.

1 **Pain:** opioids are the mainstay of treatment of pain and dyspnoea in the dying patient

    i Fentanyl: short half-life, rapid onset of action. Should be administered as a continuous infusion in this setting

    ii Morphine: often the agent of choice in palliative care due to its efficacy, low cost and familiarity with healthcare staff

    iii Diamorphine: more rapid onset of action than morphine and more potent. Can be administered IM or by subcutaneous infusion

2 **Sedation:**

    i Benzodiazepines:

      – Midazolam: most rapid onset of effect (max response at 5–10 minutes following IV administration)

      – Lorazepam: requires 20–25 minutes for maximum effect following IV administration

    ii Propofol: Rapid onset and offset and is easily titrated to desired level of sedation

3 **Delirium:** haloperidol – can be administered IV or subcutaneously via syringe driver

4 **Nausea and vomiting:**

    i Dopamine receptor antagonist, e.g. levomepromazine and haloperidol for metabolic/biochemical disturbance

    ii Prokinetic, e.g. metoclopramide for motility disorders

    iii Anticholinergic or antihistamine, e.g. cyclizine and dexamethasone for intracranial disorders, raised ICP, vestibular dysfunction

5 **Excess secretions and colic:** hyoscine butylbromide – can be administered IV, IM or subcutaneously by syringe driver

Further Reading

Cook D, Rocker G. Dying with Dignity in the Intensive Care Unit. *N Engl J Med* 2014; **370**(26): 2506–2514

General Medical Council, 2010. Treatment and Care Towards the End of Life: Good Practice in Decision Making [online]. London: GMC. Available at: www.gmc-uk.org/End_of_life.pdf_32486688.pdf (Accessed: 7 December 2016)

Winter B, Cohen S. Withdrawal of treatment. *Brit Med J* 1999; **319**(7205): 306–308

Bibliography

Al-Shaikh B, Stacey S. *Essentials of Anaesthetic Equipment*. Philadelphia, PA: Churchill Livingstone Elsevier, 2007

American Psychiatric Association. *Diagnostic and Statistical Manual of Mental Disorders: DSM-IV-TR*. Washington, D C: American Psychiatric Association, 2000.

Anderson C S, Heeley E, Huang Y, et al. for the INTERACT2 Investigators. Rapid blood-pressure lowering in patients with acute intracerebral hemorrhage. *N Engl J Med* 2013; **368**(25): 2355–2365

Andrews P J, Sinclair L, Rodriguez A, et al. for the Eurotherm3235 Trial Collaborators. Hypothermia for intracranial hypertension after traumatic brain injury. *N Engl J Med* 2015; **373**(25): 2403–2412

Asfar P, Meziani F, Hamel J F, et al. for the SEPSISPAM Investigators. High versus low blood-pressure target in patients with septic shock. *N Engl J Med* 2014; **370**: 1583–1593

Altman D, Carroli G, Duley L, et al. The Magpie Collaborative Group. Do women with pre-eclampsia, and their babies, benefit from magnesium sulphate? The Magpie Trial: A randomised placebo-controlled trial. *Lancet* 2002; **359**(9321): 1877–1890

Bellomo R, Cass A, Norton R, et al. for the RENAL Replacement Therapy Study Investigators. Intensity of continuous renal-replacement therapy in critically ill patients. *N Engl J Med* 2009; **361**: 1627–1638

Bernard G R, Vincent J L, Laterre P F, et al. for the PROWESS Study Group. Efficacy and safety of recombinant human activated protein C for severe sepsis. *N Engl J Med* 2001; **344**(10): 699–709

Bickell W H, Wall M J, Pepe P E, et al. Immediate versus delayed resuscitation for hypotensive patients with penetrating torso injuries. *N Engl J Med* 1994; **331**: 1105–1109

Brunkhorst F M, Engel C, Bloos F, et al. for the German Competence Network Sepsis (SepNet). Efficacy of Volume Substitution and Insulin Therapy in Severe Sepsis (VISEP). *N Engl J Med* 2008; **358**: 125–139

Caironi P, Tognoni G, Masson S, et al. The ALBIOS Study Investigators. Albumin replacement in patients with severe sepsis or septic shock. *N Engl J Med* 2014; **370**: 1412–1421

Carson J L, Terrin M L, Noveck H, et al. Liberal or restrictive transfusion in high-risk patients after hip surgery. *N Engl J Med* 2011; **365**: 2453–2462

Casaer M P, Mesotten D, Hermans G, et al. Early versus late parenteral nutrition in critically ill adults. *N Engl J Med* 2011; **365**: 506–517

Child C G, Turcotte J G. Surgery and portal hypertension. *Major Probl Clin Surg* 1964; **1**: 1–85

Choudhury A, Kedarisetty C K, Vashishtha C, et al. A randomised trial comparing terlipressin in patients with cirrhosis and septic shock. *Liver Int* 2017; **37**(4): 552–561

Cook S-C, Thomas M, Nolan J, Parr M, eds. *Key Topics in Critical Care*. London: JP Medical Ltd, 2014

Cooper D J, Rosenfeld J V, Murray L, et al. The DECRA Trial Investigators. Decompressive craniectomy in diffuse traumatic brain injury. *N Engl J Med* 2011; **364**(16): 1493–1502

Dutton R P, Mackenzie C F, Scalea T M. Hypotensive resuscitation during active haemorrhage: impact on in-hospital mortality. *J Trauma* 2002; **52**: 1141–1146

Faisey C, Meziani F, Planquette B, et al. for the DIABOLO Investigators. Effect of acetazolamide vs placebo on duration of mechanical ventilation among patients with chronic obstructive pulmonary disease. *J Am Med Assoc* 2016; **315**(5): 480–488

Ferguson N D, Cook D J, Guyatt G H, et al. for the OSCILLATE Trial Investigators. High frequency oscillation in early acute respiratory distress syndrome. *N Engl J Med* 2013; **368**(9): 795–805

Finfer S, Bellomo R, Boyce N, et al. for the SAFE Study Investigators. A comparison of albumin and saline for fluid resuscitation in the intensive care unit. *N Engl J Med* 2004; **350**(22): 2247–2256

Finfer S, Chittock D R, Su S Y, et al. for the NICE-SUGAR Study Investigators. Intensive versus conventional glucose control in critically ill patients. *N Engl J Med* 2009; **360**: 1283–1297

Frat J P, Thille A W, Mercat A, et al. for the FLORALI Study Group and the REVA Network. High-flow oxygen through nasal cannula in acute hypoxemic respiratory failure. *N Engl J Med* 2015; **372**:2185–2196

Gordon A C, Mason A J, Thirunavukkarasu N, et al. for the VANISH Investigators. Effect of early vasopressin vs norepinephrine on kidney failure in patients with septic shock: The VANISH randomized clinical trial. *J Am Med Assoc* 2016; **316**(5): 509–518

Gordon A C, Perkins G D, Singer M, et al. Levosimendan for the prevention of acute organ dysfunction in sepsis. *N Engl J Med* 2016; **375**(17): 1638–1648

Guérin C, Reignier J, Richard J C, et al. for the PROSEVA Study Group. Prone positioning in severe acute respiratory distress syndrome. *N Engl J Med* 2013; **368**(23): 2159–2168

Hajjar L A, Vincent J L, Galas F R, et al. Transfusion requirements after cardiac surgery: the TRACS randomized controlled trial. *J Am Med Assoc* 2010; **304**: 1559–1567

Hebert P C, Wells G, Blajchman M A, et al. for the Transfusion Requirements in Critical Care (TRICC) Investigators, Canadian Critical Care Trials Group. A multicenter, randomized, controlled clinical trial of transfusion requirements in critical care. *N Engl J Med* 1999; **340**: 409–417

Hernández G, Vaquero C, González P, et al. Effect of post-extubation high-flow nasal cannula vs conventional oxygen therapy on reintubation in low-risk patients. A randomized clinical trial. *J Am Med Assoc* 2016; **315**(13): 1354–1361

Heyland D, Muscedere J, Wischmeyer P E, et al. for the Canadian Critical Care Trials Group. A randomized trial of glutamine and antioxidants in critically ill patients. *N Engl J Med* 2013; **368**: 1489–1497

Holcomb J B, Tilley B C, Baraniuk S, et al. The PROPPR Study Group. Transfusion of plasma, platelets, and red blood cells in a 1:1:1 vs a 1:1:2 ratio and mortality in patients with severe trauma: The PROPPR randomized clinical trial. *J Am Med Assoc* 2015; **313**(5): 471–482

Holcomb J B, del Junco D J, Fox E E, et al. for the PROMMTT Study Group. The Prospective, Observational, Multicenter, Major Trauma Transfusion (PROMMTT) study: Comparative effectiveness of a time-varying treatment with competing risks. *JAMA Surg* 2013; **148**(2): 127–136

Holst L B, Haase N, Wetterslev J, et al. for the TRISS Trial Group; Scandanavian Critical Care Trials Group. Lower versus higher hemoglobin threshold for transfusion in septic shock. *N Engl J Med* 2014; **371** (15): 1381–1391

Hutchinson P J, Kolias A G, Timofeev I S, et al. for the RESCUEicp Collaborators. Trial of decompressive craniectomy for traumatic intracranial hypertension. *N Engl J Med* 2016; **375**(12): 1119–1130

Jakob S M, Ruokonen E, R M Grounds, et al. Dexmedetomidine vs midazolam or propofol for sedation during prolonged mechanical ventilation: Two randomised controlled trials. *J Am Med Assoc* 2012; **307**: 1151–1160

Jaber S, Lescot T, Futier E, et al. Effect of non-invasive ventilation on tracheal reintubation among patients with hypoxemic respiratory failure following abdominal surgery. *J Am Med Assoc* 2016; **315**(13): 1345–1353

Joannes-Boyau O, Honoré P M, Perez P, et al. High-volume versus standard-volume haemofiltration for septic shock patients with acute kidney injury (IVOIRE study): A multicentre randomized controlled trial. *Intensive Care Med* 2013; **39**(9): 1535–1546

Kacmarek R M, Villar J, Sulemanji D, et al. Open lung approach for the acute respiratory distress syndrome: A pilot randomised controlled trial. *Crit Care Med* 2016; **44**(1): 32–42

Kar P S, Ogoe B, Poole R, Meeking D. Di-George syndrome presenting with hypocalcaemia in adulthood: Two case reports and a review. *J Clin Pathol* 2005; **58**: 655–657

Keh D, Trips D, Marx G, et al. for the SepNet-Critical Care Trials Group. Effect of hydrocortisone on development of shock among patients with severe sepsis: The HYPRESS randomized clinical trial. *J Am Med Assoc* 2016; **316**(17): 1775–1785

Kirkpatrick P J, Turner C L, Smith C, et al. for the STASH collaborators. Simvastatin in aneurysmal subarachnoid haemorrhage (STASH): A multicentre randomised phase 3 trial. *Lancet* 2014; **13**(7): 666–675

Lacroix J, Hébert P C, Fergusson D A, et al. for the ABLE Investigators and the Canadian Critical Care Trials Group. Age of transfused blood in critically ill adults. *N Engl J Med* 2015; **372**: 1410–1418

Martin J N Jr, Blake P G, Perry K G, et al. The natural history of HELLP syndrome: patterns of disease progression and regression. *Am J Obstet Gynecol* 1991; **164**: 1500–1513

Meduri G U, Golden E, Freire A X, et al. Methylprednisolone infusion in early severe ARDS: results of a randomised controlled trial. *Chest* 2007; **131**(4): 954–963

Mendelow A D, Gregson B A, Fernandes H M, et al. for the STICH investigators. Early surgery versus initial conservative treatment in patients with spontaneous supratentorial intracerebral haematomas in the International Surgical Trial in Intracerebral Haemorrhage (STICH): A randomised trial. *Lancet* 2005; **365**: 387–397

Mendelow A D, Gregson B A, Rowan E N, et al. for the STICH II Investigators. Early surgery versus initial conservative treatment in patients with spontaneous supratentorial lobar intracerebral haematomas (STICH II): A randomised trial. *Lancet* 2013; **382**: 397–408

Mendelow A D, Gregson B A, Rowan E N, et al. Early Surgery versus Initial Conservative Treatment in Patients with Traumatic Intracerebral Haemorrhage (STITCH[trauma]): the first randomised trial. *J Neurotrauma* 2015; **32**(17): 1312–1323

Mijzen E J, Jacobs B, Aslan A, et al. Propofol infusion syndrome heralded by ECG changes. *Neurocrit Care* 2012; **17**(2): 260–264

Molyneux A, Kerr R, Stratton I, et al. International Subarachnoid Aneurysm Trial (ISAT) of neurosurgical clipping versus endovascular coiling in 2143 patients with ruptured intracranial aneurysms: A randomised trial. *Lancet* 2002; **360**: 1267–1274

Morrison C A, Carrick M M, Norman M A, et al. Hypotensive resuscitation strategy reduces transfusion requirements and severe postoperative coagulopathy in trauma patients with haemorrhagic shock: preliminary results of a randomised controlled trial. *J Trauma* 2011; **70**(3): 652–663

Mouncey P R, Osborn T M, Power S, et al. for the ProMISe Trial Investigators. Trial of early, goal-directed resuscitation for septic shock. *N Engl J Med* 2015; **372**: 1301–1311

Murphy G J, Pike K, Rogers C A, et al. for the TITRe2 Investigators. Liberal or restrictive transfusion after cardiac surgery. *N Engl J Med* 2015; **372**: 997–1008

Myburgh J A, Finfer S, Bellomo R, et al. for the ANZICS Clinical Trials Group. Hydroxyethyl starch or saline for fluid resuscitation in intensive care. *N Engl J Med* 2012; **367**: 1901–1911

Nielsen N, Wetterslev J, Cronberg T, et al. for the TTM Trial Investigators. Targeted temperature management at 33°C versus 36°C after cardiac arrest. *N Engl J Med* 2013; **369**(23): 2197–2206

Papazian L, Forel J M, Gacouin A, et al. for the ACURASYS Study Investigators. Neuromuscular blockers in early acute respiratory distress syndrome. *N Engl J Med* 2010; **363**: 1107–1116

Parsons P, Wiener-Kronish J P, eds. *Critical Care Secrets*. Missouri: Elsevier Mosby, 2013

Peake S L, Delaney A, Bailey M, et al. for the ARISE Investigators and the ANZICS Clinical Trials Group. Australasian resuscitation in sepsis evaluation randomised controlled trial. Goal-directed resuscitation for patients with early septic shock. *N Engl J Med* 2014; **371**(16): 1496–1506

Peck T, Hill S, Williams M. *Pharmacology for Anaesthesia and Intensive Care*. Cambridge: Cambridge University Press, 2014

Peek G J, Mugford M, Tiruvoipatti R, et al. Efficiency and economic assessment of conventional ventilatory support versus extracorporeal membrane oxygenation for severe adult respiratory failure (CESAR): A multicentre randomised controlled trial. *Lancet* 2009; **374**(9698): 1351–1363

Perner A, Haase N, Guttormsen A B, et al. for the 6S Trial Group and the Scandinavian Critical Care Trials Group. Hydroxyethyl starch 130/0.42 versus Ringer's acetate in severe sepsis. *N Engl J Med* 2012; **367**(2): 124–134

Qureshi A I, Palesch Y Y, Barsan W G, et al. for the ATACH-2 Trial Investigators and the Neurological Emergency Treatment Trials Network. Intensive blood-pressure lowering in patients with acute cerebral hemorrhage. *N Engl J Med* 2016; **375** (11): 1033–1043

Ranieri V M, Thompson B T, Barie P S, et al. for the PROWESS-SHOCK Study Group. Drotrecogin alfa (activated) in adults with septic shock. *N Engl J Med* 2012; **366**(22): 2055–2064

Reade M C, Eastwood G M, Bellomo R, et al. The DahLIA Investigators. Effect of dexmedetomidine added to standard care on ventilator-free time in patients with agitated delirium: A randomised clinical trial. *J Am Med Assoc* 2016; **315**: 1460–1468

Rice T W, Wheeler A P, Thompson B T, et al. for the ARDS Clinical Trials Network. Initial trophic vs full enteral feeding in patients with acute lung injury: the EDEN randomized trial. *J Am Med Assoc* 2012; **307**(8): 795–803

Rice T W, Wheeler A P, Thompson B T, et al. Enteral omega-3 fatty acid, γ-linolenic acid, and antioxidant supplementation in acute lung injury. *J Am Med Assoc* 2011; **306**(14): 1574–1581

Rivers E, Nguyen B, Havstad S, et al. for the Early Goal-Directed Therapy Collaborative Group. Early goal-directed therapy in the treatment of severe sepsis and septic shock. *N Engl J Med* 2001; **345**(19): 1368–1377

Roberts I, Yates D, Sandercock P, et al. for the CRASH Trial Collaborators. Effect of intravenous corticosteroids on death within 14 days in 10 008 adults with clinically significant head injury: randomised placebo-controlled trial. *Lancet* 2004; **364** (9442): 1321–1328

Russell J A, Walley K R, Singer J, et al. for the VASST Investigators. Vasopressin versus norepinephrine infusion in patients with septic shock. *N Engl J Med* 2008; **358**: 877–887

Sandercock P, Wardlaw J M, Lindley R I, et al. The benefits and harms of intravenous thrombolysis with recombinant tissue plasminogen activator within 6 hours of acute ischaemic stroke (the third international stroke trial [IST-3]): A randomised controlled trial. *Lancet* 2012; **379**: 2352–2363.

Singer P, Anbar R, Cohen J, et al. The tight calorie control study (TICACOS): A prospective, randomized, controlled pilot study of nutritional support in critically ill patients. *Intensive Care Med* 2011; **37**(4): 601–609

Sprung C L, Annane D, Keh D, et al. for the CORTICUS Study Group. Hydrocortisone therapy for patients with septic shock. *N Engl J Med* 2008; **358**:111–124

Steinberg K P, Hudson L D, Goodman R B, et al. Efficacy and safety of corticosteroids for persistent acute respiratory distress syndrome. *N Engl J Med* 2006; **354**(16): 1671–1684

Steiner T, Poli S, Griebe M, et al. Fresh frozen plasma versus prothrombin complex concentrate in patients with intracranial haemorrhage related to vitamin K antagonists (INCH): A randomised trial. *Lancet Neurol* 2016; **15** (6): 566–573

Taylor F B, Toh C H, Hoots W K, et al. for the Scientific Subcommittee on Disseminated Intravascular Coagulation (DIC) of the International Society on Thrombosis and Haemostasis (ISTH). Towards definition, clinical and laboratory criteria, and a scoring system for disseminated intravascular coagulation. *Thromb Haemost* 2001; **86**(5): 1327–1330

Thachil J, Hill Q A, eds. *Haematology in Critical Care: A Practical Handbook. John Wiley & Sons Ltd*, 2014

The Acute Respiratory Distress Syndrome Network. Brower R G, Matthay M A, Morris A, et al. Ventilation with lower tidal volumes for acute lung injury and the acute respiratory distress syndrome. *N Engl J Med* 2000; **342**: 1301–1308

The CRASH-2 Collaborators. Shakur H, Roberts I, Bautista R, et al. Effects of tranexamic acid on death, vascular occlusive events, and blood transfusion in trauma patients with significant haemorrhage (CRASH-2): A randomised, placebo-controlled trial. *Lancet* 2010; **376**: 23–32

The Hypothermia after Cardiac Arrest (HACA) Study Group. Mild therapeutic hypothermia to improve neurologic outcome after cardiac arrest. *N Engl J Med* 2002; **346**(8): 549–556

The ProCESS Investigators. Yealy D M, Kellum J A, Huang D T, et al. A randomized trial of protocol-based care for early septic shock. *N Engl J Med* 2014; **370**: 1683–1693

Vasilevskis E E, Ely E W, Speroff T, et al. Reducing iatrogenic risks: ICU-acquired delirium and weakness – crossing the quality chasm. *Chest* 2010; **138**(5): 1224–1233

Waldmann C, Soni N, Rhodes A, eds. *Oxford Desk Reference Critical Care*. Oxford: Oxford University Press, 2008

World Health Organisation. *ICD-10 Classifications of Mental and Behavioural Disorder: Clinical Descriptions and Diagnostic Guidelines*. Geneva: World Health Organisation, 1992.

Young D, Lamb S E, Shah S, et al. for the OSCAR Study Group. High frequency oscillation for acute respiratory distress syndrome. *N Engl J Med* 2013; **368**(9): 806–813

Young D, Harrison D A, Cuthbertson B H, et al. for the TracMan Collaborators. Effect of early vs late tracheostomy placement on survival in patients receiving mechanical ventilation: The TracMan randomized trial. *J Am Med Assoc* 2013; **309**(20): 2121–2129

Index

Printed in the United States
By Bookmasters